Burdens of War

RECONFIGURING AMERICAN POLITICAL HISTORY
Ronald P. Formisano, Paul Bourke, Donald DeBats,
and Paula M. Baker, Series Founders

Burdens of War

Creating the United States Veterans Health System

Jessica L. Adler

Johns Hopkins University Press
Baltimore

This book was brought to publication with the generous assistance
of the Columbia University Bancroft Dissertation Award.

Johns Hopkins University Press
2715 North Charles Street
Baltimore, Maryland 21218-4363
www.press.jhu.edu

Library of Congress Cataloging-in-Publication Data
Names: Adler, Jessica L., 1978– author.
Title: Burdens of war : creating the United States Veterans Health
    System / Jessica L. Adler.
Description: Baltimore : Johns Hopkins University Press, [2017] |
    Includes bibliographical references and index.
Identifiers: LCCN 2016041512 | ISBN 9781421422879 (hardcover :
    alk. paper) | ISBN 9781421422886 (electronic) | ISBN 1421422875
    (hardcover : alk. paper) | ISBN 1421422883 (electronic)
Subjects: LCSH: Veterans—Medical care—United States—History—
    20th century. | World War, 1914–1918—Medical care—United
    States. | World War, 1914–1918—Veterans—Medical care—United
    States—History—20th century. | Disabled veterans—
    Rehabilitation—United States—History—20th century. | Veterans'
    hospitals—United States—History—20th century. | United States.
    Veterans Bureau—History. | Veterans—Services for—United
    States—History—20th century. | Medical policy—United
    States—History—20th century.
Classification: LCC UB369 .A475 2017 | DDC
    362.1086/970973—dc23
LC record available at https://lccn.loc.gov/2016041512

A catalog record for this book is available from the British Library.

*Special discounts are available for bulk purchases of this book. For more
information, please contact Special Sales at 410-516-6936 or specialsales@
press.jhu.edu.*

Johns Hopkins University Press uses environmentally friendly book
materials, including recycled text paper that is composed of at least
30 percent post-consumer waste, whenever possible.

Contents

Acknowledgments

I am indebted to teachers, archivists, colleagues, friends, and family and am grateful for the opportunity to thank them. Scholars at the University of Rochester and Columbia University provided perspective on the rigors and rewards of studying history. Daniel H. Borus and Robert B. Westbrook awakened me to the wonder of leafing through old documents and working to make sense of them. They are inspirational mentors, writers, researchers, and men, and I would doubtless be on a different life course had I not been fortunate enough to encounter them. The magnanimous and productive David K. Rosner ignited my interest in the history of public health and in so doing helped shape my research path. I learned much about the study of US political history during seminars and meetings with Alan Brinkley, who took the time and care to discuss some of the ideas contained in this book at an early stage. After introducing me to important sources in the literature of the American welfare state and public health, Samuel Kelton Roberts offered incisive advice on initial iterations of this project. Finally, Alice Kessler-Harris is a ceaselessly devoted mentor and confidante, who has a keen sense of when to offer positive reinforcement or a kick in the pants. She has pushed me to do better and do more, and also encouraged me to post a note on my computer containing two words: "Have Fun."

Learned archivists and librarians who translate finding aids, share insights about collection contents, and locate boxes in the catacombs of the stacks shape history books, and this one is no different. Doran Cart, senior curator at the National World War I Museum and Memorial, offered useful perspective on— of all things—military-issued underwear. Columbia University reference librarian Mary Cargill tirelessly fielded my requests for assistance locating obscure congressional documents and always came through. I am grateful to James Chaney and Alice Bersch, who granted me the privilege of looking through unsorted files at the Disabled American Veterans headquarters and provided copies of the organization's early meeting minutes. Howard Trace and staff at the American Legion headquarters' library, too, were very accommodating and helpful hosts. At the Cincinnati Museum Center, Sarah Staples ably assisted with the Robert S. Marx papers. In his post at the US Army Medical Department's Office of Medical History, Sanders Marble took the time not only to gather a fat pile of documents but also to lend me an open ear and useful advice as I began pursuing research. David Keough offered a wealth of information and served as a patient guide at the US Army Heritage and Education Center. Also at AHEC, Richard Sommers patiently discussed my project and shared helpful feedback. At the National Archives and Records Administration in College Park, Maryland, Mitch Yockelson and Haley Maynard provided expert assistance with World War I–era government records. Juliette Arai and Paul Harrison offered valuable guidance at the National Archives in Washington, DC, especially as I attempted to decipher the complex finding aids of Record Group 15. Likewise, Richard McCulley and Kate Mollan helped me navigate House and Senate records at the Center for Legislative Archives in Washington.

Gracious scholars shared invaluable perspective and feedback. Rosemary Stevens, whose early work on veterans' health care offered me a guiding light, is the model of a generous intellectual. I am fortunate to have been enriched by her unflagging support. Stephen Ortiz offered insightful critical comments during conferences and demonstrated on numerous occasions that he is selflessly committed to educating junior colleagues. When I began studying military and veterans' health issues, John R. Pierce was kind enough to meet with me and provide references he had gathered during his many years researching Walter Reed Army Medical Center. Around the same time, Beth Linker and Carol R. Byerly generously pointed me to useful sources that shed light on the institution's early years. Jeffrey M. Berry, Jerry Lembcke, and Theda Skocpol also offered helpful feedback and ideas. At Walter Reed, Sherman Fleek, Lt. Col. US Army (Ret.), allowed me access to unsorted files of the Public Affairs office, which yielded, among other things, a photo of soldier-patients preparing to be fit with prostheses (figure 2.4). Jesse Tarbert kindly shared scans of *PM* magazine articles cited in the conclusion. Since our graduate school days, Thai Jones and Tamara Mann have pushed me to be a better analytical thinker and, every once in a while, have a good time; I am honored to benefit from their scholarly prowess and enjoy their loyal companionship. Edward D. Berkowitz, Alice Kessler-Harris, Tamara Mann, Sanders Marble, April Merleaux, Wendy Moffat, Samuel Kelton Roberts, David Rosner, Dale Smith, and Rosemary Stevens read portions of this work and offered trenchant feedback. Though I did not take all of their advice, I am deeply indebted to each of them.

Discussions with veterans have reminded me that a health system is not only a political and bureaucratic mechanism; it touches the lives of those it is intended to serve. During conversations with Peter Harlem, Timothy F. Kavanaugh, Jack Meeder, Leonard Poirier, members of the Student Veterans of America-FIU chapter, and the participants of Talking Service Miami, I learned much about how men and women recall their experiences of military service and homecoming. I also came to recognize that some aspects of war are unique to a particular time period or conflict, but at least one is timeless: long after fighting ceases, veterans and their families are among those who work to shoulder the powerful, pervasive health effects of mass conflict. I thank these men and women for sharing their time and stories with me, and for enriching my perspective.

Support from institutions, colleagues, editors, and friends facilitated research and writing. Grants from the Doris G. Quinn Foundation, the Institute for Political History, the US Army Military History Institute, and Columbia University helped make research for the project possible. Christina Ching, Thomas Darke, Michael Lisman, and Michael and Gwyneth Neuss welcomed me in their homes during research and conference trips and shared the gift of their warm hospitality and friendship. At Florida International University, I am privileged to be part of a community of accomplished scholars in the Departments of History and Health Policy and Management. I thank my colleagues for their intellectual support. Johns Hopkins University Press editor emeritus Robert J. Brugger has been a patient, steadfast, and encouraging force. I have benefited from his expertise and counsel. I am grateful for the guidance of Johns Hopkins senior acquisitions editor Elizabeth Demers and freelance copyeditor Glenn Perkins.

Finally, my family has given me love and then some. I am grateful for the loyalty and generosity of Seth Adler, my brother and my first friend. On numerous occasions, he has entertained his nephew and niece, alongside the stellar Magdalena Plicha, to help ensure I had time to work on this book. My mother, Laura Adler, was a dedicated educator, a zealous reader, and a devoted family woman. Her work as a public school teacher and advocate and her thoughtful notes to friends and family made me realize that writing could be worthwhile—even powerful and magnificent. In addition to teaching me how to throw and catch a baseball, my father, Edward Adler, helped me recognize the art of asking questions, the importance of seeing things from multiple perspectives, the complexity of presenting arguments, and the rewards that come from engaged listening. I learn from him still. My daughter and son, Lael and Samuel, remind me to examine insects, find delight in storybooks, participate in dark dance parties, and prioritize. Aaron Mattfeld, my husband, partner, and advocate, motivates, calms, and sustains me. From Miyagi-ken to Miami and everywhere in between, he has made adventures great, tragedies bearable, joys intense, and challenges surmountable. He shares wisdom patiently, modestly, and unassumingly, and every day makes me realize the beauty in open-mindedness.

Abbreviations Used in the Text

AEF	American Expeditionary Forces
AHA	American Hospital Association
AL	American Legion
BWRI	Bureau of War Risk Insurance
CND	Council of National Defense
DAV	Disabled American Veterans
DPR	Department of Physical Reconstruction (US Army)
FBH	Federal Board of Hospitalization
FBVE	Federal Board for Vocational Education
OT	occupational therapy
PHS	Public Health Service
VA	Veterans Administration/Department of Veterans Affairs
VB	Veterans Bureau
WRIA	War Risk Insurance Act

Burdens of War

War and Federally Sponsored Health Care

One night in 1974, Leonard Poirier sat up in bed and started to strangle his wife. Four decades later he recalled that he had no idea what he was doing; he had been having a nightmare about Vietnam. During the day, Poirier could drink at the Veterans of Foreign Wars or American Legion post and "store it in the back of [his] mind"—the memories of his assistant machine gunner loading thousands of rounds while he "put the lead out," the thoughts of going out on a mission with forty guys and coming back with twelve. But nighttime was different.

"You need to get help or I'm outta here," Poirier's wife told him.

He was already visiting a Veterans Administration (VA) outpatient clinic near his Somerville, Massachusetts, home every couple of months to receive treatment for the lingering effects of malaria and the ringing in his ears caused by exposure to the sounds of explosions and gunshots. The strangling incident convinced him to attend regular counseling sessions with a VA doctor, which helped him cut back on drinking and feel "straightened out." After a couple of years, he stopped the therapy.

In 2006, as a new generation of service members fought wars in Iraq and Afghanistan, Poirier was about to retire from a career as a letter carrier with the US Postal Service and begin spending his days with his wife, babysitting his grandkids. But even after so many years, the nightmares were relentless. A fellow Vietnam veteran suggested that someone at the VA hospital in Bedford, Massachusetts, could help. Ten minutes into Poirier's first conversation with a primary care doctor, the physician recommended that he meet with a therapist. "Guess I was pretty screwed up," he reflected. Now he goes to the VA to be treated for service-connected conditions, including post-traumatic stress disorder (PTSD) and heart troubles traceable to the effects of the chemical weapon Agent Orange.[1]

It is fitting that the hospital where Poirier accesses care is named for Edith

Nourse Rogers, a Massachusetts congresswoman who was a fierce proponent of veterans' rights following World War I.[2] In the interwar years—decades before PTSD or Agent Orange became part of the American lexicon—the federal government made an expansive commitment that shaped a century's worth of postwar experiences for veterans like Leonard Poirier, their families, and their nation: to provide access to professionally administered health care as a primary means of alleviating the human consequences of war. This book reveals how that commitment materialized and how it fostered the development of a massive government-funded health system. High-minded ideals—a societal commitment "to care for him who shall have borne the battle," a decree that "the nation has no more solemn obligation than healing the hurts of our wounded"—are only one part of a multidimensional story.[3] The veterans' health system became a lasting reality, and a pillar of American health and social policy, because of circumstances specific to the reformist Progressive Era, the socially turbulent 1920s, and the economically troubled 1930s. Its establishment marked a reimagining of modern veterans' benefits and signaled a pathbreaking acceptance of the validity and power of professionalized institutional medical care. It also indicated an uneasy recognition—in a country with a long tradition of skepticism about federal intervention in the health and welfare of individual citizens—that the government could fund and administer a selective and conditional entitlement program.[4]

Reimagining Veterans' Benefits

At the turn of the twentieth century, the US military received an increasing share of the federal budget as the nation established itself as a world power. For the first time, many Americans accepted the notion of a peacetime standing army.[5] In this period of growing ambitions, the government revamped domestic health facilities for service members. The army had long provided wounded and ill soldiers with first aid on the battlefield or in temporary field and camp hospitals intended to return them intact to their units. But by the World War I era, military personnel could receive multifaceted treatment in large general hospitals. Those institutions laid the foundations of the modern military health care system.[6] They also raised expectations among discharged service members that their government would provide them with relatively comprehensive health services as they transitioned to civilian life.

The growth of the military and its medical infrastructure helped lay the groundwork for the rise of the veterans' health system and a larger shift from nineteenth-century benefits centered on pensions and domicile care in Soldiers' Homes, to a twentieth-century model that relied on modern institutions and services to foster economic independence.[7] Even though some Soldiers' Home campuses had long contained hospitals, those institutions were designed to serve primarily as *homes*, not medical care facilities, and many Great War veterans resisted being sent to them.[8] Policy makers of the World War I era created veterans' hospitals, in part, as a response to that hostility. They hoped to ensure that the newest generation of veterans would be cured by modern medicine rather than face the prospect of becoming enmeshed in a benefits system that symbolized long-term dependency.[9]

The medicalized system that took root during World War I influenced veterans' benefits during the interwar years and the century to come.[10] When the United States mobilized for World War II in the 1940s, approximately 58,000 former service members were patients in more than fifty veterans' hospitals, where doctors, nurses, social workers, therapists, and other professionals managed their care and researched their health conditions.[11] During and after World War II, policy makers relied on the infrastructure created to serve approximately 4 million Great War veterans to manage a bevy of new entitlements for more than 16 million Good War veterans.[12] Building on the existing bureaucracy, they envisioned veterans' benefits not just as piecemeal measures to stave off economic dependency but as a systemic means of improving the health of former service members and ushering them into the middle class.[13] Like their World War I–era counterparts, they were guided by the edict that modern medical facilities and professional caregivers could assuage the long-term health impacts of war.

The veterans' health system established after the Great War continues to exist in expanded form, as a crucial modern institution. It is part of the US Department of Veterans Affairs, which now oversees the provision of health services for more than 9 million beneficiaries through the Veterans Health Administration (VHA).[14] As a legal scholar observed in 2015, "The veterans benefits system that we have today is, with modest changes, the same one that was created in 1917 for the veterans of World War I."[15] Indeed, some of the questions and controversies facing the VHA in the twenty-first century—regarding, for example, long wait times for appointments, whether illnesses and injuries are service connected, and quality of care—echo concerns voiced nearly a hundred years ago.

Entrenching Professionalized, Institutionally Based Health Care

That access to health care became a veterans' benefit had much to do with changing perceptions of curing and caring. In the years surrounding the Great War, medical and education experts began to view disability as a temporary condition that an individual could "rise above."[16] The massive World War I military hospital–based rehabilitation effort that preceded the establishment of the veterans' health system encapsulated that perspective. It "symbolized a dream, a hope that physical 'handicaps,' 'pauperism,' and 'defects of manhood' could all be conquered on the home front."[17] Some veterans living with long-term health maladies challenged those lofty ideals, argued for enhanced services and programs, and leveraged emerging military and veterans' health systems in order to ensure their financial, occupational, and physical well-being.

The drastic change that took place in the nature of veterans' benefits—and the enthusiastic fight for hospitals that propelled that change—was due in no small part to the dynamic state of American medicine and health care. In the first two decades of the twentieth century—thanks to advocacy efforts of professionals in the field, industrialization, and urbanization—public perceptions of health and hospitals were in transition. The germ theory of disease absolved individuals of blame for their ailments and took away the shame of seeking care; illnesses such as tuberculosis were gradually seen largely as products of one's environment, as opposed to a form of punishment for individual moral transgressions. At the same time, chronic illnesses overtook epidemics as the leading cause of death among Americans and gained credence as medical ailments best treated by professionals.[18] Amid those drastic changes, doctors and administrators self-consciously ensured that hospitals boasted new technologies such as X-ray machines and amenities including well-appointed private rooms. By the second decade of the twentieth century, middle- and upper-class Americans increasingly sought medical care at such institutions, rather than in their homes. Health care, in other words, was professionalized and commodified.[19]

The veterans' health system reflected those larger changes. Medical professionals and bureaucrats conceived of a nationwide network of hospitals not only to provide for the relatively small number of former service members who endured acute injuries and illnesses but also to serve a larger population of veteran-patients with mental illnesses and tuberculosis, whom, they believed, needed care in institutions where they would not pose a health threat to fellow citizens.[20] That was, in part, because disease was the leading health threat for World War I–era soldiers.[21] By 1919, more than 80 percent of the approximately 205,000 soldiers discharged from the army with disabilities had been released due to disease. Tuberculosis was the most common diagnosis, constituting approximately 21,600 discharges.[22] The second-most common was "mental deficiency," which led to approximately 10,000 discharges.[23] About 12 percent, or 25,000 soldiers, were discharged with a disability due to wounds received in action.[24] Many more soldiers were treated for diseases and wounds while enlisted than were discharged with disabilities: more than 3 million (in the United States and abroad) were excused from military duty for a day or more due to disease (influenza, bronchitis, and gonorrhea were common diagnoses), and 224,000 were temporarily excused from service, but not discharged, after being wounded in action.[25] Some who left the military due to disability never sought care as veterans, and many who were judged to be healthy upon their release from service later requested treatment, but data regarding discharges provide a picture of the diverse ailments that warranted care during and after the war.

Many injured and ill doughboys who demobilized in an era of rising faith in professional medicine viewed services previously available to veterans—the convalescent care offered in Soldiers' Homes being a primary example—as inadequate. But proponents of medicalized care could hardly predict the financial commitment it would entail. The veterans' health system arose at a time when few fully comprehended, or prioritized, the potential long-term costs of professionally administered health services.[26] By the 1930s, as the war receded from view, the Great Depression took hold, and social scientists undertook formal studies of financial burdens associated with medical care, an increasing number of health professionals and bureaucrats came to see the fully integrated, federally funded veterans' health system as an expensive and unwieldy commitment.

Building Expansive Social Policy in an Amorphous State

The widespread acknowledgment that the federal government should play some role in funding hospital care sprang from a Progressive Era conviction that the state should help citizens navigate the health- and work-related challenges of urban industrial life.[27] Formative prewar policies such as the 1917 War Risk Insurance Act, which offered service members access to disability and life insurance, envisioned military personnel first and foremost as employees of the federal government.[28] Similar principles shaped workers' compensation and occupational health measures emerging in the same period: laborers, whether they were employed by the federal government as privates and lieutenants or by business owners as machine operators, deserved certain rights. Not least of all, they deserved compensation and, in some cases, health services if their work led to illness or injury. In this respect, the World War I–era veterans' health system represented an attempt by the government to offer special services to a particular group of high-risk workers.[29]

Beyond showcasing how contemporary debates and values shaped health policy, the story of the beginning of the veterans' health system reveals intricacies of policy machinations. There was no single piece of legislation—no "comprehensive reform"—that established state-sponsored veterans' health care. Instead, it came about incrementally.[30] The 1917 War Risk Insurance Act made the government liable to care for veterans, but it contained few details regarding how that responsibility would be fulfilled. Over the next decade, bureaucrats, legislators, and professionals addressed questions about implementation, setting rules regarding access, federal oversight, and institution building while aiming at economic and operational efficiency. The early years of the veterans' health system show that "legislation cannot hard-wire administrative outcomes."[31] Elected officials, bureaucrats, and beneficiaries shaped (and consistently reshaped) how veterans' health care worked. As a result of their actions, veterans in the World War I era became part of a "protected public"—a clearly defined interest group that won government assistance in accessing health care, strengthening a trend of "rationing" that would continue in the decades to come.[32]

While the advent of a veterans' health system indicated a massive expansion of the reach of the state, it also illustrated the wider tendency of the government to award health entitlements selectively—to individuals based on their social standing and membership in a clearly definable group.[33] In the eighteenth century, the federal government established the Marine Hospital Service so that sailors, who were seen as potential threats to public health, could receive care in institutions.[34] In the nineteenth century, former slaves, people with developmental disabilities, people with mental illnesses, and American Indians also received government aid to access services. Care for each of those populations was often far from generous; it was based not solely on humanitarianism but on the goal of relieving local governments of burdens that community officials argued should be shouldered by the nation.[35] Federal involvement in increasing access to health care expanded in the twentieth century with the advent of Medicare and Medicaid in 1965.[36] But a century after it was established, the veterans' health system remains the largest integrated system of care in the United States—meaning, the government both funds and organizes service provision.

To say that the veterans' health system is integrated is not to say that it is, or has ever been, all-inclusive. World War I–era debates about veterans' worthiness for benefits highlighted enduring questions about how to administer public aid in a diverse society skeptical of centralized social assistance programs.[37] Ideological battles regarding the merits of a government-sponsored health system highlighted a long tradition of disdain toward "means-tested relief" and reverence for social insurance offered to groups based on "fixed, objective criteria such as age, disability, or unemployment."[38] Advocates of expanding veterans' access to hospital care argued in the 1920s and 1930s that it could "help people help themselves" and should be viewed as an entitlement—to be granted regardless of income.[39] But the story of the advent of a veterans' health system in the World War I era demonstrates that veterans' benefits often could not be so simply classified. Policies enacted throughout the 1920s stipulated that while veterans with service-connected disabilities could access publicly sponsored hospital care as social insurance with no means test, those with non-service-connected disabilities officially qualified for it as public assistance—if enough facilities existed, and if they demonstrated financial need. In the 1930s, when the latter group constituted more than 80 percent of veterans' hospital patients, government officials, doctors, and the general public expressed deep hostility toward a system they viewed as exorbitant and unproductive. Meanwhile, many veterans argued that their injuries and illnesses were definitively due to service, and that they had earned the right to publicly sponsored care.

Social conditions—not least of all considerations about the worthy poor, race, and gender—shaped veterans' health policies, as well as individuals' experiences of them.[40] Members of minority groups demanded quality health services but faced major barriers in accessing them, both in the military and veterans' health systems.[41] Deciphering who was entitled to receive treatment in publicly sponsored hospitals proved exceedingly complex.

The veterans' health system conditionally offered federal assistance with the end goal of self-reliance. As such, it foreshadowed watershed New Deal programs of the 1930s.[42] President Franklin D. Roosevelt and other elected leaders argued that the veterans' benefits system was too costly and wrongly privileged one group over the larger population. But they supported a signature piece of American social policy legislation—the Social Security Act—that provided old age and unemployment benefits to industrial and commercial workers, with some common motivations and goals. Although structured and funded differently than veterans' health care, the Social Security program was initially relatively selective and represented the hope that a large-scale system of federal assistance could serve as a safety net.[43] During debates about Social Security legislation in the 1930s, the veterans' health system served as a policy chameleon. Skeptics of increasing governmental provisions represented it as a showcase of wastefulness and bureaucratic failure while supporters argued that it rested on a noble American ideal: certain citizens could (and should) earn entitlements.

Soldiers, veterans, advocacy organizations, caregivers, reformers, and policy makers had distinct perceptions of the meaning and purpose of a veterans' health system. The dynamics of its creation and growth demonstrate that policy formation is "interactional"—a product of historical circumstance, grassroots-level experiences and activism, and the shape of the state and of political parties.[44] Hospital newspapers, transcripts of veterans' organizations' meetings, and letters, memoirs, and disability claims of former service members help explain why people felt compelled to join groups like the American Legion and the Disabled American Veterans in the interwar years and why they fought for—of all things—access to institutional health care.[45] While many veterans viewed health care as an earned right, government correspondence and congressional debates reveal that other political actors supported the expansion of health entitlements for reasons ranging from promoting social progress to staving off radicalism.[46] As such, the veterans' health system established in the interwar years fit larger tenets of social welfare policy: its multifaceted aims, which included "relief of misery" and "appeasing protest," appealed to diverse groups.[47]

Although the veterans' health system was a product of the interwar years, it has proven lasting and resilient, in part because the United States has spent the century since its creation in the "shadow of war."[48] At the Edith Nourse Rogers Memorial Veterans Hospital, Leonard Poirier receives medical care, but he also acts as an advocate for a younger generation. He and other veterans recently created the Consumer Council for Post-Traumatic Stress Disorder, focused on topics ranging from the need for more handicapped parking to ensuring that patients maintain communication with a therapist, even during annual summertime staffing transitions. Poirier points out that the group's regular troubleshooting meetings with VA personnel are not primarily geared at the needs of his cohort of Vietnam veterans. "We're dying off . . . we're all done," he says. Instead, Poirier's group is focused mainly on those who served in wars in Afghanistan and Iraq. "Now," he says, "we're fighting for them."[49]

In his quest, Poirier aims to enhance a system with a dynamic history.

CHAPTER ONE

An Extra-Hazardous Occupation

Preparing for the Health Outcomes of War

In the summer of 1918, as Allied and German troops endured mustard gas and shell explosions in northern France, Spanish-American War veteran Patrick O'Donnell penned a letter from his house in Massachusetts to the Eastern branch of the National Home for Disabled Volunteer Soldiers in Maine. He wondered whether his application to the facility, which offered domicile care and medical services to war veterans, had been approved. "They doctors around Boston doesn't seem to help me any," he explained. Plus, the 36-year-old former service member noted of his efforts to seek treatment, "I cannot afford to keep it up as I have a wife and 4 children and I haven't worked since last September."[1]

Two weeks later, Togus staff completed O'Donnell's admission forms, indicating that he had chronic gastritis and tabes dorsalis, a degenerative nerve condition in the spine that could cause shooting, burning pains, incontinence, and a variety of other symptoms. Paperwork from an earlier visit listed another condition: locomotor ataxia, which typically led to a loss of gross motor control and sensory perception and made the sufferer walk with jerking, lurching motions.[2]

At Togus, O'Donnell joined residents like Alonzo Nichols, a 70-year-old Civil War veteran who had worked as a cook before being admitted in April 1916. Nichols, too, suffered from a variety of debilitating heart conditions: myocarditis, cardiac hypertrophy and dilation, and arteriosclerosis. He was also missing parts of three fingers and had varicose veins and eczema on both legs.[3]

The cases of Nichols and O'Donnell foreshadowed the fates of millions of US service members who mobilized in 1917. In addition to harboring injuries that seemed directly attributable to war, both men suffered from chronic conditions that some would argue had little to do with military service. In O'Donnell's case, tabes dorsalis and locomotor ataxia likely resulted from untreated syphilis.[4] And Nichols's heart trouble was probably, at least in part, a product of old age.[5]

But both had served their country. And both had few alternatives to seeking care from the government.

In the months surrounding the 1917 declaration of war by the United States, policy makers, civilian advisers, military officials, and medical professionals readily acknowledged that wounded and ill soldiers were an inevitable consequence of raising an army. They knew about Soldiers' Homes like the one at Togus. They were well aware that thousands of service members had been treated in England and France since 1914 for a variety of ailments, from psychological conditions and tuberculosis to amputations and gunshot wounds.

But they hoped to quell some of the dire consequences of war through smart, efficient planning. As the United States mobilized forces, policy makers were determined to create self-sufficient soldiers and veterans—rehabilitated, trained to work, and able to provide for their families. In this hopeful model, planning for long-term care in hospitals was as abhorrent as planning for cash pensions: it signified that former service members might become facile, unproductive, and dependent on their government.

There were hints in 1917 of problems to come. Although some forecast that soldiers would demand medical services following their discharge, the framers of the War Risk Insurance Act, members of the Council of National Defense Medical Board, army officials, and others focused on the more immediate—and in some ways less amorphous—matter of planning for the rehabilitation and care of military personnel. But even as they reached a general consensus that the army should oversee a wide-ranging rehabilitation program, there were delays in implementing a definitive plan. Army officials and policy makers faced difficult questions about the nature of care for service members, especially those who suffered from mental illness and exposure to poison gas. When should personnel be discharged? Where might they turn for assistance as civilians? Policies established by social reformers, doctors, and army officials of the Progressive Era set parameters during and after the war, as bureaucrats, caregivers, legislators, and veterans debated what the government owed to its former service members.

"Fitting him for a life of activity and usefulness"

It had been about a month since President Woodrow Wilson had declared war, and now the western Pennsylvania town of Philipsburg was rallying support for the mobilization effort with a patriotic parade. Eighteen-year-old Cornelius

Vernoy Davis joined the festivities as memories of summers spent in the local "Boy's Brigade" ran through his mind. Organized by a local Spanish-American War veteran named Mr. Graffius, the group wore khaki uniforms, learned about arms and close-order drill, and participated in mock battles. During those events, Davis recalled, participants who were "designated to fall wounded or dead" were wrapped in "red stained bandages" and carried off the field by "stretcher-bearers." Around a campfire at night, after the younger children were asleep, Mr. Graffius would talk about the "horrors of the Philippine campaign."

"Is there any wonder," Davis later reflected, "that many of us were inspired with the desire to go to war?"

Within a few days of the parade, Davis received assurances from the local school board that he would be awarded a high school diploma even if he enlisted and shipped out before the end of classes. As he said his goodbyes to his family, his mother and sisters urged him to reconsider; his father, a local storeowner who regretted that he had not served during the Spanish-American War, did nothing to discourage him.

On May 14, 1917, Davis joined other young men at the local train station and headed to the nearest recruiting office. There, he chose to enlist in the US Army's Field Artillery because he wanted to "operate a big gun rather than use a rifle." Next, the cohort went by ferry to Fort Slocum, New York, where they stripped down for showers then lined up to be examined by doctors who would determine if they were fit to serve. After their physicals, they "were sent thru a gantlet of needles, like sheep through a dip," as Davis put it. Some "passed out cold" before receiving the injections. As some of the first combatants in a major war to have access to a typhoid vaccine and tetanus and diphtheria antitoxins, they learned early that medicine and technology could minimize the risk of harm.[6] After the young men got dressed, they lined up again and prepared to take the Oath of Allegiance: "I, Cornelius Vernoy Davis, do solemnly swear that I will support and defend the Constitution of the United States against all enemies, foreign and domestic; that I will bear true faith and allegiance to the same."[7]

Davis likely did not know that philosophical and legal debates were under way in Washington, DC, regarding the government's obligations to him as a soldier and future veteran. But as he and other early recruits received their uniforms, Woodrow Wilson and his underlings were calling on their Progressive allies to help conceive of orderly and rational plans for mobilization and beyond.

The War Risk Insurance Act set the tone for the legislative conceptualization of the treatment of Great War soldiers and veterans—wounded, ill, or healthy.

The original act, passed soon after the outbreak of war in Europe in 1914, provided $100,000 for the establishment of a Bureau of War Risk Insurance in the US Treasury Department, which would administer an insurance program for "American vessels, their freight, and passage moneys, and cargoes shipped or to be shipped therein, against loss or damage by the risks of war."[8] When the United States declared war in April 1917, it became clear that human beings, not just materiel, would be mobilized in the conflict, and policy makers expanded the law to include protections for men and women who served in the armed forces.

The revised War Risk Insurance Act indicated that the United States had an expanded agenda when it came to ensuring the security of those who served, as well as their families. It contained plans for three types of assistance and protection. First, all male service members who had "Class A dependents"—a wife, a child under 18, a child of any age who was "insane or permanently helpless," or an ex-wife who had not remarried and had been granted rights to alimony payments—were obliged to allot half of their monthly $30 pay to familial support. For the purposes of the act, a dependent was a person who was "compelled to rely, and the relations between the parties are such that he has a right to rely in whole or in part on the other for his support." The federal government supplied an "allowance" that was contingent on the number of dependents and was at least equal to, if not greater than, the service member's contribution. The second form of support offered by the War Risk Insurance Act was government-funded compensation for death and disability. Regardless of income, a service member who incurred a disability "in the line of duty" would receive monthly payments while he was physically unable to earn a living. The amount of the payment would be based on "the size of his family." A variety of conditions might preclude him from receiving payment: for example, receiving a dishonorable discharge, registering as a conscientious objector, or bearing an injury that resulted from willful misconduct. Finally, the act laid plans for a non-compulsory life and disability insurance scheme. Within 120 days of enlistment, service members could purchase a policy worth $1,000 to $10,000; the government would deduct from their monthly paychecks 63 cents to $3.35. In the event of death or total permanent disability (according to the act, "an impairment of the mind or body which renders it impossible for the disabled person to follow a gainful occupation") service members or their beneficiaries could receive up to 240 payments in monthly installments.[9]

In addition to serving as the basis for an allotment, allowance, and insurance system, the War Risk Insurance Act vaguely guaranteed that those who needed medical care could receive it. "The injured person shall be furnished by the United States," it said, "such reasonable governmental medical, surgical, and hospital services and with such supplies, including artificial limbs, trusses, and similar appliances, as the director (of the Bureau of War Risk Insurance) may determine to be useful and reasonably necessary."[10] The law offered no explanation of how such ideals would become a reality.

It was a remarkable oversight, considering that medical care was, at the time, viewed as an occasionally costly commodity. Included in discussions of the War Risk Insurance Act were excerpts of a 1917 report to the Dallas, Texas, Wage Commission, which analyzed city residents' cost of living. It noted that medical costs as well as "loss of time through . . . sickness" could represent "a double loss" for an employee.[11] Paying heed to that fact, in the second decade of the twentieth century, the American Association of Labor Legislation undertook campaigns across the country to advocate for compulsory health insurance for workers. Their efforts, inspired in large part by recently enacted policies in England and other European countries, gained support from some civic-minded doctors and public health advocates, but were opposed by medical societies fearing a loss of control over treatment, labor unions dreading diminished wages, and large corporations hoping to engender worker loyalty through the pursuit of welfare capitalism.[12]

Policy makers of 1917 devised a unique system of assistance and protection, in part as a means of distancing their efforts from previous initiatives surrounding veterans' entitlements. The Revolutionary War Pension Act of 1818 served as a poor law of sorts for veterans who could demonstrate financial need. After the Civil War, federal pensions were refigured with the intention of limiting the number of potential beneficiaries: lawmakers mandated that benefits would be contingent on the degree to which a malady limited an individual's ability to work. But thanks in no small part to the eagerness of politicians to gain the favor of veterans as a voting bloc, they gradually expanded coverage; by the late 1880s, more than one-third of all elderly men living in the North, as well as men, widows, and dependents of veterans across the nation, received quarterly payments from the US Pension Bureau.[13] The nineteenth-century laws set a precedent that veterans could receive government payments by virtue of the fact that they had served. The fact that they were passed demonstrated the potential political power of a veterans' lobby.

As they debated the contents of the War Risk Insurance Act in the summer of 1917, politicians, insurance experts, and social reformers supported the ideal of rehabilitation as an alternative to the legacy of dependency they felt had arisen from Civil War veterans' pensions, which had been subsuming more and more of the federal budget since the late nineteenth century. Secretary of the Treasury William J. McAdoo, a former businessman, called pensions, "a helpful measure of justice" for a former service member but argued that "rehabilitation and reeducation, fitting him for a life of activity and usefulness" was a societal "obligation." Crucially, although such ideals were central to the contents and general structure of the War Risk Insurance Act, McAdoo pointed out that "the bill does not attempt to cover the matter of means and methods of effecting this."[14]

In many ways, for those devising the War Risk Insurance Act, aftercare was an afterthought. In a report evaluating a draft of the act, a committee of insurance experts noted that, in general, "the benefits are fair and liberal." As for injured veterans, the report noted, "if the man has a mother or wife, the necessary care will be provided by the family, and if the man is alone he will live at some home or hospital provided for such cases."[15]

As they discussed the War Risk Insurance Act, McAdoo and his colleagues were pondering a deeper question, one that had come to the fore in the past and would arise again in months after the Armistice: should soldiers and veterans receive government entitlements strictly by virtue of past military service, or should the nature of that service and other considerations apply? Selectivity, they decided, was preferable. "The great outcry against the [Civil War] compensation system had not been due to the moneys that were paid to the men who died or were disabled because of injuries received while serving this country," declared Julian Mack during War Risk Insurance Act hearings. "The outcry," he said, came with the establishment of the service pension legislation in the 1890s, which "aims to give a man a pension because he was a soldier, and sometimes a soldier for 30 days, and sometimes not much of a soldier at that for 30 days."[16]

The perspective that a service member's social status and background should determine his level of compensation was firmly rooted in the Progressive Era ideologies of Mack and his fellow reformers. A lawyer and judge by trade, Mack helped manage the affairs of "the first children's court in the world" in Chicago. There, one of his obituaries noted, he implemented his credo that a child accused of a crime "should, of course, be made to know that he is face to face with the power of the state, but he should at the same time, and more emphatically, be made to feel that he is the object of its care and solicitude."[17] In juvenile cases, Mack wrote in 1909, "the problem for determination by the judge is not, Has this boy or girl committed a specific wrong, but What is he, how has he become what he is, and what had best be done in his interest and in the interest of the state to save him from a downward career."[18] The government, Progressives like Mack strongly believed, could be a force for good not only in regulating industry but also in reforming the behavior of individuals—not least of all of those who were poor or not fully "Americanized."

In addition to harboring reservations about a pension system, Mack and his colleagues were skeptical about the future of another staple of the existing veterans' welfare state—a national system of Soldiers' Homes. Serving as social service institutions above all, the Homes were intended to provide somewhat domestic environments for war veterans like Alonzo Nichols and Patrick O'Donnell, who may have had few other options. By June 1917, ten branches of the homes housed approximately 20,300 veterans—a massive increase over the June 1890 population of about 13,000. Hospitals stood alongside residences and workshops at Soldiers' Homes, but were not the primary focus of the institutions. In the summer of 1917, of more than 20,000 home residents, approximately 2,700 were being treated in hospitals. Another 1,800 were considered "sick" in their quarters.[19] Even as the homes provided an important institutional precedent for future veterans' hospitals, World War I–era policy makers pointed to them as symbols of economic and social dependency, and as the antithesis of modern health care. A February 1918 account of the virtues of the War Risk Insurance Act noted that "the soldiers' home will not reappear after this war if the spirit of this measure is carried out." Instead, the government would rely on "allotments and allowances," insurance payments, and "re-education and vocational training." The latter effort, the report suggested, might take place in hospitals overseen by the War Department, which had "large plans underway for putting into operation the best methods of dealing with injuries of varying character."[20] In this model, modern military hospitals would be the antithesis of—and render unnecessary—Soldiers' Homes.

The War Risk Insurance Act contained a stipulation that veterans would be provided with "hospital services and supplies" because hospitals were, in the lead-up to World War I more than during any other conflict, viewed as ideal sites of treatment. In the nineteenth century, prior to the acceptance of the germ theory of disease, such institutions were the province of poor and working-class patients who could not afford home-based care. But by the turn of the twentieth century, many believed they provided certain amenities unattainable in the home, such as a sanitary environment and access to new technologies like the X-ray. In 1873, 178 hospitals existed in the United States. By 1909, there were more than 4,300. The institutions were products of new understandings of disease pathology, the professionalization of medicine, changing socioeconomic conditions, and the advent of an urban, industrial economy.[21]

In addition to being shaped by larger social and demographic realities and transformations in the world of professional medicine, the War Risk Insurance Act was practically and ideologically modeled on contemporary legislation focusing on various aspects of workers' rights. In the first decades of the twentieth century, a "coalition of radicals, reformers, labor leaders, and . . . business representatives" who believed the newly powerful United States was "woefully behind the industrialized European community" looked to the government to create a rational system to manage workplace hazards.[22] Among other things, they fought for legislation to establish an eight-hour workday, limitations on child labor, and workers' compensation laws that would provide payment and, in some cases, medical services, to an employee following a workplace accident. By 1920, forty-two states had workers' compensation laws on the books.[23] According to one insurance expert of the time, compensation laws, whether administered by private companies or state or federal governments, were centered on "earning power"; they were intended to serve as a safety net when beneficiaries experienced "the loss of ability to earn money."[24] The general theory behind them, a 1920 report said, was that "instead of the least able unit of industry (the worker) assuming . . . risks, the consuming public, acting through the employer, furnishes relief to injured workers by fixed awards."[25] Likewise, the War Risk Insurance Act offered soldiers and veterans some security based on the fact that they were, on the simplest level, employees of the federal government. A 1918 journal article noted that the legislation was predicated on the idea that "the government of the United States is the employer and the nation or the people of the United States are the consumers or those for whom the operation of war are carried on."[26]

The War Risk Insurance Act reflected an increasing reliance on workers' compensation and occupational safety laws for security in a modernizing economy, as well as the mainstreaming of modern life insurance policies. Well before World War I, life insurance had become common among middle-class Americans. By 1870, the US life insurance industry was worth $1.3 billion, and one in three northeastern families owned a policy.[27] In a sense, the shape of the act indicated an acceptance—and adoption—by the American government of private business practices and trends.

The composition of the army was also an important factor in the shaping of the War Risk Insurance Act, whose authors argued that conscripted soldiers, in many respects, deserved more than volunteers or career soldiers or officers. Because the United States was "drafting men and compelling them to make, if necessary, the supreme sacrifice for their country," Secretary McAdoo maintained, "a higher obligation . . . rests upon the government to mitigate the horrors of war . . . through compensations, indemnities, and insurance." Dramatically driving the point home, McAdoo argued, soldiers "should know that if they are disabled, totally or partially—if they come back armless, legless, sightless or otherwise permanently injured—definite provision is made for them, and that they are not going to be left to the uncertain chances of future legislation or to the scandals of our old pension system." Such guarantees should not be construed as "charity," McAdoo noted, but "part of his deserved compensation for the extra-hazardous occupation into which his government has forced him."[28] Julian Mack agreed with the premise that conscripted soldiers deserved more comprehensive guarantees than volunteers. He argued that men who enlisted voluntarily in the armed forces as individuals could be "dealt with . . . alone" by the government, through the provision of compensation for injuries and illnesses. "But in these days of the draft and conscription, when you take a man away from his family against his will the family ought to be considered."[29]

Although debates about the War Risk Insurance Act, and the ideals it contained, focused mainly on male service members, the law's conditions applied to a limited number of women. As a result of hard-fought battles by women nurses at the turn of the century, which led to the establishment of a permanent Nurse Corps in the army in 1901 and the navy in 1908, military nurses by the outbreak of World War I were no longer considered civilian personnel, but instead appointees of the military branch with which they served. According to the act, women could make allotments to dependents, but unlike male service members, they were under no obligation to do so.[30] Section 300 of the act stipulated that compensation rules applied to "any commissioned officer or enlisted man or . . . any member of the Army Nurse Corps (female) or of the Navy Nurse Corps (female)."[31] Though such measures were, in many respects, relatively egalitarian, they did not include thousands of women who worked with volunteer organizations such as the Red Cross and YMCA, and with the army in roles still considered "civilian," such as occupational and physical therapists. In the 1920s and 1930s, women who served in various capacities—including nurses who argued that the government was not fulfilling its obligation to them—would fight for an expansion in access to compensation and care.[32]

As policy makers debated the War Risk Insurance Act in the summer of 1917, some predicted future problems, worrying that the legislation would lead to subsequent demands for more generous benefits. John A. Key (D-OH), chairman of the Committee on Pensions, believed that "should the pending bill be enacted with its present provisions . . . within a year from the date of its passage, Congress will be flooded by bills, seeking by special acts of Congress individual cases to adjust, rectify, and remove the inequalities and injustice."[33] In fact, by guaranteeing "reasonable governmental medical, surgical, and hospital services," the act paved the way for a flood of complaints during and after the war. Although it certainly did not establish a veterans' hospital system, the rights it guaranteed eventually helped bring about federally sponsored medical care for millions of veterans. Key's words proved prophetic.

In 1917, however, others took the stance that the pace of mobilization made decisive action necessary. Supporters of the War Risk Insurance Act argued that unique times called for drastic—and hasty—measures. "When it comes to saying exactly what should be offered at the end of the war, it is a little difficult to formulate it in two or three weeks, and to say exactly what is practicable," noted Philemon Tecumseh Sherman, a New York lawyer who specialized in workmen's compensation, unemployment, and old-age insurance, and served during the war as a government adviser. "We left the exact formulation of that to be determined later."[34]

The "family-focused" nature of the War Risk Insurance Act helps explain why legislators overlooked—or left to the discretion of others—details regarding how soldiers and veterans could access care following military discharge. According to the act, a service member was not a man alone but a husband, father, and provider. Indefinite post-service incapacitation—whether at a hospital or any other institution—was contrary to one of its paramount goals: "keeping the family together."[35] The idea made perfect sense to commentators eager to find an alternative to poverty and pensions. The War Risk Insurance Act, according to the editors of *Outlook* magazine, represented "the last word in scientific, thoughtful, and wise care for the soldier by the people of the country through its Government."[36]

"The problem is military and should be under military control"

While Julian Mack, William McAdoo, and others pored over statistics and debated legal terms, C. Vernoy Davis was learning how to ride a horse at Fort Sam Houston in Texas. The beginning of training, he wrote in his diary, was "a circus," especially since he had never so much as sat in a saddle. The oppressive weather did not help any; trainees often became overheated, fainted, and were "placed in the shade of one of the buildings and left to revive . . . while the drill continued without interruption."[37]

On one such warm summer day, after two weeks of riding practice, Davis was feeling confident enough to request an especially spirited horse for a cross-country trek. He was having "the time of (his) life," galloping at a clip, when the horse caught his back legs on a fence and fell to the ground, throwing Davis over his head in the process. As the animal struggled to get up, he rolled over a still crouched Davis. "It was a terrible crushing feeling," the young trainee recalled. "And I found that I could not move my legs."[38]

Davis was several miles away from camp, and, at first, there was little his captain could do but offer him a cigarette. When the trainee refused it and also refused the offer of chewing tobacco, his superior quipped: "What the hell are you going to do in the army if you don't smoke or chew?" He soon had the young soldier placed on his horse for a long ride—"agony," as Davis recalled—to the camp medic.[39]

The doctor rushed Davis to the Fort Sam Houston hospital, where he spent the next five weeks. The base hospital, which had been enlarged during battles along the Mexican border in 1916, was one of many army institutions undergoing a war-related expansion in the summer of 1917. Davis might have witnessed workers constructing ten new pavilion wards, a new kitchen, an X-ray room, and a ward for women patients. In the year to come, Fort Sam Houston would see the addition of new roads, two psychiatric wards, and Red Cross and YMCA recreation buildings. Even in July 1917, before the extensive work was complete, patients in the main building of the hospital had access to well-ventilated rooms and electricity—amenities that were luxurious in comparison with those available in smaller post and camp hospitals. While in many ways, things could have been worse, Davis's personal situation posed substantial challenges. He was initially unable to get off his back and passing "a great quantity of blood," the result, he soon learned, of a ruptured left kidney. After two weeks, he determinedly became more upright—moving from bed to wheelchair to crutches to his own two feet. Army officials offered Davis an honorable discharge with disability, but he turned it down, eager to join his unit, which he had learned was soon to embark for Europe.[40]

By August 16, 1917, less than a month after being released from the hospital, Davis was standing watch for German submarines aboard a ship bound for France. After a stint on all-night duty took a toll on his damaged hips, he reported for sick call to ask for something to relieve the pain. But he found little sympathy and no relief. "We will be in France in a few days and then it may not be too long until you are killed in action and your pains will be over," a doctor told him. At that point, Davis made a decision: "That was the last time I ever reported for sick call, how ever sick I was." Years later, Davis would learn that his pain was more than justified. In addition to the ruptured left kidney, the fall at Fort Sam Houston had brought about fractures in both of his hips, an internal hernia, and damage to several discs in his neck. Meanwhile, as his ship neared the front lines, his medical troubles were about to multiply.[41]

Several parties attempted to coordinate efforts to ensure that Davis and other soldiers had access to medical and rehabilitative services. While the War Risk Insurance Act laid the legislative foundation for soldiers' and veterans' entitlements, government officials, military personnel, doctors, and other professionals deliberated complex health-related questions outside the halls of Congress. How and to what extent would the medical profession be mobilized? How would a variety of federal agencies and organizations—military branches, the Public Health Service, the American Red Cross—divide responsibilities and coordinate their activities? What role would private medical schools and hospitals play? What services would be offered at hospitals like the one at Fort Sam Houston? Should wounded and ill service members remain enlisted while they were being treated? As civilian and military personnel discussed options at the height of the mobilization efforts, they focused on the immediate and pragmatic goal of ensuring that service members had access to care. What would happen to them once they became veterans remained, in many respects, unclear.

Meetings of the Council of National Defense Medical Board provided an important forum for discussion. Created by an act of Congress in August 1916, and fully organized in March 1917, the CND was charged with the "coordination of industries and resources for the national security and welfare" and the "creation of relations which will render possible in time of need the immediate concentration and utilization of the resources of the nation." It included the secretaries of war, the navy, agriculture, commerce, and labor, who were responsible for electing seven representatives "with special knowledge" of a specific industry or natural resource, or who were "otherwise specially qualified." The first annual report of the CND, released in June 1917, made a self-conscious declaration: "It has become a truism that no past war has been so essentially a war of the mechanic and the machine, and it is the realization of this truth that has been the inspiration of the policy pursued by the council."[42] As such, the bulk of CND activities had to do with industry—for example, coordinating railroad operation and "managing" conflicts between labor and capital. The seven council representatives included the civic and business elites of the day: Daniel Willard, president of the Baltimore & Ohio Railroad, oversaw transportation and communications; Julius Rosenwald, president of Sears Roebuck & Co., was in charge of supplies; banker Bernard M. Baruch coordinated raw materials, minerals, and metals; American Federation of Labor president Samuel Gompers dealt with labor issues. Never before had the government played such an active role in managing the economy.[43]

Among the "industrial" representatives on the CND, Chicago surgeon Franklin H. Martin headed the efforts concerning medicine. A personal friend of army surgeon general William C. Gorgas, Martin personified "a virtual revolution" taking place in the medical profession and its affiliated institutions. At the turn of the twentieth century, the increasingly powerful American Medical Association promoted the implementation of universal standards for medical education, as specialization increased and surgery—separate and apart from general practice—gained respectability.[44] During those years, Martin helped establish the journal *Surgery, Gynecology and Obstetrics* and served as an active member of local and state medical societies. In 1913, he helped to found, and became director-general, of the American College of Surgeons, an organization that had a mission ranging from hospital standardization to passing guidelines for the proper care of injuries and chronic diseases.

Martin did not have to search far for the personnel or structure of his CND General Medical Board; he had a prototype in the Committee of American Physicians for Medical Preparedness, which was formed in April 1916 by joint action of the presidents of the American Medical Association, the American Surgical Association, the Congress of American Physicians and Surgeons, and the Clinical Congress of Surgeons of North America. Members of the committee, aware that Congress was debating the National Defense Act, quickly organized nine-member state groups with two overarching duties: to obtain information regarding medical resources in local communities and to secure applicants for the Army Medical Reserve Corps. When the Committee of American Physicians for Medical Preparedness offered its services to Woodrow Wilson soon after its formation, the president replied that he was "regretful that existing laws did not permit the acceptance by the federal government of gratuitous services." But the administration managed to get around the problem by asking the committee to do its work under the auspices of the CND, thus capitalizing on the power and considerable reach of the private sector group. With the formation of the CND Medical Board, prominent American medical professionals went from meeting and corresponding privately to serving as officially sanctioned experts for the federal government. Professors of medicine, municipal health officials, and officers of professional organizations oversaw a variety of subcommittees focused on topics such as shell shock, ophthalmology, surgical methods, cardiovascular impairment, drug addiction, tuberculosis, public health nursing, and alcohol, among others.[45]

Throughout 1917, questions regarding how the war would affect health professionals dominated CND General Medical Board meetings. Its members lobbied congressional representatives to exempt medical students from the draft and to offer higher rank and pay for enlisted doctors. The medical board also attempted to establish professional standards for those who remained at home. It ordered doctors who maintained private practices to cap their fees and abstain from attempting to permanently win over patients of colleagues who were serving. Board members also spent much time organizing state committees to coordinate enlistment drives. Civilian professional groups thereby assisted the army in reaching its quota of wartime doctors. Further to this cause, the board assisted with the staffing of a Medical Reserve Corps, which allowed medical students an alternative to being drafted into enlisted service. In addition, it helped to devise standards for medical suppliers who intended to do business with the government.[46]

Meetings of the medical board also served as forums for the exchange of information and requests. The surgeons general of the army, navy, and Public Health Service (PHS) each provided concise reports of their activities surrounding physical examinations of soldiers, base camp and ship sanitation, and staffing of medical personnel. Occasionally, they revealed their prewar professional passions. PHS surgeon general Rupert Blue, for example, was a long-time advocate of compulsory sickness insurance and advancement of workers' health; he lobbied actively at CND meetings for a comprehensive study of the health of industrial workers in war industries, which he argued was necessary for efficient mobilization. Many understood that with the frenzy of war came opportunity. Professional advancement, for example, was a priority of women physicians, orthopedists, and dentists, all of whom participated in CND meetings and argued that they should enjoy equal access to work as part of the US military effort.[47]

Organizing care for soldiers with chronic conditions and wounded and ill veterans was hardly a top priority for organizations focused on mobilizing forces, but various parties rightfully predicted that there would be some demand for long-term care. In April 1917, a member of the board's hospital committee noted that a "previous report" had recommended that the CND be "given authority to consider the ultimate need of special hospitals or facilities for the care of special groups of cases such as neurological, orthopedic, mental, those suffering from shell shock, etc." But "in order to guard against the duplication of work, it was voted that the chairman be requested to determine whether or not they [*sic*] desire this committee to take up this problem and to organize these special hospital facilities." To be sure, the representative noted, "the committee is ready to be of service in every possible way, in undertaking constructive work, but it wishes to avoid duplication of work which may already be provided for in some other way."[48] In its May 13, 1917, report to the medical board, the CND hospital committee acknowledged that "a study of the ultimate need of convalescent hospitals, and a large group of special hospitals such as shell shock, orthopedic, cardiac, etc." was "of such magnitude and requires so much detailed and special information, most of which can only be obtained from the sanitary service of our allies, that your committee feels this work is quite beyond this committee." The group thus rescinded the responsibility of deliberating the provision of long-term health services and suggested that the issue be addressed by the Army Surgeon General's Office.[49] In the winter of 1917 and the spring of 1918, the general topic of hospital aftercare rarely came up in CND Medical Board meetings.

Although the CND medical board was focused primarily on governmental efforts and institutions, some advocated for deeper civil-military coordination. In December 1917, Sigismund Shulz Goldwater of the American Hospital Association told the CND Medical Board that his organization "deplored" the fact that the army did not want to utilize "existing institutions." Given the fact that the "Army must be sure of preparation, must have absolute control of everything it does," Goldwater conceded that it was "easy to understand" why it must "oversee care of its own personnel." Still, "there are instances in which private institutions and hospitals can be utilized to advantage." He urged the medical board not to "assume that the hospitals already existing have nothing to contribute."[50]

Goldwater elaborated on the point in the pages of *Modern Hospital* magazine, where articles demonstrated that the range of questions faced by officials planning for the treatment of soldiers—regarding ideal hospital design and the usefulness of various clinical specialties, for example—also shaped debates taking place in the broader civilian health care world. In mid-1918, Goldwater sat on the editorial board of *Modern Hospital* with Henry M. Hurd, Winford H. Smith, and other physicians who constituted a tight circle of some of the most prominent civilian hospital policy makers of the day.[51] Smith, for example, had succeeded Hurd as the superintendent of the prestigious Johns Hopkins Hospital, serving in that post from 1911 through 1946. All the while, he assisted in planning and organizing some of the country's most prominent medical centers: Duke, Cornell, Vanderbilt, and Yale Universities, as well as the Universities of Chicago and California. He also served as a medical adviser in both world wars. Around the outbreak of World War I, Smith, Goldwater, and their colleagues were especially concerned with ensuring that the general public ceased viewing hospitals as dens of dependency and began to see them as embodiments of the great promise of professional medical care—a "necessary factor in the preservation of health."[52]

Goldwater hoped that service members would enjoy the fruits of modernizing institutions and be treated among their fellow citizens. "The time of military officers would be wasted," he argued, "if devoted to the care of physical wrecks returned from France, this being a job for a civilian, not a military man." Goldwater did not take issue with the idea that the Army Medical Department should maintain control of some cases—soldiers who fell ill at cantonments, for example, or those who were being cared for at or near the front lines. He was concerned mainly with the domestic care of the severely wounded and seriously ill. "The extension and development of existing civil hospitals and sanatoriums under government direction, in accordance with a Government program, and with the support of Government funds," he argued, "may conceivably be a better way of providing the additional facilities required than the purchase of hospital sites in localities remote from the centers of population, and the erection, upon such sites of costly 'special military hospitals.'" The latter, Goldwater said, would have difficulty attracting "competent staffs" that could be retained after the war. Goldwater urged the government to undertake a comprehensive study of domestic civil hospitals to ascertain how they could serve in the war effort.[53] Thomas W. Salmon, chief of psychiatry for the American Expeditionary Forces (AEF), also doubted that army rehabilitation and medical efforts could completely alleviate the need for care after individuals were discharged. "Few who we fail to cure here will recover under *any* military treatment," he wrote from France during the war. "Those who must be evacuated to the United States should find Homes of Recovery . . . perhaps those homes later might serve for treating neuroses among the poor and moderately well off."[54] Salmon, like many others, recognized the need for civilian aftercare but remained focused on the all-encompassing and more immediate problem of rehabilitating soldiers.

Conversations about hospital care for soldiers—and who should oversee it— often centered on vocational education, which prewar planners included as a crucial aspect of an injured patient's "cure." "The establishment of reconstruction hospitals, or hospital schools, for the repair of cripples and disabled persons is essential," one report to the CND Medical Board maintained. Such institutions should be aimed at ensuring that the soldier-patient would be "self-supporting or partly self-supporting." They should also be "under military control" since it had been observed in Europe that, once discharged, "many disabled soldiers . . . would not undertake reeducation, and apparently preferred to be permitted to remain helpless and, thus, a social liability." CND representatives pointed out that in England, participation in vocational rehabilitation programs was optional, and only about 15 percent of all eligible service members enrolled.[55]

That was unfortunate and avoidable, according to council representatives. Jefferson R. Kean, director of military relief for the American Red Cross, noted that while treating soldiers abroad, "it was impossible to accomplish anything . . . unless they were under military discipline and treated as soldiers until repair work has been completed." As such, Kean argued, "The problem is military and should be under military control."[56] In March 1918, Charles H. Mayo, chairman of the CND Committee on Surgery, former president of the American Medical Association, and co-founder of Minnesota's famed Mayo Clinic, voiced his support for that policy. "The Surgeon General has full control of the men in the army until they are discharged," he said. "This is exactly as it should be and it is fortunate for us. So, military medical and surgical service will reconstruct disabled men."[57] In other words, the United States should keep men soldiers until they could be discharged as workers, or at least as semi-independent.

One problem with such a policy was that it required the acquiescence of individual service members, including many who sought discharge as soon as possible, regardless of their physical state. "Many will want to go out of the army," Frank Billings, who oversaw the army's rehabilitation program, told the medical board. "They have been abroad for months in an unusual environment and want to get out—they are homesick." But such an impulse, Billings argued, must be discouraged. "We must create a sentiment to educate that soldier. He must not return to his home until he can make a living for himself better than he did before—until he can enjoy life."[58]

Others rightfully predicted that the rehabilitation project would gradually expand, and gain import among various groups as time passed, but most fingers pointed to the Army Medical Department as the proper entity to oversee hospital care for ailing soldiers, regardless of the likelihood that they would return to duty. Rehabilitative treatment "would have to go on for years after the war" and necessitate the establishment of "a considerable number of hospitals," Army Surgeon General William Gorgas said at a CND meeting in October 1917. But the long-term vision of such institutions was hazy, if not completely lacking. "Some provisions will have to be made for these great hospitals after the war is over." But, he added, "we concluded to let that go and not decide the exact means of taking care of them until the time comes." Gorgas remained focused on the massive problem of care for soldiers, though he did share his belief that, "it seems to me if we get these [hospitals] organized and running, it will be natural for the War Department to continue afterward these hospitals."[59] Like the head of the CND hospital committee and those who debated the War Risk Insurance Act, the army surgeon general knew that postwar hospital care and rehabilitation programs for veterans would be necessary, but he pushed the matter aside as he concentrated on more pressing concerns.

Planning for the postwar care of veterans was ideologically problematic and fell outside of everyone's purview. Hospitals focused on aftercare were costly, they symbolized a lack of faith in the broader military-based rehabilitation and reconstruction project, and they could lead to the onset of "hospitalization of the patient"—a condition believed to promote laziness and complacency.[60] Meanwhile, the "patchwork of public and private institutions" helping to stock and sanitize military camps and train and examine soldiers focused primarily on their own organizational goals.[61] Government officials and doctors pointed out the need for nonmilitary institutions that could address the specific health problems of former service members, but they argued that the issue was too complex to be handled hastily or piecemeal. Many acknowledged the problem, but no one directly addressed it in practical terms.

"Functionally restored as far as possible"

It had been a long journey to the front for the 7th Field Artillery of the First Division, but a year after he set sail for Europe, C. Vernoy Davis was a weathered soldier. He had spent the early fall of 1917 training at a camp in Valdahon, on the western border of France, and the winter marching into battle, sleeping in barns in small towns, and hearing horror stories about young women being raped by German soldiers. Along the way, the number and frequency of the gas and shell attacks he endured and executed increased. By the summer of 1918, Davis could report that seeing a "man with his head blown off" was "not a pretty sight." He had come to believe that his oilskin slicker could protect him from being burned during a mustard gas attack. He had been amused one morning as a shell hit the breakfast that sat inches away from him and oatmeal splashed his face. When he was buried with his gun crew after an explosion brought the ground in from around their pit, he watched his friend and fellow soldier John McMahon become a "raving maniac." Once the young men were dug out, he saw "Mac" get shipped out to a nearby hospital for treatment for shell shock.[62]

Shortly before he made his way to the Second Battle of the Marne in July 1918, Davis could state in no uncertain terms that his bold actions—emerging from a foxhole during heavy fire to repair his gun, running across a "hot" area so he could retrieve water—were motivated not by bravery but instead by a firm conviction that he would not live through the war anyway. During the fierce fighting at the Marne, he observed that, viewed from a distance, a field covered with dead bodies could appear to be moving by virtue of the number of maggots wriggling about. From time to time, he and his fellow soldiers retched from the stench of decaying flesh. In these otherworldly conditions, Davis and his comrades might kill a group of German soldiers, then search their gear for food and souvenirs—watch chains, belt buckles, uniform buttons and shoulder straps. One of the most horrific memories of this time, for Davis at least, were the "pop" and "tssss" sounds he heard after battle, "like the removing of a cork from a bottle of warm champagne." It was some time before the young soldier learned that the bodies of recently fallen fighters "had filled up with gas as they lay in the hot sun and when their bellies burst, the escaping gas made the hissing noise."[63]

Davis was finally hit on July 21, 1918. He and his gun crew were in the middle of an open field, completely exposed to German airpower. At about 8:30 at night, he ran for a foxhole as a German plane broke formation to rain machine-gun fire down on what remained of his unit. Finding a fellow soldier already occupying the hole, Davis lay down beside a pile of shells, shooting up at the plane with his .45 pistol. As he trained his eyes on the sky, the ground to his left "flew into the air, accompanied with a deafening explosion." Davis was "rolled over and over by the concussion." Only as the plane flew on and he got up did Davis realize he had been injured. A stream of blood gushed from the sleeve of his jacket, and his left arm and hand were numb. A medic swiftly made his way over and tied a tourniquet between Davis' shoulder and elbow to stop the bleeding near the point of impact. Soon the numbness wore off, and intense pain shot down his arm. As German planes resumed bombing, Davis made his way to the field dressing station with the aid of a YMCA worker. "I did not care whether I was killed or not," Davis said. As for his helper from the YMCA, "I gave no thought to his safety."[64]

At the dressing station, Davis witnessed "the most pitiful sight that could be imagined . . . There must have been an acre or more of ground covered with wounded, lying on blankets." But, again, it was the sounds that were most disturbing. "The moans, groans, shrieks, and crys was heart-rending."[65] That scene marked the beginning of the army medical care experience for many fellow service members who were wounded in battle.

Both the War Risk Insurance Act and the policies of the CND were based on the assumption that Davis and other ex-soldiers would be discharged from the military only after they were medically rehabilitated. That weighty mandate required a transition within the Army Medical Department, which had a mission at the end of the nineteenth century centered on disease-focused research rather than on the administration of specialized health services for soldiers. Army officials faced questions regarding how and to what extent to expand the military hospital system; when injured and ill service members may be discharged; what the nature of military rehabilitation efforts might be; and how those efforts could be coordinated. Plans for military health care helped determine the experiences of individuals both as service members and as veterans.

In the years leading up to World War I, the Army Medical Department focused primarily on public health rather than on individualized medical care.[66] Following the Spanish-American War, when deaths due to disease far outnumbered deaths due to battle, medical officers argued successfully that they needed more resources to offer preventive care and stave off epidemics. As diseases like typhoid, yellow fever, and hookworm were increasingly viewed as barriers to empire building and trade, and US soldiers were stationed in Cuba, Puerto Rico, and the Philippines, the Army Medical Department spearheaded fruitful campaigns aimed at the eradication of some of the major epidemic threats of the time. While pursuing international public health missions, department physicians completed coursework in military and tropical medicine at the Army Medical School, established in Washington, DC, in 1893. They also had limited opportunities for field- and hospital-based training during hostilities along the Mexico-US border in 1916. But in 1917, on the eve of mobilization, the Army Medical Department was generally unprepared for a massive modern war.[67]

World War I necessitated a major expansion of its mission and resources. In April 1917, there were 9,530 hospital beds contained in 131 post hospitals ranging in size from twelve to forty-eight beds; five larger base hospitals, like the one where C. Vernoy Davis was treated at Fort Sam Houston; and four general hospitals, which offered specialty care for especially complex cases. The conditions in at least some of the facilities were subpar. Post hospitals especially were severely underfunded, often in ill repair, and lacking in such basic sanitary measures as clean drinking water.[68] The number and quality of domestic hospital beds would have to grow exponentially, and quickly, as the United States mobilized forces. Using the experiences of France and Britain as a guide, Army Medical Department officials calculated that enough military hospital beds should exist to cover 3.5 percent of AEF soldiers.[69] In 1917 and 1918, Congress appropriated more than $37 million and $200 million respectively for the construction and repair of hospitals. That was a vast increase over the average annual expenditure of $400,000 in each of the ten years prior to the war.[70]

Many army officials—like their counterparts on the Council of National Defense, and the architects of the War Risk Insurance Act—were determined to ensure that service members would not be placed in civilian institutions, which they felt could be technically and organizationally inferior to those of the military. Also, they believed, civilian facilities were needed for the care of the general population and could hardly be adapted to military needs; they contained no living quarters for staff and were too small and geographically disbursed to be managed efficiently by the military. As one army report put it soon after the war, "after due consideration, it was decided that the use of civil hospitals for the care and treatment of troops was not feasible because of the uncertainty of the supply of beds, the impracticability of taking over entirely civil hospitals in sufficient number without creating a hardship on the civil population, and the difficulty in operating a military and civil organization in the same institution."[71]

The Hospital Division of the Army Surgeon General's Office, created in July 1917, was charged with, among other things, devising formulas and methods for increasing domestic bed capacity and obtaining buildings for post, camp, and general hospitals, as well as hospitals for treating soldiers who had served overseas. Its primary aim was to locate facilities close to soldiers' homes and families, so numbers of necessary beds were calculated within each of sixteen regions that had been used to organize the military draft.[72] Plans called for meeting the increased need by utilizing military post hospitals and temporarily leasing privately owned land and buildings. Each of the institutions would be under military control. Funding and construction plans for leased or newly purchased facilities had to be approved by various War Department divisions. In spite of bureaucratic "red tape," by August 1918, the Hospital Division had successfully made available approximately 95,000 beds at general, port, and base hospitals.[73]

In the summer of 1917, the hospital unit was one of more than twenty divisions within a highly compartmentalized Army Surgeon General's Office. Titles of divisions indicated that ensuring the well-being of soldiers was a complex, multifaceted pursuit: the Division of Finance and Supply, the Division of Food and Nutrition, the Museum and Library Division, the Division of Gas Defense, and the Board of Publications. The office also contained sections centered strictly on burgeoning medical specialties, including the Divisions of Neurology and Psychiatry, Orthopedic Surgery, and Internal Medicine.[74]

Early in the war effort, the Army Surgeon General's Office played an active role in rehabilitation—beyond the expansion of hospitals and the provision of strictly medical therapies. In the summer of 1917, as C. Vernoy Davis trained at Fort Sam Houston, Lt. Col. Theodore Lyster, a career Army Medical Department doctor with a long list of professional and research accomplishments, recommended that Army Surgeon General Gorgas appoint one person to spearhead efforts surrounding "reconstruction, reeducation, and aftercare of disabled soldiers."[75] Gorgas heeded Lyster's call by establishing in August 1917 a Division of Physical Reconstruction (DPR).

He chose as its head physician Frank Billings, who was deemed one of the "foremost medical men of the country" when he first accepted a commission in 1908, along with fellow prominent colleagues, to the newly established Army Medical Reserve Corps.[76] Billings received his medical degree from Northwestern University in 1881 and underwent subsequent training in Vienna, Paris, and London, then served as an attending physician at various Chicago hospitals between 1890 and 1920. Credited with helping to shape medical education standards, he served as dean of Rush Medical College and president of the American Medical Association, the Association of American Physicians, the National Association for the Study and Prevention of Tuberculosis, and, later, the Institute of Medicine.[77]

Prominent doctors who worked with the Army Medical Corps during the war saw their military endeavors both as a patriotic duty and as highly relevant to their civilian careers. Most applied for commisions in 1917—between April and October 1917, the staff of the Medical Corps grew from slightly less than a thousand to more than fourteen thousand.[78] A commission allowed doctors to avoid conscription and serve somewhat on their own terms. At least some viewed their military experiences as valuable training. "One may not contemplate the physical and mental rehabilitation of disabled soldiers," Billings wrote in 1919, "without a consideration of the past and present neglect of the disabled men in the great industrial armies of the world." General rehabilitation principles, he argued, "should be the same as that applied in military organizations, but the program should be modified to meet civilian demands and conditions."[79]

Billings's DPR cooperated with the surgeon general's Hospital Division, as well as clinical divisions such as General Surgery and Neuropsychiatry, but it had a general mission that was, at the outset, "not well defined" and occasionally controversial, according to a 1923 army report.[80] Surgeon General Gorgas instructed his new department head to "take immediate steps to coordinate all activities of both military and civilian interests relating to physical reconstruction."[81] In other words, the DPR was to ensure that disabled and ill soldiers received the therapies and vocational training necessary to become self-supporting civilians.

In November 1917, the Army Surgeon General's Office released an auspicious and all-encompassing "plan for physical reconstruction and vocational training." Physical reconstruction, as Gorgas later defined it, was "the completest [*sic*] form of medical and surgical treatment carried to the point where maximum functional restoration, mental and physical, may be secured." Informed by research findings regarding other countries' rehabilitation efforts, the program's ultimate goal was to return the patient to service or civilian life "with the full realization that he can work in his handicapped state, and with habits of industry much encouraged."[82] The surgeon general's plan stipulated that each of the country's sixteen military draft districts would contain both general and reconstruction hospitals. The latter would be equipped with special physical and occupational therapy curative workshops. The connected "matter of training men in professional lines," the report conceded, "is partially worked out but not completed." Some military hospitals would contain commercial schools offering an array of classes, including English, mathematics, salesmanship, advertising, and bookkeeping, among others. In the most general sense, Gorgas's rehabilitation plan was aimed at "making [the wounded soldier], in so far as possible, an independent, wholly self-supporting, self-respecting workman." It was based on the firm belief that "the returned soldier's claim on an opportunity to earn a livelihood is not to be considered a concession to be granted, but rather a right to be recognized." In some cases, the government could pay for courses at existing schools while attendees remained under the oversight of army officers. By retaining men in service, the government would ensure that they were "comfortably cared for" and that they would expeditiously complete their training.[83] It would also be following the mandate of section 304 of the War Risk Insurance Act, which stipulated that as injured soldiers followed rehabilitation courses "a form of enlistment may be required which shall bring the injured person into the military or naval service."[84]

A subsequent surgeon general's report intended to clarify the reconstruction plan broached the familiar question of whether the military should control rehabilitation. It noted the same concern discussed at CND Medical Board meetings: in England, where vocational training was offered after soldiers had been discharged only 15 percent of patients were choosing to complete the courses. The report emphasized that soldiers under military control would be subject to "strict Army discipline." The soldier simply had to "be made to understand that before he is discharged from the army he is to be functionally restored as far as possible and is to receive proper training that will enable him to overcome his handicap." According to the report, medical and surgical work, as well as vocational training, "rightfully" should be handled by the Army Surgeon General's Office.[85]

By the winter of 1917–1918, the Army Medical Department was pursuing many of its goals, requesting approvals for actions piecemeal, even as a comprehensive rehabilitation plan remained unapproved. By early 1918, reconstruction work had begun at Fort McHenry in Baltimore, Fort McPherson in Georgia, and Walter Reed Army General Hospital in Washington, DC. There was no shortage of need: influenza and pneumonia were ravaging domestic camps, and ill and wounded soldiers were arriving from overseas. As late as July 1918, the surgeon general requested that the secretary of war lend legitimacy to the rules he was passing down to hospital personnel via his own office. Could a "general order be issued," Gorgas asked, "stating the policy of the War Department in regard to the physical reconstruction of soldiers and including rules for the transfer of such sick soldiers from different camps to special hospitals?"[86] Around the same time, the surgeon general also requested that the definition of physical reconstruction—"complete medical and surgical treatment, carried to the point where maximum functional restoration, mental and physical, has been secured" —be published as a general order.[87] After the war, Frank Billings recalled his frustrations with delays within the military bureaucracy. "Memoranda requesting approval of needed hospital construction, equipment for physiotherapy, for occupational therapy and for a qualified personnel," Billings recalled, "were disapproved wholly or in part or were returned for additional information from the General Staff."[88]

In addition to logistical and administrative challenges to the implementation of an army rehabilitation policy, a vexing question remained: when did a wounded soldier become a rehabilitating veteran? In the winter of 1917 and 1918, civilian vocational educators challenged the predominant view that the army—and doctors—should maintain control over rehabilitation. The educators argued that they were best suited to return disabled and ill soldiers to productive citizenship, since their craft promoted independence whereas continued medical treatment and long-term hospitalization promoted the opposite. Frank Billings and other volunteer army doctors took issue with the portrayal of medicine as such a limited field, and with civilian educators' depictions of them as "martinets" blindly attempting to keep all rehabilitation efforts under the control of the military.[89]

At a moment when hospitals and specialty medical care were becoming more accepted, but were hardly well-defined, the vocational educators' arguments proved powerful and appealing. In April 1918, the army dictated that the Federal

Board for Vocational Education, which had been created approximately a year earlier to provide aid to state vocational schools training conscripts, would oversee the educational aspect of rehabilitation.[90] Legislative approval came in July 1918, with the passage of the Smith-Sears Act, which appropriated $200 million for the rehabilitation of disabled veterans, and placed the FBVE in charge of oversight.

Throughout the spring of 1918, as it became clear that the FBVE would gain control of vocational education efforts, some army officials questioned the surgeon general's proposed reconstruction policy, wondering where "medical reconstruction" (the province of the Army Medical Department) ended and "physical and mental rehabilitation" (which the FBVE was to oversee) began.[91] Col. E. D. Anderson, chairman of the army's Equipment Branch, noted that, according to the originally proposed reconstruction plan, it was unclear "where the Surgeon General intends to draw this line of distinction." Anderson took issue with the surgeon general's stipulation that prior to discharge, "work, mental and manual" should be used to ensure that "maximum functional restoration, mental and physical has been secured." Such an order, he argued, conflicted with the province of the FBVE.[92] Representatives of the Army Surgeon General's Office also expressed worry that discharged soldiers—"disheartened men"—would not, of their own volition, apply for aid or obtain the help they needed once the FBVE assumed control.[93] It was imperative, these army rehabilitation advocates argued, to at least begin practical rehabilitation work while soldiers were still enlisted.

To these ends, Col. James E. Russell, dean of the Teachers' College of Columbia University, was appointed director of the Education Division of the army's Department of Physical Reconstruction. His efforts were guided by the belief that "mental depression and indisposition to respond to medical and surgical treatment on the part of the wounded men covered [by the Smith-Sears Act] is particularly active owing to the seriousness of their injuries and the consequent lack of hope of being of future use to the community." Russell suggested that "cheer-up" work begin in army hospitals, in the form of "real education," to help lay the groundwork for later work by the FBVE.[94] In formal outlines of the work to be completed by the Education Section, submitted in the spring and summer of 1918, Russell defined "real education" in broad terms, encompassing everything from musical entertainment, handiwork, lectures, sports, and elementary classes for those who were illiterate to technical and academic classes in subjects such as drawing, applied science, and agricultural work. In large army general hospitals, plans of the Education Division guided occupational therapy and recreational programs and constituted a major thrust of the army's attempt to ready soldiers for civilian life.[95]

"When the nature of his disability is considered"

The reconstruction tactics bolstered by the Department of Physical Reconstruction were intended to serve patients with a variety of what were later termed "medical" conditions; they were based largely on the predicted needs of soldiers with visible bodily wounds. But what of other major health problems—tuberculosis, mental illness, exposure to chemical weapons—that afflicted thousands of service members and, later, veterans? During mobilization and war, there were hints that those conditions would pose major challenges in the decades to come.

In 1917, the army mandated that recruits undergo medical exams to ensure that individuals with tuberculosis and a supposed predisposition to psychological issues would be barred from the ranks, but the exams achieved limited success. Families and local communities protested when potential recruits were diagnosed by military examiners with tuberculosis and shipped back home with the potential of spreading the disease. During a hasty mobilization effort, the army accepted plenty of recruits who had tuberculosis but who exhibited minor or no symptoms. Army policy also allowed physicians with tuberculosis to serve "on a case by case basis." In general, medical officers used a relatively "narrow definition" of tuberculosis when deciding whether an individual should be barred from service and also "explicitly allowed men with healed lesions in their lungs to serve."[96] It would prove especially difficult to apply principles of military medical care, including the army reconstruction plan edict regarding "maximum functional restoration," to service members suffering from such chronic conditions. Later, many veterans with tuberculosis who requested government-sponsored medical care faced questions about whether the illness had originated in service.

The same held true for service members with a variety of mental illnesses. In 1917, Thomas W. Salmon, chief consultant in psychiatry for the American Expeditionary Forces, pressured army brass to avoid "careless recruiting" prior to the war and supported "rigidly excluding insane, feebleminded, psychopathic and neuropathic individuals from the forces which are to be sent to France and exposed to the terrific stress of modern war." Like specialists of various types, he based his prescriptions on observations of the medical challenges faced by fellow belligerent nations, which struggled to meet the mental health needs of their forces.[97]

In August 1917, the surgeon general mandated that four neurological conditions served as grounds for rejection from military service: "organic nervous diseases," "mental defect," "mental disease and pathological mental states," and "confirmed inebriety (alcohol or drugs)." But definitions of those ailments were vague at best. "Mental defect or deficiency" was "a defect in general information with reference to native environment, ability to learn, to reason." Medical examiners who may have had little familiarity with—or active skepticism about—mental illnesses were advised that dementia praecox (one type of "mental disease and pathological mental states") could be exhibited as "indifference, apathy, withdrawal from environment." Given those somewhat subjective characteristics, army psychiatrists later acknowledged that "many of the mentally and nervously unfit are border-line cases" with "actual symptoms [that] are not always definite." Whether or not a recruit was rejected often depended on "the judgment of the examiner."[98]

The screening process was imperfect. In March 1918, Secretary of War Newton D. Baker ordered that "no officer or man who is physically unable to perform full military duty will be permitted to accompany his organization to France unless it is believed by the medical officers ... that he will be able to perform full duty within two weeks from date of departure." Others, Baker said, would be transferred to depot brigades or US-based organizations.[99] But mental illness and other chronic conditions were more difficult to assess than visible injuries. Early in the war effort, only recruits who were referred by general medical examiners underwent psychiatric evaluations; those who did not have "evident defects" were admitted to serve. As such, according to a report published in 1929 (as numbers of hospitalized veterans were rising), "a considerable number of men unfit for military service, because of nervous or mental condition, were carried overseas." Many had a "history of illness of from one to five years' duration previous to their entrance into the Army."[100]

The problem became pronounced enough that the army instituted a new screening policy: psychiatrists—some with no military training—were stationed in camps to conduct survey examinations of previously accepted recruits. In one day, these special officers might observe and have brief conversations with up to 150 recruits, then recommend rejection or discharge to a general disability board. The recommendations, however, were no guarantee of action: a disability board might disagree with the assessment, or the results of the psychiatric evaluations may not be received until a division shipped out. In one case, up to three hundred privates of the New York National Guard were deemed unfit to serve when they were examined in New York, but psychiatrists' recommendations for discharge were delayed, and the supposedly "unfit" service members were shipped to training in South Carolina. Only after their arrival there did they receive their discharges.[101] After the war, members of Congress and others were troubled to find that individuals like these—who had been accepted for service but then discharged because of purported previously existing conditions—were eligible for veterans' health and other benefits.

In addition to the so-called weaknesses in constitutional make-up that might be overlooked or ignored during pre-entry exams, according to Thomas W. Salmon, "a very striking fact in the present war is the number of men of apparently normal mental make-up who develop war neuroses in the face of the unprecedentedly terrible conditions to which they are exposed." Salmon and his colleagues therefore hoped the government would prepare "in advance of an urgent need, a comprehensive plan for establishing special military hospitals and using existing civil facilities for treating mental disease in a manner that will serve the army effectively and at the same time safeguard the interests of the soldiers, of the government and of the community."[102]

Civilian psychiatrists like Salmon, who went on to play a crucial role in laying plans for veterans' care after the war, attempted to make the military a testing ground for an ongoing transition in the perception and treatment of mental illnesses. The army, they maintained, should focus on prevention and therapies rather than only guarded institutionalization. He and other adherents of a "mental hygiene" movement were motivated by the belief that "overwork, congestion of population, child labor . . . and the hundred economic causes which increase the stress of living for the poor" might awaken "weaknesses in constitutional makeup," which "would have remained undiscovered under happier circumstances."[103] One's environment, in other words—in civilian or military life— could increase the risk of the onset of mental illness.

Much to Salmon's chagrin, in spite of the surgeon general's July 1917 approval of the formation of a Division of Neurology and Psychiatry, efforts to recruit "officers with special experience in nervous and mental diseases," and the institutionalization of screening exams, the United States seemed destined to follow the path of its fellow belligerents.[104] "War neuroses cases were appearing in increasing numbers in base hospitals throughout the American Expeditionary

Forces," Salmon later reported, "where they were treated without special facilities and in accordance with many different clinical points of view." In the spring of 1918, a hospital specially designed to treat such cases—Base Hospital No. 117—was established relatively close to the French front. By May 1918, it was full to capacity and ceased accepting new patients.[105] Additional hospitals, both in the United States and overseas, admitted service members who were thought to have a variety of illnesses ranging from psychosis and epilepsy to mental deficiency and alcoholism. Between April 1918 and June 1919, more than 6,200 "mental and nervous patients" who served abroad were admitted to forty army hospitals throughout the United States.[106] In spite of the numerous admissions, according to Thomas Salmon, "a large number of men were restored to duty who otherwise would have required a considerable period of treatment."[107] Early oversights and shortfalls in care hinted at some of the root causes of a torrent of demand for psychiatric services among veterans—those who had received treatment in army hospitals and those who had not—in the years following the war.

Soldiers' exposure to chemical weapons also posed special challenges for the army and, later, the veterans' health program. Chemical agents had been a part of warfare for thousands of years, but their large-scale use during World War I was unprecedented. Armies endured chlorine, phosgene, lewisite, and most prevalent in campaigns involving US soldiers—and "most violent and destructive"—mustard. Like chlorine and phosgene, mustard caused pain and damage to lungs but also seared into the skin, potentially causing blisters and damage to eyes. The extent of mustard's impact was dictated by the amount one was exposed to and the duration of exposure; battle-weary soldiers became schooled at hastily evacuating sites of attacks and removing their uniforms. Between February and November 1918, more than seventy thousand US service members were admitted to hospitals for gas poisoning.[108]

In a 1919 memoir, Martin Joseph Hogan recalled the feeling: "The gas takes its victim unawares. The first thing I noticed in my excitement was that the water was streaming from my eyes almost as though they were hydrants. I could not see my hand before my face. A gray, impenetrable mist closed thickly around me and I fell upon my knees to steady myself. Crawling I knew not in what direction, I was starting to feel my hands and knees stinging as though they had been burned. I had crawled into mustard gas." By the time Hogan arrived at a dressing station, he was blinded. The pain in his eyes and head "had grown intolerable . . . and the water flowed in such a stream down my cheeks that I began to fear that my eyes themselves were running out." After two months in the hospital, Hogan's sight had returned and his burns had healed. He was swiftly shipped back to the front, only to be gassed again shortly before the Armistice.[109]

Between 1916 and 1918, Army Medical Department officials researched the experiences of other Allied armies and learned about the immediate dangers of gassing. They distributed gas masks, devised plans for removing clothing to minimize risks of extensive burns, and designed "motorized mobile degassing plants" that could be used to cleanse bodies exposed to toxins. But like proposed rehabilitation plans, well-intended measures were often held up within a vast military and governmental bureaucracy. Specifications for mobile degassing stations, for example, were only approved at the end of August 1918 and never employed in combat. When it became clear that "the rank and file were not properly instructed in gas matters," each division was assigned a trained gas officer and a Medical Gas Warfare Board was created. Both of those developments occurred in October 1918—about one month before the Armistice.[110] Just as best practices were being established, major fighting—and, by extension, the justification for funding medical initiatives and retaining personnel—had passed.

The comprehensive reconstruction plan finally approved by the surgeon general on August 1, 1918—sixteen months after the United States declared war and approximately three months before the Armistice—made few distinctions between the variety of health conditions endured by service members. It stipulated three types of cases to be treated in military hospitals: those able to return to full military duty, those fit for limited service, and those eligible for discharge due to disability. Fifteen hospitals across the country were designated as reconstruction hospitals, where the surgeon general's recommended discharge policy would be in effect: that "no member of the military service disabled in line of duty, even though not expected to return to duty, will be discharged from service until he shall have attained complete recovery or as complete recovery as may be expected when the nature of his disability is considered." Although soldiers who would be able to return to duty constituted the highest priority in military hospitals, those who might serve in a limited capacity or be discharged due to disability, the plan said, should "have, while in the hospital, such physical training and general education as will best promote their physical reconstruction."[111]

In spite of their shapers' best intentions and attempts to be proactive, the army's policies were, in many ways, too slow in coming. The number of soldier-patients in army general hospitals had increased dramatically during the year the secretary of war and army surgeon general debated a reconstruction policy.

For example, at Walter Reed Army General Hospital, admissions increased from approximately 4,300 in 1917 to more than 14,400 in 1918.[112] Thousands of patients thus received treatment before a comprehensive plan existed regarding their rehabilitative care.

Within three and a half months of the passage of the reconstruction plan, the Armistice brought about new questions. The official declaration of peace in November 1918 marked only the beginning of a massive demobilization effort. Reconstruction hospitals in the United States, for example, did not see peak populations until May 1919. But once fighting ceased, many approved hospital projects were abandoned, and the army relied on expanded base and general hospitals.[113] The mind-set of the government and public was shifting toward peace, and resources for army rehabilitative care were more difficult to attain even before many soldiers had made their way home from abroad. That helps explain why service members, administrators, and medical professionals experienced confusion and redundancies during and after the war.

C. Vernoy Davis spent a little over a year in base hospitals in France and a rehabilitation hospital in Cape May, New Jersey, before being honorably discharged with a certificate of disability in August 1919. In army facilities, he underwent multiple surgeries to repair nerve damage in his arm, but by the time he was released from service, he still had limited movement in his thumb and forefinger. Davis refused the army's offer to remain enlisted to undergo more treatment, asking instead to be discharged so he could attend university. In August 1919, he visited a Bureau of War Risk Insurance office and was told that the agency would pay for two years of schooling. As the prospect of discharge became more real, Davis found himself "over joyed at the thoughts of . . . getting back to civilian life" and "being free to come and go" as he pleased.[114] The young veteran went on to attend Pennsylvania State University, marry, buy a home in a central Pennsylvania town not far from where he grew up, and make a good living with the Bell Telephone Company.

Still, Davis's freedom was, in some ways, limited. Like Patrick O'Donnell and Alonzo Nichols, who applied for entry into the Togus, Maine, Soldiers' Home around the time the United States declared war in 1917, the physical impact of Davis's wartime service remained with him for the rest of his life. He never regained the use of all the fingers on his left hand and, more than seventy-five years after the war, he told a local newspaper reporter that he thought World War I veterans had been "all but forgotten." It was evident during the interview that he felt the impact of his year in France with almost each passing breath. Because of mustard gas inhalation, he was constantly forced to pause mid-sentence to "gather his second wind."[115]

In spite of those long-term effects, Davis's case encapsulated a primary hope of prewar policy makers: that veterans would leave the military and become self-sufficient. Prewar federal policies surrounding the health of soldiers were characteristic of a Progressive Era dominated by the idealization of industrial productivity and efficiency, individual and familial responsibility, and selective governmental protections for citizens. The highest aspiration of policy makers was to stave off long-term dependency on the government—for pensions or services—among a new cohort of veterans. As such, government officials established a massive insurance scheme modeled on state workers' compensation programs and a rehabilitation plan that would be largely overseen by the military. According to their rationale, by the time most service members were discharged as civilians, they would be relatively healthy and independent. Some in the medical profession and beyond noted that soldiers would eventually become wounded and ill civilians in need of extended care. But that problem was both daunting and unpredictable in scope, and efforts to establish formal plans for extended aftercare were haphazard and limited.

As army officials devised an expansive rehabilitation plan, there were signs that many important questions remained unanswered. At what point would a wounded soldier be discharged as a civilian? What was the government's obligation once service members resumed their place in society? Who would manage and fund medical services for discharged soldiers? Prewar policies regarding soldiers' care were, in many respects, vague and impractical. Yet within a decade they would justify demands for a vast national network of federally funded hospitals tailored to veterans' needs.

The relative brevity of US involvement in the war meant that the army rehabilitation program was nascent even as the country demobilized. Nonetheless, the Army Medical Department eagerly built reconstruction programs at US hospitals, and thousands of ill and injured soldiers, like C. Vernoy Davis, adapted to their health circumstances in domestic military institutions. Those facilities faced major challenges as they undertook the complicated mission of healing.

CHAPTER TWO

A Stupendous Task

The Challenges of Domestic Military Health Care

Paul A. Bazaar recalled spending his early days at Walter Reed Hospital in "sober reflection." The long, bed-lined wards were a world away from the front, where Bazaar lost both of his hands when a grenade detonated prematurely. At Walter Reed, he said, "I painfully nursed the birth of a new hope, I made that little sphere the starting point of a new and brighter life." Bazaar was discharged in February 1919, after being fitted with metal prostheses. By January 1921, he had graduated from business school and was making a living in Rochester, New York, assisting people with their income-tax returns. "I am doing quite well," he reported in a letter to the hospital. "I find the going exceedingly rocky at times, and the obstacles many, but my philosophy, a light heart and a smile, helps to surmount most difficulties."[1]

Of the approximately 224,000 American Expeditionary Forces soldiers wounded abroad, more than 51,000, like Bazaar, received treatment in US military hospitals.[2] The army sent patients with the most complex conditions to general hospitals, which offered relatively advanced medical technologies and procedures, as well as extensive rehabilitation options, including occupational and physical therapy, and academic and commercial training courses. The fact that Bazaar could be fitted for, and trained to use, prosthetic hands while remaining under the care of the Army Medical Department indicated just how far the military had gone in its mission to help disabled soldiers become productive citizens. In terms of prewar policies, Bazaar's was a model case: he had used his hospital time wisely, coming to terms with his injury instead of resenting it. He had even gone on to obtain professional training and become a working member of society.

In some ways Bazaar's experience was typical, but in others, it was unique. Walter Reed served as "a starting point" for many of its thousands of patients during and immediately after World War I. But not all soldiers were, by their own standards, or those of the army and the government, successful in planting roots there for a "new and brighter life."

Prewar health policies affected domestic military hospitals, which devised extensive rehabilitation programs and contributed to an expanded vision of a "new army": one that not only trained service members to fight but also shaped citizens. Indeed, as the case of Paul Bazaar demonstrates, military-based medical and rehabilitation efforts of World War I went well beyond measures of the past, capitalizing on and, in many ways, advancing contemporary health care innovations. The army initiated a host of specialty services during the war, including a program in occupational therapy (OT), which aimed to allow injured and ill service members to begin preparing for post-discharge work and life. Early in the war effort, however, there were hints that the ambitious goal of containing the healing process within military institutions was unrealistic. Tensions developed between patients and practitioners, based on social backgrounds and professional and service records. Army officials and doctors voiced skepticism about whether service members who had never shipped abroad, or had ailments that were difficult to trace to battle, were worthy of treatment. Meanwhile, soldier-patients grew dissatisfied with aspects of military hospital life, including strict discipline, the nature of rehabilitation tactics, and fluctuating discharge policies. There were logistical problems as well, as army officials attempted to treat patients with long-term needs in institutions that were designed for very different purposes.

The tensions that arose between patients and caregivers, and the dissatisfaction that mounted in military hospitals during and after the war, could be traced, in part, to disparate goals and expectations. Patients' and caregivers' perceptions of military health care were predicated on how they answered at least two thorny questions: (1) What were the nature and extent of health-related military obligations? (2) Should hospital staff treat soldier-patients who would likely never return to duty as service members or honored civilians? While the army's health program saw many successes during and after World War I, it was also challenged by vaguely defined mandates.

Implementing and Experiencing Rehabilitation at Walter Reed Hospital

The health mobilization effort of the US Army during World War I, and the treatment rendered to Paul A. Bazaar and thousands of others, was part of an organizational culture in transition. When Walter Reed General Hospital opened its doors in 1909, the Spanish-American War had been over for a decade, World War I was in the unforeseeable future, and army hospital admission rates were steadily decreasing. A symbol of the country's heightened imperial ambitions, the changing infrastructure of the US military, and emerging ideas about the prospective role and possibilities of professional medicine, funding for the institution was included in a 1905 civil appropriations bill under a section entitled "Miscellaneous Objects, War Department." The bill allotted $100,000 for the purchase of the site and $200,000 more for hospital construction.[3] When the Georgian-style main building containing eighty beds was erected in 1908, the *Washington Post* praised it as being "modern in every detail" and "of stately Colonial style."[4]

In its early years, Walter Reed operated as the post hospital for Washington Barracks and as a general hospital for the United States east of the Mississippi. Between 1911 and 1916, the number of patients admitted increased from 565 to 1,350 per year as staff worked to fulfill one of its founding missions: "to save the men to the service, to reduce the pension list, and to give men disabled in the service of their country the benefit of the most advanced medical and surgical knowledge."[5] Reasons for admission were highly varied. Venereal disease was a common ailment among patients, as were tonsillitis and appendicitis. Throughout the period, the Washington, DC–based Army Medical School maintained an active relationship with Walter Reed Hospital, processing thousands of Wasserman tests each year to ascertain whether patients had syphilis, in addition to blood cultures and "laboratory examinations of pathologic specimens." Walter Reed's Commanders also worked to ensure that the hospital would grow—aesthetically—"into a general hospital that shall be a credit to the army." They reported that enlisted men helped plant hundreds of trees, bushes, and flowers, and undertook infrastructural improvements such as road repair and installing new outdoor light fixtures. In 1916, the hospital was still somewhat of a small operation: it had a 180-bed capacity and an average of 9 medical officers on duty, along with 26 nurses (figure 2.1).[6]

The number of army general hospitals grew exponentially during World War I—from four in 1916 to an eventual peak of more than fifty.[7] Some specialized in treating patients with particular conditions, such as tuberculosis or shell shock. One—General Hospital No. 7 in Baltimore, Maryland—provided care for patients who were blind. But most of the facilities were focused on the general mission of meeting "any surgical or medical requirement."[8] In May 1919, there were about forty thousand beds available in general hospitals across the

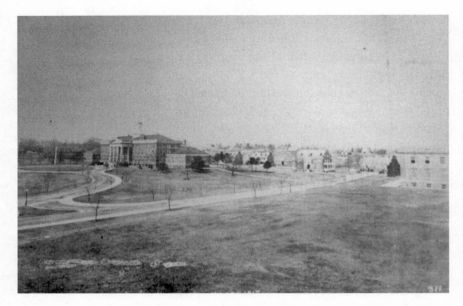

Figure 2.1. Exterior view of Walter Reed Army General Hospital, 1917. OHA 355: Walter Reed Historical Collection, box 11, folder 143. Otis Historical Archives, National Museum of Health and Medicine, Silver Spring, MD

country (figure 2.2).[9] Among these many institutions, Walter Reed Army General Hospital in Washington, DC, was a flagship.

The army planned to move patients like Paul Bazaar from their locations relatively near the front to base hospitals in France then transport them by train to embarkation hospitals at French ports. A naval ship or army vessel would then bring them to US ports and debarkation hospitals where medical officers determined which domestic base or general hospital was best suited to care for them. Although the army attempted to locate ill and wounded patients close to their homes, their medical conditions were the most important factors when it came to determining where they would be treated.[10]

During the Great War, Walter Reed Hospital transitioned from being a new facility that provided treatment for a relatively small number of service members to a destination institution for the personnel of a large and hastily assembled army. In June 1917, construction of temporary buildings began, including additional nurses' quarters, barracks, a mess hall, a store house, and a guard house, among other structures. That year, approximately 4,300 patients were admitted and the hospital staff averaged 23 medical officers and 44 nurses.[11] In 1918,

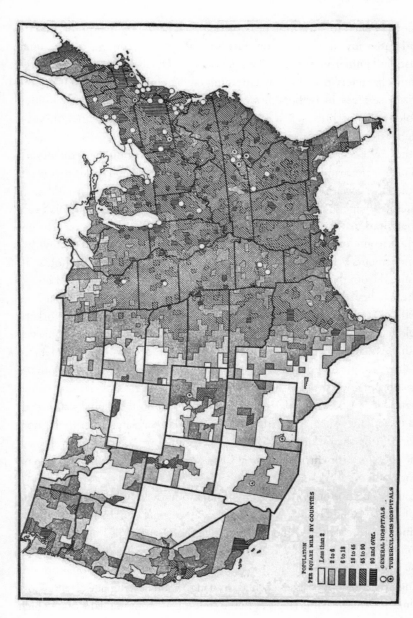

Figure 2.2. General hospitals superimposed on Bureau of Census population map of 1910. Frank W. Weed, *Military Hospitals in the United States,* vol. 5 of *The Medical Department of the United States Army in the World War,* ed. M. W. Ireland (Washington, DC: GPO, 1923), 36

admissions swelled to a wartime peak of 14,435 patients. By that point, 86 officers and 148 army nurses were on duty, in addition to about 34 occupational therapists and numerous other civilian personnel.[12] During the war, Walter Reed had many characteristics of newly emerging civilian medical centers. It offered specialized services in orthopedics, neurosurgery, amputations, dermatology, and urology, among others. It was also home to the new Army School of Nursing, a laboratory with bacteriological, chemical, and pathological sections, and physiotherapy, occupational therapy, and vocational education departments.[13]

A glance at the army's occupational therapy (OT) program reveals that ideals expounded by prewar planners regarding the importance of long-term independence helped shape the implementation and perception of military hospital care and rehabilitation. Occupational therapy was rooted in the late nineteenth century, when women reformers involved in the settlement house and mental hygiene movements viewed arts and crafts as a means of combating the social ills that resulted from the mechanization of industry. Staff at Chicago's Hull House and others believed weaving, design, and other handiwork—activities that later qualified as OT—could quell the revolutionary impulses of disaffected workers, who held factory jobs that precluded them from overseeing a project from start to finish. Arts and crafts could also, they maintained, allow the "leadership class"—increasingly entering white collar and managerial jobs removed from the industrial production process—to experience the satisfaction of creating something tangible.[14] Likewise, doctors found that allowing ill hospital patients to partake in activities such as sewing and woodworking assisted with their "normalization."[15] By the outbreak of World War I, clinics using crafts for the treatment of patients with chronic physical illness existed in San Francisco, upstate New York, and New York City.[16]

The army's bellwether OT program began modestly in February 1918, in the home of Walter Reed Hospital's handyman, who instructed patients in "the simplest kind of carpentry." Within two months, the Division of Physical Reconstruction of the Surgeon General's Office allotted $3,000 for therapy tools and staff. By the end of 1918, the hospital boasted a variety of educational options including arts and crafts classes such as drawing, wood carving, jewelry making, engraving, and rug weaving. (It also offered training in "commercial work," which consisted of more vocationally centered activities: bookkeeping, typewriting, automobile repair and "truck farming out of doors.")[17] The Walter Reed program was a model for other army institutions; approximately 350 occupational therapists had served in 52 army hospitals by mid-1919.[18]

Practitioners argued that OT could prime both bodies and minds for economic self-reliance and productivity. "The specific purpose," according to a report from Walter Reed's Occupational Therapy Department, was "to help each patient find himself and function again as a complete man, physically, socially, educationally and economically." OT could help a soldier "restore his body so far as possible to its normal condition ... enabling him to feel that despite his physical handicap he may still be a self-reliant and self-respecting member of the community ... providing him a means of earning a comfortable livelihood so that with his return to civil life he may be an economic asset instead of a liability."[19] Herbert J. Hall, who would serve as president of the American Occupational Therapy Association from 1920 to 1923, argued, "Idleness means degeneration of body and spirit." As such, "the best way to bring back courage to a wounded soldier and the best way to restore the use of a stiff elbow is to employ the man and his elbow in useful work, naturally taking care not to overdo the process."[20]

Efforts to recruit occupational therapists reflected those lofty goals. Stated qualifications for the job were based on both education and personal grace, though most calls for applicants emphasized the latter. "A young woman entering the profession should be a person of both academic and manual ability," one pamphlet said. "She should possess tact—initiative—a strong sense of responsibility —good poise—a good sense of humor—excellent physical health and emotional stability."[21] The prospective therapist "must be patient and cheerful and like to work with people." She should also possess some artistic ability, like to work with her hands, and be between 21 and 50 years old. "Other personal qualities which are most desirable," another pamphlet noted, "are tact, resourcefulness, a sympathetic attitude, and a love for the work."[22] As Herbert J. Hall put it, "It is a serious business, this good start on the right road for the crippled soldier." Aides should, he said, avoid "a too-technical or matter-of-fact approach," and "have charm and appeal."[23] Recruitment literature often overlooked the matters of pay and rank. Occupational therapists, along with army physical therapists, dieticians, and many other women war workers, were subject to military orders but served in military hospitals at home and abroad as civilians, which meant they had limited access to government-sponsored benefits after the war.

Part of a larger wave of women who sought to capitalize on wartime professional opportunities, Lena Hitchcock was less attracted by the army's request for women with tact, cheerfulness, and appeal than she was by the prospect of personal betterment and following in the footsteps of her mother, who had been a

Red Cross nurse.[24] "Long before the United States declared war on Germany, I wanted to go overseas," she recalled after the war: "Probably my motives were mixed. The tremendous odds against the allies appealed to all the chivalry of youth, sense of romance and adventure. The military atmosphere in which I was steeped at that time also undoubtedly influenced me. Then also I very probably entertained a vain desire to prove my courage and achieve heroic deeds. I need not point out that the dreams engendered by my childhood diet of tales of heroism and patriotism never materialized but, whatever the motives, I was determined somehow to get there."[25] Prior to departing for service, Hitchcock paid a visit to her grandfather. Since she was the "only one in the family who the army wants and will take," he told her, she "must hold the banner high as the men and women of [her] family had always done." As Hitchcock's grandfather bid her farewell, he added, "May God bless you and keep you and help you to fulfill your duty," then he handed her a check. Across the bottom he had written "For Patriotism." When the army assigned Hitchcock to Walter Reed General Hospital in early 1918 as one of the US Army's first occupational therapists, she was determined to "prove [her] courage and achieve heroic deeds."[26]

While fulfilling daily duties, she and other occupational therapists acquired a somewhat pragmatic view of the goals and prospective benefits of their service and of soldiers' hospital-based work. "So far, none of our occupational therapy is orthopedically corrective," Hitchcock reported in 1919, after she had been shipped from Walter Reed to a hospital in France, "but at least it prevents the boys from drinking too much and losing all their money shooting craps."[27] Alberta Montgomery, who began working at Walter Reed as a reconstruction aide in August 1918 and served as the hospital's director of occupational therapy from January 1922 through 1933, was likewise focused on the immediate mental benefits of OT.[28] Her notes on patient treatment in early 1919 documented her assessment of various patients. Among her weekly observations: "work keeps him more quiet"; "work keeps him from thinking about his troubles"; "work makes him less restless"; "work makes him more ambitious"; "work makes him concentrate on plans for future"; "work makes him more contented"; and "work keeps him happy—makes him forget his condition."[29] According to the assessments of Montgomery and Hitchcock, OT could, at the very least, spur optimism, character development, and perhaps even industriousness.

Soldier-patients, for their part, viewed hospital-based classes as a means of availing themselves of a professionally oriented education. In December 1918, commercial work attracted large numbers of the 1,449 patients participating in OT at Walter Reed; traditional arts and crafts activities were less popular: 142 patients partook in courses such as typewriting and bookkeeping while only seven were enrolled in jewelry, four in engraving, and five in clay modeling.[30] Having access to a diverse menu of formal classes was likely a unique experience for many patients. Results of army intelligence tests indicated that 21.5 percent of all white soldiers and 50.6 percent of all black soldiers were officially illiterate.[31]

Indeed, soldiers could be openly skeptical of OT offerings that they interpreted as impractical. "Just as at Walter Reed," Hitchcock wrote from France, "the men were suspicious and scoffing—'women's work'—they called it." Alberta Montgomery's notebook was replete with accounts of soldiers who resisted participating in bedside activities like knitting and jewelry making. According to Montgomery, a soldier named Burns reported that he "does not want to do anything that would look, as he says, 'the least bit feminine.' " So he was assigned to "sawing and making equipment." Merlin Meyhard, who was in the hospital with a gunshot wound to his left hand and had been crafting a cord belt during visits to the OT shop, told Montgomery that he preferred auto repair work. Jerome McGinn, also in the hospital with a gunshot wound and working on a cord belt, told the reconstruction aide he was more interested in academic work than crafts: "Wants to complete his belt later—is working on electricity now and is interested in that." Similarly, Montgomery reported that Verne Caldwell, hospitalized for a gunshot wound in his forearm, "wants to take full advantage of the opportunity for education offered by the government." When Caldwell did partake in a cord belt project, Montgomery said, "he did this only to show someone else how and did not use the injured arm." Instead, Caldwell devoted his intellectual and physical efforts to drafting classes.[32]

Patients' resistance to some army rehabilitation tactics prompted practitioners to search for cause. To Grace Harper, chief of the Bureau of Reconstruction and Re-education of the American Red Cross, it seemed as though "Many wounded men are somewhat like children." In rehabilitation efforts, she said, "ignorance is our stumbling block."[33] In an address before the National Society for the Promotion of Occupational Therapy in November 1918, Columbia University Teachers' College dean James E. Russell, who was serving with the Army Surgeon General's Office's Division of Physical Reconstruction, alleged that many military hospital patients had not seen battle and were predisposed to tuberculosis and heart conditions—"weaklings and not soldiers." "Some of these men are not worthy of the efforts being expended upon them," Russell maintained. Men "who were just no good and never will be any good," he said, were "hardly worth saving." Russell also distinguished between extent of disability. There were, he suggested, some patients who were "so nervously broken down that the stringing of beads or some such simple occupation is all that can be expected of them." Others, he noted, were "full-blooded men": "Many are only slightly weakened by their wounds; their disabilities are of a kind that do not tend to break them down physically, maybe an amputation of one leg, maybe an arm off, maybe the loss of sight or hearing or any other accident that may come to any individual leaving him still strong and physically fit to work if the right work can be found."[34]

Patients and Practitioners

The impressions that individuals like James Russell formed in military hospitals helped shape opinions about the merits and future of government-sponsored care. During and immediately after the war, in institutions like Walter Reed, disabled soldiers and their caregivers evaluated not only treatment methods but also each other. Their reviews were mixed. Although there may have been vast differences in their educational and cultural backgrounds, practitioners and patients who encountered each other on surgical tables and at bedsides near the front lines reported feeling great respect for one another. But in other circumstances judgments could be less favorable.

Sick and wounded World War I–era military personnel—the people most likely to fill military and, later, veterans' hospital beds—could be classified in at least three broad categories. Local draft boards accepted thousands of recruits who were deemed physically or mentally unacceptable for service upon their arrival at training camps.[35] One official explained the numbers by noting "the hasty and superficial examinations given by inexperienced and indifferent medical examiners for enlistment, immediately following the declaration of war."[36] It did not help that standards for acceptance into the army changed over time and that local draft boards were "overworked and undermanned in the face of a large flow of recruits."[37] A sampling of approximately 52,600 of these accepted-but-later-rejected men showed that almost 9,000 were denied entry into the army due to "diseases of bones and organs of locomotion." Eye, digestive, and circulatory system diseases each accounted for between 7,000 and 8,000 rejections. Another 4,700 accepted by local draft boards were found to have tuberculosis;

3,500 were diagnosed with "mental diseases." Slightly more than 2,000 were rejected on the grounds that they had venereal diseases.[38]

There was uncertainty and disagreement about whether this group was entitled to the compensation and medical care that had been guaranteed to veterans by the War Risk Insurance Act. The army judge advocate general initially ruled that "a man who has been accepted by a draft board and dispatched to a camp had been drafted into active service" and was therefore eligible for benefits. But the Bureau of War Risk Insurance, the government agency responsible for allocating the entitlements of the War Risk Insurance Act, held that "the man did not actually enter active service until he was accepted by the medical officers of the army."[39] Public Law 104, passed December 24, 1919, settled the matter. Much to the chagrin of some members of Congress and medical professionals, it stipulated that thousands of soldiers were eligible for compensation and medical care in spite of never having rendered service in any official capacity. They were, the law held, officially hired by the US government once they were accepted by their local draft boards and therefore were deserving of subsequent benefits.[40]

A second group eligible for care as soldiers, and later as discharged veterans was the contingent that had garnered such skepticism from James E. Russell: those who never saw service abroad but who fell ill while stationed in the United States. In October 1918, when the army was at its peak strength, there were approximately 1.9 million soldiers serving in Europe, 1.6 million in the United States, and 300,000 in other countries.[41] About 75 percent of discharges for conditions such as tuberculosis, venereal diseases, and "mental deficiency" were among those who never left the country.[42] Between April 1917 and December 1918, the Army Medical Department added about 2.57 million patients to the sick report. 2.4 million of them were serving in the United States while 873,816 were serving abroad.[43]

When army higher-ups and medical practitioners considered questions regarding the treatment and rehabilitation of soldiers who had not shipped abroad, impressions of heroism were replaced with more tenuous opinions. In March 1918, one army doctor held that 10 percent of those reporting to sick call and the camp dispensary were "pure malingering" while "40 percent exaggerate symptoms, which would not be sufficient to cause a cessation of work in civil life, [and] 40 percent [were] somewhat sick and would stop work in civil life, but would not send for a doctor." That left only 10 percent who were "quite in need of attention and in civil life would stop work and procure medical attendance."[44]

In order to eliminate waste and determine if a soldier was being truthful about his condition, the Army Surgeon General's Office encouraged doctors to ask and ponder a litany of questions about a soldier-patient's work, family, and personal life. Without indicating that the individual was "under suspicion," doctors should try to ascertain how successful he was prior to service in school and at work. Had he deserted wives and children? Had he been a "good mixer" or was he "solitary, secretive, and morose"? Did he "bear grudges" against people? What did other people think and say of him? Did he "think the world a good place to live and enjoy"? What were his "views as to war and the rights of the individual"? A patient's answers to such questions, "will often flatly contradict the possibility that his present claims are genuine." As many soldiers as possible should be kept out of hospitals, the Army Surgeon General's Office noted, but those admitted who might be feigning their maladies should not be told exactly *why* they were admitted and could be offered a "light diet" and "disagreeable medications." Additionally, patients could be given "anesthetics for diagnostic purposes . . . as, during semi-consciousness, the patient often says things which contradict previous statements." Hospital staff could also make stays of supposed malingerers less pleasant if "visits of family and friends were discouraged" and if the soldier-patient was "confined to his quarters when not on duty."[45]

Suspicions of malingering were not limited to the home front. One study of 281 patients being treated in a field hospital in France for gas exposure found that fewer than one-third were actually suffering from poisoning. While the rate of mortality due to gas exposure was 3 to 4 percent in the British and French armies, the rate in the US Army was 1.7 percent. According to a postwar analysis from the Army Medical Department, that was "not believed to be due to any better treatment received in our hands than that given by our Allies, but due wholly to the fact that a large number of reported gas casualties were suffering from other causes." While the report maintained that some soldiers "claimed they were gassed in order to get out of the front lines," it also noted that "a still larger number thought they were gassed and were suffering from conditions which might be called gas mania."[46] Similarly, soldier-patients suffering from various types of "neuropsychiatric diseases" (which encompassed conditions ranging from psychoneurosis and epilepsy to mental deficiency and hysteria) "could not altogether escape being regarded in a sense as malingerers," according to a 1929 report co-written by former chief consultant for the American Expeditionary Forces, Thomas W. Salmon. While most army doctors did not reject the idea that some might truly suffer from mental ailments, the report noted, "there was some feeling on the part of Army surgeons that such soldiers did not play the game quite fairly, that they could have done more if they would."[47]

Even if ailing soldier-patients were not feigning their maladies, some commentators felt that since many likely had illnesses before enlisting, it was inappropriate to treat them in an army hospital. In his postwar statistical analysis of wartime casualties, Albert Love argued that a large number of soldiers eventually discharged due to disease were ill upon enlistment, seeing as a "great majority" never saw overseas service.[48] The 1921 surgeon general's report likewise quoted base commanders, who lamented, "Never in the history of the army has its ranks been filled with such poor physical specimens and such young lads so susceptible to disease." The commanders noted that "a large majority of cases . . . have disabilities which existed prior to enlistment, and a number . . . have been previously discharged from the military service with the same disability." Ultimately, they concluded, "it would seem that a great deal of laxity existed in the recruiting system which permitted the enlistment of these men."[49] A postwar report about drafted men who were eventually rejected from service supported the argument that many eligible recruits had long-standing health issues, including bone and joint issues, hearing and sight problems, tuberculosis, cardiovascular limitations, and venereal diseases.[50] But assertions about the poor prior health status of those who did actually serve were difficult to prove, given that military camps were breeding grounds for injuries as well as influenza, tuberculosis, and other diseases. Still, as the war effort waned and funds dried up, many would argue that the lack of glowing service records among some of those who sought medical care, and the prospect that they might have entered the military ill, justified a lessened government responsibility.

A third group of military personnel treated for injuries and illnesses comprised those who served abroad. Approximately 224,000 soldiers were wounded in action during World War I, in addition to almost 10,000 Marines. More than 65 percent of injuries resulted from gunshot wounds and about 32 percent from poisonous gases.[51] Contrasting with tenuous opinions about supposed malingerers, doctors and army officials reported being overwhelmed by the heroism and grace of many of their patients wounded in action. "I wish you could accompany me through my wards on any old morning and see these boys paying the price of war without any brass bands or speeches to cheer them on, yet doing it gladly and without complaint," wrote New York surgeon Condict Cutler to a colleague in June 1918 from a field hospital in France.[52] Cutler further reported having a tremendous "admiration for their spirit" and a desire to "do everything I can for all my patients."[53] Arthur Purdy Stout, a professor of pathology at Columbia University and an army volunteer in France, had similar feelings. "It is particularly hard to see the wounded die," he wrote in his diary. The dead and wounded were "fine lads who started out so bravely to this land of France and have to leave so many loved ones behind."[54] Nurse Nettie Trax, who also served in a hospital in France, reported that her soldier-patients were "absurdly grateful." "Never before have I felt a sense of achievement nor felt that my own bit of work was worth something to somebody," Trax said. "But it is here."[55]

Soldiers, for their part, passed their own judgments of caregivers—both at home and abroad. John V. Hawley, who served as a cook in a convalescent hospital in France referred to the doctors he worked alongside, as "gentlemen." They were "dedicated" to the cause, he said, and some were "family men that left a fine practice to help out when their country needed them. THEY WERE TOPS."[56] When Martin Joseph Hogan was treated for gas poisoning at a "battered chateau" in France, he recalled, doctors and orderlies "wasted few moments and the perspiration glistened on their foreheads as they hurried from case to case."[57]

Joseph W. Bubendorf had similar recollections of his experiences working at a hospital in France, and very different ones while serving stateside. Near the front he had seen medical staff giving injured patients hot showers and careful, tender treatment. But things were different at Camp Merrit, in New Jersey, where he fell and developed an abscess on his hand. "They had medical inspection once a day at 5pm and the officer in charge, if you could call him such—stuck his head in the door and called—'is everybody all right?' hoping he would have nothing to do—so I called out—'no—I need attention' so he pulled out his jack knife and drained the abscess with no sign of a dressing. I recovered eventually."[58] In the army medical system, treatment procedures depended on the origins and seriousness of one's injury—including its potential impact on a military campaign—and the approaches and perspectives of individual patients and caregivers.

"Fair play was we should have our clothes washed"

Bubendorf's sense of disappointment with perceived varying standards hints at some of the tensions that pervaded the World War I army health system. Patients and caregivers often had different impressions of what the army and the government owed ailing service members. How far should the army push soldier-patients to proactively achieve self-betterment? Should they be subject to maximum discipline with limited rights or viewed as venerated citizens who had done their bit and deserved special treatment?

A January 1919 *Washington Evening Star* exposé and follow-up investigation regarding laundry service at Walter Reed Hospital tacitly broached those questions. Some patients, the paper reported, wore unwashed undergarments—military-issued wool pants and shirts—for weeks because they lacked the physical ability, due to incapacity from injury or illness, to clean them. Since Walter Reed's laundry service washed only hospital pajamas and bedsheets for patients, some sent their clothing and wool underwear to be professionally cleaned at their own expense. Others, lacking the funds to do so, were compelled to do their own laundry in bathtubs. Still others, according to the *Star*, wore only cotton pajamas, and abandoned wearing undergarments altogether.[59]

After the release of the *Star* story, the Inspector General's Department conducted a follow-up investigation. Of the 1,881 patients in the hospital, the investigation found, 1,054 were ambulatory and being treated for injuries or illnesses that did not involve amputations; they were fully capable of doing their own laundry. Of the patients surveyed—267 with arm amputations and 332 with leg amputations—450 were considered ambulatory. The Inspector General's Office ultimately collected testimony from forty-five patients, including those who had been the focus of the *Star* story.[60] Some had few complaints. Private Jim Pares, whose right arm and right leg had been amputated, said he wore pajamas because they were more comfortable given his physical condition. But he had no qualms with Walter Reed or its staff: "They treat me good," he said. "I can only kick for this leg, that is all." Private Joseph Thibodeux said he would have preferred to wear his wool undergarments instead of hospital pajamas, mostly because the former were warmer, but they had disappeared after he washed them in the latrine and left them there to dry. Since then, he had been unable to secure others. Private Edward Stubbs, whose left arm was amputated, said he was able to wash his handkerchiefs and socks but that washing underwear, because it was comparatively larger, was impossible. Private Ernest E. Birge, who had both of his legs amputated at the thigh, reported that it was "perfectly alright" that he had to wear pajamas temporarily while he awaited his laundry. He was fortunate enough to have his washing done by a local volunteer who decided to do her bit for wounded soldiers by washing their clothes.[61]

But a few who had not happened on such resources spoke less blithely about their feelings. Private Samuel Ellis, a soldier whose right arm was amputated, explained to the inspector general that he was wearing pajamas because his only pair of underwear had disappeared after he washed them "with my one hand" and left them to dry. Following his detailed account, the inspector bluntly asked him: "What did you report to me for?" Ellis answered with equal abruptness: "My complaint is no clothes, no underwear, no socks, bought my own socks and got no way to wash my clothes and can't wring them out with one hand and there is no place to dry them in the ward." Private Owen McMahon, whose right leg had been amputated, spoke with similar urgency directly to the issue of whether patients should be held accountable for doing their own washing at all: "I thought that we had done our bit," he said, "and fair play was we should have our clothes washed."[62] According to the inspector general, twenty amputees were, like McMahon and Ellis, doing their own laundry—mostly while seated at hospital bathtubs—while others either sent it out to be washed at their own expense or opted to wear pajamas (figure 2.3).[63]

Even as hospital staff and army officials recognized the problem and vowed that immediate action would be taken, it was clear that some harbored ideals

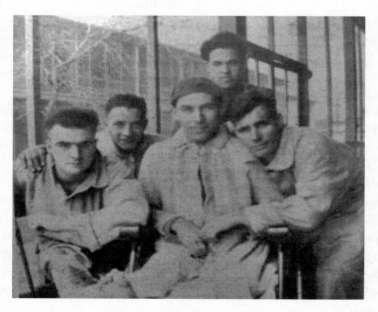

Figure 2.3. Patients at Fort McHenry, MD. Photo #3. OHA. 200: Lynch Collection, box 1, Otis Historical Archives, National Museum of Health and Medicine, Silver Spring, MD

regarding governmental responsibility that clashed with the expectations of soldier-patients like Ellis and McMahon. Maj. Francis Christian, hospital quartermaster, noted that in January and October of 1918, E. R. Schreiner, the commander of Walter Reed, had requested that the surgeon general authorize the expansion of laundry facilities at the hospital. Although the "laundry was built," Christian told the inspector general, "no machinery [was] authorized."[64] Schreiner himself reported the same, adding that prior to the publication of the story in the *Star*, "no information of maimed patients doing their own washing had come to my attention." Following the article's publication, he noted, he had worked with Christian to arrange for patients' laundry to be sent to Fort Meade in Maryland.[65] Still, hospital staff did not necessarily believe that the government should foot the bill. In fact, Schreiner had considered utilizing a private laundry service at the expense of the soldiers themselves but thought the record keeping involved in such an endeavor would be overwhelming.[66]

The American Red Cross was eager to help—with some conditions.[67] Along with a variety of civilian groups like the YMCA, Knights of Columbus, and Jewish Welfare Board, the Red Cross played a prominent role in the expansive wartime projects of mobilization and rehabilitation. Its wartime funding drives helped bring in a total collection of more than $169.5 million for relief work, almost a quarter of which was devoted to providing services at domestic hospitals.[68] At institutions like Walter Reed, the organization sponsored a plethora of services and activities, including movie screenings, dances, and sightseeing trips.[69] It also helped hospitalized soldiers and sailors who were "worried about their home affairs" connect with their families by providing stationery, stamps, telegrams, and, in some cases, financial assistance for visits home.[70] In so doing, Red Cross staff and volunteers aimed to contribute to the government's mission to, as one commander put it, "send [soldiers] back home better men than they were when they came into the Army."[71]

During the investigation into laundry services at Walter Reed, Edith Oliver Rea, field director of the Red Cross post at Walter Reed, expressed regret that neither she nor the women under her charge who visited patients in wards daily were aware of the situation. "Of course, we listen to a great many complaints of different kinds, but my orders to all my ladies have been not to encourage [patients] in their grouches but to do everything in their power to help them; and I assure you that this thing was not brought to our attention," she told a representative of the Inspector General's Office. As hospital higher-ups like Schreiner and Christian planned to offer a new laundry service through Camp Meade, Rea said the Red Cross would take written requests from patients for assistance with washing. It was important to get the requests in writing, Rea said, to avoid abuse of the system by "some of those lazy men who would want to have their's done—you know, there are a great many men who want to accept favors without doing anything in return."[72]

Rea, a devoted wartime volunteer who is credited with caring deeply about her patients and organizing a nursing service at Walter Reed, was pragmatic, not heartless.[73] Her statement alluded to a central principle of World War I–era reconstruction: caregivers felt they had an obligation to help wounded and ill soldiers get physically better, but they faced a conundrum regarding the prospective role they should play in promoting self-reliance and a quick return to noninstitutional life. Lt. Willard A. Widnew of the Sanitary Corps at Walter Reed, for example, realized that the act of doing one's washing was a "hardship" for some soldiers, but "our attitude—at least my attitude—in regard to the one-armed men has been to regard them as nearly as I was able to as whole men and . . . able to do what other men were able to do, and although I have seen men have difficulty with their washing . . . I felt that they would devise a way to do it and it was an instrument to assist us in the rehabilitation of the men."[74]

The investigation into laundry service at Walter Reed reveals that as soldiers like Paul A. Bazaar and Samuel Ellis reckoned with the long-term impact of their injuries and illnesses, hospital staff faced the difficult question of how to treat them, not just medically but socially. Ill and injured soldiers believed they had earned the right to a certain level of care and services from their government, and when they did not receive them they felt unjustly disregarded. The military hospitals where they were treated were not designed, and their staffs not trained, to handle the needs of long-term patients. Caregivers could interpret rehabilitation tactics as constructive even as service members viewed them as quite the opposite.

A few months after the appearance of the *Washington Evening Star* story, during extensive congressional hearings in the summer of 1919, soldier-patients brought up similar questions about the extent and nature of military discipline in hospitals. Sergeant Greenleaf B. Johnson was one of multiple patients who reported being punished after leaving hospital grounds without permission. Johnson, who had served before World War I on the Mexican border with his Nebraska National Guard Unit, was struck in the abdomen by a grenade in France. "My entrails protruded," he recalled, "and I bandaged it with a legging." The battalion surgeon told Johnson it would be "impossible to get . . . to a hospital," so, he said, "I did the heavy marching with my wound like it was" from Argonne to Verdun (a journey of more than 20 miles). Around the first of August, the soldier said, he was gassed, before finally being placed in French then American base hospitals for treatment. Eventually, he was shipped to Walter Reed Hospital.[75]

Johnson told legislators that he was the victim of several injustices at Walter Reed because he had gained a reputation as a vocal critic of the hospital. His visitors were denied the privilege of seeing him, he said, and his letters to friends and family were routinely discarded instead of mailed. Finally, hospital staff sent him to "Ward B," a 20-by-20-foot basement room where patients with a variety of ailments—contagious diseases, amputations, wounds—were indiscriminately placed together as punishment for disciplinary infractions. Officials detained him there, Johnson believed, because he left the hospital without permission in order to see his only surviving sister—three others had recently died. At the congressional hearings, Johnson explained that he had requested leave but had been denied. When one legislator pedantically questioned whether Johnson realized that his actions would have consequences, the soldier replied, "I weighed it carefully . . . it was a deliberate act." He elaborated: "After I had had three deaths in the family and I had been so cruelly treated in Walter Reed and this one sister that I had left—my love for her was stronger than my fidelity to this institution of torture, and I went to see her and took the chance."[76] Johnson was pained and apoplectic—not mainly because he was "spitting blood and passing blood from the bowels" but because he felt cheated. "I live in the country, and if the flag is good enough to live under it is good enough to die for," he told congressional representatives. "But I do believe if a man is patriotic enough to die for a flag, the country ought to guarantee the protection of its laws and protect him against the criminal treatment that is practiced in Walter Reed Hospital." Johnson argued that his claims of neglect were hardly unique. Plenty of soldier-patients, he maintained, had been, "pulled out of bed and run up and down the ward there when they were not able."[77]

Reports of treatment in the disciplinary ward of Army Hospital No. 21 in Aurora, Colorado, likewise showed that ailing patients resented having little control over their fate. Army Medical Corps doctor Neill Duncan MacArten, a "strapping six-footer" who oversaw the ward, was unapologetic, if not slightly defiant, when Rep. William Vaile (R-CO) questioned him about patients' allegations of abuse. MacArten reported that one soldier, Roy Parks, "became insubordinate . . . and cursed me and the hospital and the Government in general."

The doctor told legislators that he told Parks to "shut up and for me not to hear another word out of him." But the soldier "continued to curse and talk right on." MacArten could not recall exactly what Parks had said because the doctor had abruptly "turned and walked out of the ward." A short while later, he directed a sergeant and two guards to place Parks in a straitjacket. MacArten told legislators that between December 1918 and January 1919, hospital staff had ordered seven patients to be placed in straitjackets as punishment for insubordinate acts, such as being absent without leave and smuggling tobacco into the disciplinary ward. The medical repercussions of such a punishment could be dire. Parks, for one, reported being bound for thirty hours. Not only did the incident bring about a hemorrhage, but it also left him unable to walk unassisted for the following ten days.[78]

Race in the Wards

The testimonies of Greenleaf Johnson and Samuel Ellis, who were both black men, indicated that rehabilitation experiences depended on preconceived notions not only about service records and health conditions but also about race. During World War I, approximately 8 percent of US soldiers were African American.[79] Official army policy dictated that white and black soldiers would be treated in the same wards according to their ailments. But in the face of rising social tensions, there were plenty of exceptions to the rule.

Medical treatment of soldiers posed a distinct challenge to the US Army's official policy of racial segregation, which remained in place through 1948. Hospital wards were different from staff quarters and army camps, where the military worked diligently to maintain segregated units and living spaces. Upholding the policy of separate quarters for black and white soldiers in health facilities was simply untenable, maintained Col. D. W. Ketcham of the War Plans Division. "In hospitals, patients have to be classified by diseases rather than with reference to other considerations," he said, "and moreover, while men are sick in bed there is scarcely any opportunity for friction due to race troubles."[80] Thus, during the Great War, hospital wards and occupational therapy workshops provided a brief foray into racial integration for at least some soldiers and caregivers (figure 2.4).[81] That stated policy pertaining to military hospitals was integration, not segregation, as it was in civilian (and, in the near future, veterans') hospitals, corresponded with the notion that military medicine was based first and foremost on efficiency.

Although it was hardly unusual at the time for white doctors and nurses to

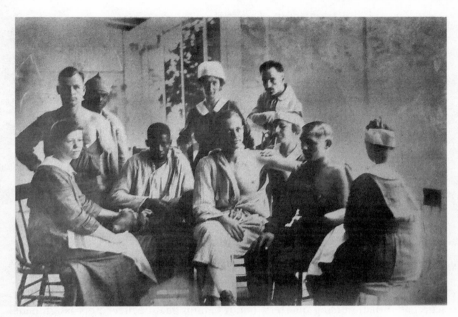

Figure 2.4. Undated photograph captioned "W.R.G.H. Artificial Limbs, massaging of stumps preparatory to fitting." Unsorted Files, Public Affairs Office, Walter Reed Army Medical Center, folder: Occupational Therapy, Old Photos—Historical, 235a. Courtesy of US Army/Walter Reed Army Medical Center

resist providing care to black patients—indeed, a variety of southern states had laws on the books stipulating that white nurses could refuse to do so if they wished—some caregivers embraced the army's approach.[82] Alice Duffield, a white nurse who spent the bulk of her wartime service treating young black soldiers diagnosed with pneumonia at Camp Pike in Little Rock, Arkansas, shrugged off the suggestion that as a working-class southern white woman she would have thought anything of bathing and taking the temperatures of African American soldiers. "Didn't bother me," Duffield said in an oral history interview recorded seventy years after the war. Family and friends "never said one thing about it," she maintained. "It was just nursing, that was all there was to it."[83]

While white nurses like Alice Duffield might be tasked with treating black patients, they did not live alongside their African American nurse colleagues. Aileen Stewart, one of approximately 1,800 black nurses certified by the Red Cross to serve with the army during World War I, reported that there was virtually no interaction between white and black nurses at Camp Sherman in Ohio.

After graduating from nursing school at the Freedmen's Hospital in Washington, DC, in 1917, she was barred from assuming a post as an army nurse but was recruited by the Red Cross to treat West Virginia miners during the 1918 flu epidemic. Only after peace was declared did the army open its doors to eighteen nurses of color. Two weeks after the Armistice, in November 1918, Stewart and her classmates received letters from the Army Surgeon General's Office offering them long-awaited positions as army nurses. One of the first African American women nurses to receive an army commission, Stewart was sent with her cohort to Camp Sherman. There, she later recalled, "we were assigned to 'separate but equal' living quarters on the base, which was the accepted system of segregated living." The home had ten bedrooms, showers, a living room, dining room, and kitchen, and, Stewart recalled, "we had a full-time Negro maid who prepared our meals and served them to us in our own dining room."[84] The segregation "didn't seem a big thing," Stewart said. "Of course, we didn't know enough to be offended. We made our own social life, didn't socialize with the white nurses."[85]

Patient care—much to the chagrin of some white service members—was less segregated than nursing quarters. James Cunningham believed his assignment to the so-called mental ward at Walter Reed Hospital qualified as an inexplicable punishment, not least because of whom he found himself surrounded by: "I am not restricted to [Ward X] as yet and I hope I won't [be] with your kind assistance," Cunningham wrote to the wife of a Marine Corps colonel in July 1918. "It will kill me if I am as I think nearly all in the ward are crazy and (50%) fifty percent of the Patients are Negroes."[86] Cunningham's claim was based on the contemporary realities of medical treatment. In the civilian world, and especially in the South, well-equipped general hospitals might turn away black patients, leaving them with few options but to seek care at underresourced institutions. It made sense then, for Cunningham to assume that if he found himself among black patients, he must be receiving substandard treatment.[87]

The inspector general duly undertook an investigation of Cunningham's sundry claims, including the one, in the words of the ensuing report, "that he was transferred from Ward 41 to 43 (formerly called X) and placed among crazy negroes as punishment." Ultimately, the inspector general's report not only concluded that Cunningham was receiving proper treatment but also reiterated Col. Ketcham's point in no uncertain terms: "It is customary to treat white and colored soldiers in the same wards at this hospital."[88]

Although integration may have been "customary," segregation was practiced throughout the war at numerous hospitals. The institutions were microcosms of an American society dominated by oppressive Jim Crow laws, racial violence, and black resistance. When the mother of an African American soldier complained about "discrimination against the colored soldiers" at Army General Hospital No. 9 in Lakewood, New Jersey, Winford H. Smith of the Army Surgeon General's Office responded that the commanding officer of the facility had been instructed to ensure that "colored soldiers are to be given the same attention."

> Over a year ago evidence of considerable friction developed in many of the hospitals particularly in the south, and numerous complaints were received because of the indiscriminate mixing of colored and white patients in the same wards. After careful consideration, and believing it to be in the interest of harmony and to the advantage of the colored soldiers quite as much as to the white, instructions were issued from this office to the effect that so far as practicable, the colored soldiers would be placed in wards by themselves, but that they would receive the same careful consideration in every detail as was accorded any other soldiers. Wherever colored soldiers were patients in the hospital in sufficient number to warrant their being placed in separate wards, this was done.[89]

The New Jersey case indicated a wider encroachment of Jim Crow. In response to claims from patients like James Cunningham, Army Surgeon General William Gorgas sent a memo to hospitals throughout the country in March 1918, declaring that "it would be a better procedure, and in the best interest of all concerned, to arrange for the care of white and colored patients in separate wards or separate rooms, so far as possible."[90] Even after Gorgas sent his memo, policies surrounding integration fluctuated from institution to institution in an "imperfectly segregated" army, but the articulated rule demonstrated the extent to which the army was willing to prioritize the social concerns of white soldiers, even if doing so might threaten the well-being of black soldiers.[91]

Although Smith of the Army Surgeon General's Office maintained that there "has been no less vigilance in the care and treatment of the colored soldiers," there were plenty of reports that African Americans encountered hostility in military hospitals, not least of all from fellow patients who were white. In the fall of 1918, two black privates at the Mineola base hospital in New York complained to local Urban League officials that a fellow African American soldier, Charles Parker, was "unmercifully beaten up by white privates from the south because he would not give his place during mess time to some white soldiers who came after him and would not get in at the end of the line." Private Parker, his peers said, would likely lose sight in one of his eyes as a result of being "attacked with white soldiers' knives and forks." The soldiers suspected of aggression were being held under arrest by the army, but the allegations were difficult to prove since "none of them will disclose the guilty ones among their number." The soldiers who reported the occurrence to Urban League officials said they were hesitant to return to camp, "and one was so downhearted that he actually shed tears," disappointed in a "government that cannot protect its own soldiers from the 'crackers,' as he phrased it."[92] The *Chicago Defender* later referred to complaints about "segregation and discrimination of the vilest sort" and hospital "treatment . . . below the standard of human endurance" as "an obvious example of a country's crime against a race that has always shed its blood that this nation might occupy the exalted place in the world of today which it now does."[93]

Efforts abounded in the African American community to provide for ill and injured black soldiers by protecting them from such injustices, celebrating their wartime efforts, and offering social options. Wartime work took place in the midst of heightened activism among a network of black club women, educators, health professionals, and advocates who had been organizing public health campaigns in black communities for decades.[94] The Circle of Negro War Relief "constituted the nearest approach to a Red Cross . . . through which the colored people cooperated during the war."[95] The group was founded in New York in November 1917 "with the idea of having the colored women of America, and some men, too . . . do as much as they possibly could for the colored soldiers." Within a few months, similar groups arose in locales "extending from New York to Utah and throughout the New England states as far south as Florida." By 1920, sixty groups of twenty-five members or more throughout the United States were affiliated with the Circle. The groups "did just what other war organizations did," according to its leaders: they arranged visits to soldiers in hospitals with baked goods and handmade knits and sponsored lectures and events. In addition, they attempted to ensure that black soldiers and veterans had social options beyond segregated military camps and tension-filled hospital wards.[96] In Baltimore, for example, the War Camp Community Club for Colored Soldiers reserved a church hall so that service members could "spend their brief furloughs in moral surroundings and away from dens of vice." The club featured a reading room, cafeteria, billiard hall, writing room, and sleeping quarters.[97] Such services were in high demand; within just a few weeks, the hall was overcrowded and the club was appealing to residents of the city to help house soldiers and veterans.[98] A prime example of how middle-class women became involved in the war effort by overseeing and joining volunteer and social service organizations, the Baltimore War Camp Club remained active throughout the fall of 1918, hosting meetings of "mothers" and "sisters" of service members.[99]

Community leaders and government officials embraced African Americans' local efforts. At the opening of a club for black soldiers in Rockford, Illinois, a prominent black physician, George C. Hall, noted the importance of contributions of African Americans to the war effort. They represented "true Americanism," as Hall put it. "All races were giving their lives and their treasures," he said, "that the benefits coming as the result of this tremendous sacrifice should know no person by race, creed or religion."[100] In the summer of 1918, the federal Committee on Women's Defense Work authorized African American educator Alice Dunbar Nelson to visit various southern cities to ascertain whether a national council of black women might be organized. By officially sanctioning local efforts and bringing them into the fold of the government, federal officials felt they could "ensure a degree of cooperation and coordination with the least likelihood of upsetting existing social relations."[101]

"Until some provision is made I do not wish to be separated from the army"

While some complained about conditions in military hospitals, and many patients pined to be discharged, others hoped to prolong their stays. In May 1920, it had been almost two years since Maj. George McAdie had helped lead New York's 165th Infantry Division in the Second Battle of the Marne, and he was finally being released from service. But he found himself disappointed and dissatisfied rather than relieved. "I was taken out of bed to be discharged," he told a government official in July 1920, referring to his recent experience at the Oteen army general hospital in Asheville, North Carolina. Still suffering from active tuberculosis, he said, he and fifteen fellow officers released at the same time "were not discharged because we had received maximum treatment, but because, under a ruling of the [War Department], we had had a years definitive treatment for tuberculosis, and were not entitled to further treatment."[102]

As the army evaluated and amended discharge policies according to fluctuating military needs and a variety of other conditions, some soldiers complained they were rushed out of the army—and its hospitals—before they were capable of supporting themselves physically or financially. Debates about discharge rules revealed that in the military health system the desires and needs of individual patients served as only one consideration in the administration of care and that policy terms such as "functionally restored as far as possible" were highly subjective.[103]

Soldiers who, unlike George McAdie, sought hasty discharges—occasionally against medical advice—not only wished to be free from army discipline and hierarchy but also wanted control over the nature of medical care they could receive. Ralph Williams, who had been wounded in France, was one of those who rejected treatment and opted to be released from the military. "When I went before the examining board, they said I was to go to Walter Reed Hospital for possible surgery," Williams reported. "I said I did not wish to have that done and explained that I had been told not to rush into it." Williams's dissent, he implied, brought about some hostility. "They informed me that I was still in the army and subject to their orders. . . . I was told that if I did not agree to the surgery I would have to sign waivers of any further claim against the government. That is what I did."[104] Jake Van Diepen, who received hospital care both abroad and in the United States because he felt nervous and fatigued after driving trucks near the front, would have done "anything to get out." When he visited the administrative offices of the Southern branch of the National Home for Disabled Volunteer Soldiers in Virginia, where his care was being paid for by the army, he observed that discharge "papers were lying on chairs, under baskets, and every other place: no system at all, it was all confusion." Van Diepen began urging hospital officials that he was well and ready to be released in June 1918. He finally received his discharge three months later.[105]

Army officials continually reevaluated the question of when the military ceased being responsible for wounded and ill soldiers, considering and amending policies regarding discharge both before and after the Armistice. In January 1918, Col. D. W. Ketcham of the Army General Staff drafted a memo to the secretary of war requesting the reconsideration of December 1917 War Department regulations that had stipulated that "when an enlisted man becomes unfitted for military service, a certificate of disability for discharge will be prepared by the soldier's immediate commanding officer and forwarded." Ketcham suggested that the policy be broadened. Echoing a recommendation by the surgeon general, he argued that no soldier should be discharged "until he has attained complete recovery or as complete recovery as it is to be expected that he will attain when the nature of his disability is considered." Ketcham justified the policy by saying "it would be most unfair" to release from service "physically unfit soldiers." Reminiscent of the sentiments of the drafters of the War Risk Insurance Act, Ketcham noted that volunteer and drafted soldiers deserved assurance, "in case they are incapacitated through injury or disease, that they will be clothed, housed, fed, and given medical treatment until as complete a cure as it is possible to attain has been effected." Retaining such soldiers in the army also alleviated the possibility that they would become "an unnecessary and unjust burden" on their relatives and communities.[106]

In February 1918, Secretary of War Newton D. Baker approved the surgeon general's recommended discharge policy, amending paragraph 159 of Army Regulations to read: "When an enlisted man becomes unfitted for military service, full or partial duty, because of wounds or disease contracted in line of duty, he will not be discharged until he has attained as complete recovery as is to be expected when the nature of his disability is considered." A certificate of disability and discharge would be prepared, the new regulation said, only "when it is believed that further treatment will not improve his condition."[107]

Army officials pondered a litany of new discharge regulations in the winter of 1918–1919, as a massive influx of sick and wounded soldiers flooded into domestic army hospitals and as doctors and patients expressed increasing eagerness to be released from service. In order to avoid the possibility that previous orders "unduly retard the discharge from the service of men clearly unfit for military service," Henry Jervey, assistant chief of staff in the office of the secretary of war, offered various clarifications to War Department policies. Cases that would not benefit from "further sojourn" in hospitals or convalescent centers, Jervey noted, "should be promptly discharged." Utilizing an iteration of the relatively vague terminology contained in an earlier army reconstruction plan, Jervey added that only the surgeon overseeing a particular case could "judge whether or not maximum restoration has been secured." Soldiers who had "funds or who have relatives or friends in position to afford them specialized care" could be discharged once a commanding officer determined that "care is assured."[108] The new rules further provided that all soldiers who had "acquired a lower physical standard than that given them when they entered the service" should be discharged once it was determined that "maximum improvement has been obtained or that physical disabilities have not been exaggerated or accentuated as a result of service in line of duty." Those whose maladies were aggravated by service were to be sent to convalescent centers; "providing further benefit can be expected by additional treatment, training and hardening processes."[109]

The War Department correspondence alludes to the fact that army officials were obliged to dictate the timing and conditions of each discharge and consider both the soldier-patient's case and the public purse. Their decisions regarding whether a service member incurred an injury or illness in the line of duty could be crucial, since those judgments could justify or call into question future claims for benefits. After World War I, countless veterans argued that their health conditions were due to service and contested the terms of army discharges that indicated otherwise.

The War Department's variable discharge policies and procedures during and immediately after the war foreshadowed the complaints to come. Between 1916 and 1918, Army Medical Department personnel could rely on two stated War Department policies when considering whether an injury or illness was service-connected. Both gave individual doctors great autonomy and power in rendering decisions. At the outset of war, they could refer to the *Manual* for the Army Medical Department, which stated that "all diseases or injuries from which an officer or enlisted man suffers while in the military service . . . may be assumed to have occurred in the line of duty; unless the surgeon knows . . . that the disease or injury existed before entering the service." In May 1918, General Order No. 47 offered more detail: the army would consider a disability to have been incurred in the line of duty "unless such disability can be shown to be the result of [a service member's] carelessness, misconduct, or vicious habits, or unless the history of the case shows unmistakably that the disability existed prior to entrance into the service."[110]

A crucial June 1918 amendment to the War Risk Insurance Act called into question the autonomy of army doctors in determining service connection. Any "officer, enlisted man, or other member," it said, "shall be held and taken to have been in sound condition when examined, accepted and enrolled for service."[111] The change had come at the behest of officials of the Treasury Department who argued that no clear definition of "line of duty" existed and that the "provision as to line of duty appears to be unsatisfactory and has already had the effect of shutting out [from receiving compensation payments] many meritorious cases."[112] In the words of a postwar report from the Army Medical Department, "This was a revolutionary change involving greatly increased obligations on the part of the Government and in consequence increasing its expenditures for compensation by millions of dollars annually."[113]

As discharge policies came under scrutiny, War Department officials debated whether military procedures should be altered based on amendments to a piece of legislation. The judge advocate general consistently argued that the army was legally obliged to honor congressionally approved changes to the War Risk Insurance Act and assume service connection for any soldier whose injury or illness was not recorded at the time of enlistment. But the surgeon general "held that the war risk insurance act was without effect as regards the Military Establishment" and that Medical Department personnel should continue to adhere to the organization's manual by basing disability assessments on independently gathered patient histories. Legislators, the surgeon general suggested, were out of bounds. Not until January 1920, with the War Department's passage of General Order No. 7, was the matter settled in any official way—and even then somewhat vaguely. In issuing certificates of disability, the order stated, army doctors should pay heed to both the War Risk Insurance Act and General Order No. 47 of 1918, authorizing them to base decisions on gathered knowledge about a patient's history.[114]

While officials in the upper echelons of the War Department debated semantics, hospital staff and commanding officers around the country daily faced the task of filling out discharge forms for service members like tuberculosis patient George McAdie. Approximately 700 of the more than 14,000 patients treated at Walter Reed Hospital in 1918 were discharged due to disability. Of those patients, 198 were reported to have incurred their injuries or illnesses in the line of duty. The great majority—147—had amputations or "injuries and diseases of organs of locomotion." Other major causes of discharge due to disability were tuberculosis, "psycho-neurosis, hysteria," and "mental deficiency, moron." But the hospital staff was much less likely to judge each of the latter conditions as service-connected. According to official discharge statuses, two of the twenty-two Walter Reed patients discharged with tuberculosis, two of the twenty-six classified as "mental deficiency, moron," and none of the fifteen discharged with "psycho-neurosis, hysteria" incurred their disabilities in the line of duty.[115] Of the 70,000 service members admitted to hospitals to be treated for exposure to gas, 2,900 were discharged with a disability.[116] Conceptions of disability, illness, and "malingering" helped shape discharge patterns, just as they played a role in influencing perceptions of service members and veterans during and after the war.

Tuberculosis among new recruits was an especially vexing problem that prompted a rethinking of army rationale regarding how to define "line-of-duty." In September 1917, Surgeon General Gorgas issued a circular stipulating that chronic tuberculosis would be considered to have existed prior to service if the ill soldier had been enlisted for less than three months, unless "exposure in line of duty" led to the condition. Eight months later, in April 1918, the Army Surgeon General's Office recommended that the policy be overturned since it had led to "considerable injustice." There was a "lack of uniformity" in how doctors judged whether cases of tuberculosis could be connected to service. For this reason, the surgeon general suggested a new blanket policy stipulating that "any soldier who shall have been accepted on his first physical examination (after arrival at a military station) as fit for service, shall be considered to have contracted any subsequently determined physical disability in the line of duty." The secretary of war approved the surgeon general's request and established that soldiers could be treated in military hospitals for tuberculosis and, by extension, other illnesses, even if they existed prior to service.[117] There was some room for judgment on the part of individual doctors: if there was evidence that the illness was "the result of . . . carelessness, misconduct, or vicious habits" or that "the history of the case shows unmistakably that the disability existed prior to entrance into the service," physicians could list the disease as having occurred not in the line of duty.[118] The relatively lenient policy made perfect sense given that before and during the war the army was attempting to retain as many people as possible. But the situation was different by the spring of 1920—around the time George McAdie was suddenly discharged. By that point, resources and personnel were considerably more limited, and there was little reason to retain men who would likely never return to active duty.

In 1920, the typical procedure for a soldier's discharge from Walter Reed, according to Maj. Lucius L. Hopwood, the hospital's supervisor of clinical records, began when the chief of the Medical or Surgical Service decided that a patient had come as close to "maximum improvement" as could be expected. The ward surgeon proceeded to seek clearance from the chiefs of various services who had been involved in treatment, then worked with the section chief to fill out discharge papers indicating, among other things, if a disability existed, "whether or not further treatment is considered necessary; whether or not the maximum degree of improvement has been attained; whether or not the patient is fit for full duty; and, in case of an officer, whether or not he wishes discharge."[119]

Soldiers and officers had limited say in the discharge process. As the section chief circulated paperwork, hospital officials sent written notice to the patient to notify him his discharge was being "contemplated." He was also told to appear before the hospital board for a physical examination.[120] In the spring of 1920, one soldier's medical board proceedings included four board members: Lucius Hopwood; William L. Keller, chief of the Surgical Service; and two other army doctors.[121] If a service member was found to have a disability, claimed to have a disability, or objected to his discharge, he could bring his case to a board of review. According to Hopwood, officers and enlisted men sat in on review board proceedings concerning their own cases and received an opportunity to share their opinions. But they were excused from the room when the doctors discussed the issues of greatest concern: whether a disability existed and whether such disability would be listed as having been contracted in the line of duty. Once the board had come to a decision regarding a soldier's release from service, he would be physically examined one last time—no more than twenty-four hours before his actual discharge.[122]

Some soldiers maintained that the process was not so systematic or fair. Complaints they filed with the inspector general hinted not simply at dissatisfaction with the quality of care offered at the hospital but, even more so, at a sense of dejection about the prospects men thought they faced following their stays there.

Lt. Arthur L. Chamberlain, for example, suffered from bronchitis, insomnia, and psychoneurosis after his boat was torpedoed off the coast of Ireland and he waded in the water for hours. Following five months of treatment at Walter Reed, the army issued Chamberlain's discharge with a disability rating of 15 percent in March 1920 (figure 2.5). Aware that the judgment would serve as one important factor in determining how much monthly compensation he could eventually receive from the Bureau of War Risk Insurance, Chamberlain balked.

A few days before his scheduled separation from service, he wrote to Hopwood: "I have asked to be discharged March 15th as I cannot see the use of staying around the hospital without improvement in my condition, however when I made this request I expected to be taken care of after leaving the service." The soldier withdrew his request for discharge, implying that his disability rating was too low. "Until some provision is made I do not wish to be separated from the army," Chamberlain wrote. "I have a wife and two children to support but as I cannot do anything for them I don't know what to do but to commit suicide and end it all."[123]

By minimizing the degree of his injury, according to Chamberlain, the army had hindered his ability to support his family. The soldier's plea was presented later to a disability board, which maintained the 15 percent decision and released him from the army. After he underwent an examination with the Public Health Service, the federal entity that assumed control of administering medical care to veterans once they were discharged from the army, Chamberlain said: "I have been told I have not reached maximum improvement, but that I was curable and would be all right in time."[124] The post-discharge review bolstered the veteran's charge that Walter Reed administrators had been unfair in their assessment.

CERTIFICATE OF EXAMINING BOARD
and
REPORT OF THE BOARD OF REVIEW.

We find that he is physically and mentally sound
with the following exceptions; Psycho-neurosis
(psychasthenia). Further hospital treatment is not
considered necessary; maximum degree of improvement
to be expected therefrom has been attained. Further
treatment by the Bureau of War Risk Insurance is not
indicated. Officer is not fit for military duty.
The board recommended the discharge of this officer
from the military service of the United States.
In view of occupation he is 15% disabled.

(signed) W. L. Keller, Colonel M.C., U.S.A.
L. L. Smith, Colonel, M.C., U.S.A.
A. E. Schlanser, Major M.C., U.S.A.

APPROVED: March 1, 1920.
(signed) J. D. Glennan,
Colonel, Med. Corps, U.S.A.
Commanding.

Figure 2.5. Certificate of Examining Board for Lieutenant Arthur L. Chamberlain, 1920. Certificate of Examining Board and Report of the Board of Review, Office of the Inspector General Correspondence, 1917–1934, RG 159, box 1110, folder 18, National Archives at College Park, MD

Lt. William H. Vail also argued that his subsequent treatment by the Public Health Service justified his claim that he had been prematurely discharged from the army. Vail, who was treated at Walter Reed from March 1919 through April 1920, had his left leg amputated below the knee and a head injury, which resulted in a depression in his skull. He was relatively satisfied with the treatment he received for his leg but reported: "The only one in the hospital operating on heads was a contract surgeon . . . [who] came to the Walter Reed Hospital only once a week, and it was not his hospital. . . . I was very much afraid of my head, knowing that it involved the brain. I wanted everything to be just as good as possible, and I felt that the conditions there were not such." Several times Vail asked for the authority to consult with specialists at Johns Hopkins Hospital. "I lost confidence in the surgeons at [Walter Reed]," he said. "They did not seem to get down to brass tacks and I was not in physical condition to force any such action." Even as Vail questioned the quality of care at Walter Reed and sought treatment outside of the military system, he protested his certificate of discharge, which he said came "out of a clear sky."[125]

Col. William L. Keller, chief of the Surgical Service at Walter Reed saw things differently. Army doctors had offered to perform the head surgery for Vail, Keller said, but the patient declined. On those grounds, officials assessed that Vail had reached maximum improvement and should be discharged from the army.[126]

Soon after the soldier's release, a Boston surgeon operated on Vail. The veteran reported to the inspector general that his medical expenses were covered by the Public Health Service, which "was all very satisfactory, but I constantly felt I should not have been discharged until this had been done."[127] Like Chamberlain, Vail believed that because he had entered the service healthy and self-sufficient, he should remain under the army's auspices—and on its payroll—until his post-service condition was unquestionably stable.

In response to the claims of premature discharge, army officials and Walter Reed doctors reported that they adhered to prewar policies regarding maximum improvement. Army Surgeon General Merritte W. Ireland shared with the inspector general his interpretation of those rules: "When it becomes clear that the condition of any officer patient is growing worse month by month, and when it is apparent for a period of several months that no improvement is being made, and when in other instance [*sic*] the patient's condition fails to furnish any grounds for expecting improvement in the future, then I believe his treatment for physical reconstruction has reached a point when further benefit can not be expected by his retention in military hospital or in the military service. Consequently his discharge is indicated under the provisions of the law."[128] Col. Keller at Walter Reed concurred, offering a further explanation, consistent with contemporary impressions of institutional care. Once medical treatments ceased being effective, he said, "the depressing atmosphere of a hospital is injurious to the patient."[129]

An Army Medical Department facing demobilization and budgetary pressures mainly deemed itself responsible for patients so long as they were receptive to prescribed treatments and demonstrating that they were being actively reconstructed. "To retain all patients indefinitely . . . would require the continued maintenance of large military hospitals with the necessary medical personnel and material; for such a procedure, the Medical Department appropriations are not sufficient," Ireland reported in a 1920 letter to a Colorado senator. Furthermore, he noted, the Bureau of War Risk Insurance boasted "abundant facilities for the care of officers and soldiers, and it is my firm belief that when the Medical Department of the Army has achieved all that can be expected in the way of the physical reconstruction of our military personnel . . . the individual should be discharged from the military service and should pass into the care of that Bureau."[130]

Army officers followed this plan in the immediate postwar years, discharging those with chronic ailments or injuries that were slow to heal to the auspices of the Bureau of War Risk Insurance and the Public Health Service, sometimes to the chagrin of patients themselves, who resisted being sent into the civilian world with what they saw as a lack of guaranteed income or follow-up medical care. While Walter Reed Hospital commander James D. Glennan argued that it was much more common for soldiers to fight to hasten discharge than it was for them to try to delay it, he did concede that it was "very common" for service members to object to their discharge and implied that such objections stemmed from fear or intimidation. "A certain type of officer after being in hospital a year or two years—sick in hospital—does not wish to leave the hospital to go into the world again to take up life outside."[131]

Ireland's point that service members could seek help through the Bureau of War Risk Insurance for continuing maladies revealed a gaping distance between soldiers' desires for and expectations of self-sufficiency, and the credo of "maximum improvement" adhered to by the Army Medical Department.[132] Keller, of the Surgical Service, frankly stated that the military hospital could only help soldiers progress up to a point, but that "it will take two years before these patients reach maximum improvement."[133] Private Jeremiah J. Hurley, on the other hand, declared that, "when I leave this hospital I do not want to have to enter any other hospital for treatment."[134] In his commentary regarding Hurley, the inspector general caustically remarked that when the veteran's disability status was raised from 100 to 200 percent (and his monthly payments thus doubled), "all his complaints seem to have disappeared."[135] In fact, Hurley, who had both his legs amputated, maintained that he sought the extra pay because he needed "a constant attendant after discharge, [and] the allowance of twenty dollars per month is not considered sufficient for one."[136]

For disabled veterans like Hurley, Vail, and Chamberlain, higher disability payments meant a higher degree of self-sufficiency and a greater chance that they could avoid institutionalization. Army officials, however, viewed them as a form of dependency and worried about the costs and implications of a prolonged rehabilitation process. The divide led to hostility and resentment from some particularly vocal soldiers, who felt that the army was cutting them off prematurely.

"The work of the War Department . . . is practically finished"

Both doctors and patients resisted embracing hospitals as ideal venues for long-term care, but an October 1920 article in the Walter Reed Hospital newspaper, *The Come-Back*, signified a turning point: "Many discharged soldiers still require hospital treatment, and many others will at some future time require treatment for conditions resulting from their military service." The administration of such care, the newspaper insisted, "does not devolve upon the War Department, but by law is placed in the hands of the Bureau of War Risk Insurance." Citing examples of the vast success of the Army Medical Department during the war—the creation of military hospital complexes that featured entertainment for soldiers and their visiting loved ones, an array of training courses, and innovations in medical treatment for amputations, speech defects, facial injuries, and training for the blind—*The Come-Back* declared: "The work of the War Department in caring for the victims of the World War is practically finished."[137]

In late 1918 and early 1919, *The Come-Back*'s news for hospitalized service members was, in many ways, positive. "This nation has no more solemn obligation than healing the hurts of our wounded and restoring our disabled men to civil life and opportunity," read a letter from President Woodrow Wilson, published in the newspaper. "The government recognizes this, and the fulfillment of the obligation is going forward fully and generously." Providing medical care and education for wounded veterans, the president argued, was not charity but "the payment of a draft of honor which the United States of America accepted when it selected these men, and took them in their health and strength to fight the battles of the nation."[138] A cartoon published in January 1919 intimated that the challenge was being met heartily by a grateful government: "Ain't it a grand and glorious feeling . . . after you've been wounded . . . and the government tells you it will teach you a new trade without charge . . . and finally you are all fixed and get a better job than you ever had—also your compensation and insurance and everything . . . oh-h-h boy!!!"[139] Similarly reassuring pieces were published throughout the postwar years. Service members' bodily sacrifice was noble, justified, and worthwhile, the newspaper argued; the US government and citizens would provide them the support necessary to facilitate their entry back into society.

As patients transitioned from soldier to veteran, their government initially conveyed the idea that they should feel both self-sufficient and entitled (figure

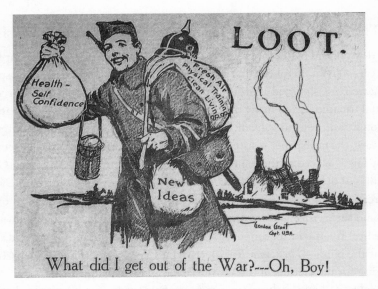

Figure 2.6. "What Did I Get Out of the War?" *The Come-Back*, Jan. 8, 1919: OHA 335:
Walter Reed Historical Collection, Otis Historical Archives, National Museum of
Health and Medicine, Silver Spring, MD

2.6 and 2.7). "Never before in the history of the world's warfare have such extensive plans been laid out for the benefit of the men disabled in conflict as those which are now in operation and others being formulated," *The Come-Back* reported in May 1920. "With practically no precedent to follow ... a stupendous task has thrust itself forward in the shape of the care of World War veterans." To deal with this "task," a "mammoth machine" had been created, which had four main parts. The first was the military hospital itself. Once a soldier was discharged from the service and that facility, he could utilize the second part of the "machine" and receive disability payments from the Bureau of War Risk Insurance. If the veteran required further medical care, he could make use of the third part of the machine: the Bureau of War Risk Insurance would cover the cost of his medical care at a Public Health Service hospital or, if geographical or hospital space constraints existed, at a civilian hospital. Finally, veterans who were well enough to work but not well enough to return to their previous occupations were free to take advantage of vocational education programs vis-à-vis the Federal Board for Vocational Education.[140]

In December 1919, *The Come-Back* reminded readers of their right to receive

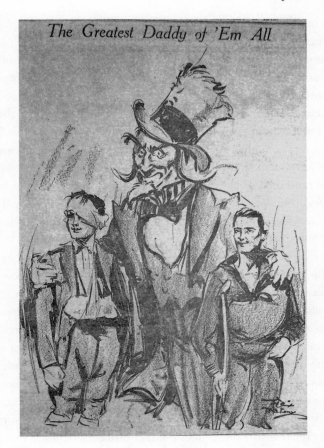

Figure 2.7. "The Greatest Daddy of 'Em All." *The Come-Back*, Feb. 5, 1919: OHA 355: Walter Reed Historical Collection, Otis Historical Archives, National Museum of Health and Medicine, Silver Spring, MD

free care in military, civilian, and Public Health Service hospitals, calling such access a "privilege" of which few were aware. Lt. Mathew C. Smith of the Army General Staff noted that discharged servicemen who felt their illness was due to wounds or other disabilities received or aggravated while in the service should arrange a physical exam with the nearest army hospital or representative of the US Public Health Service. Smith advised them to bring their discharge papers showing that their disability existed at the time of separation from the military. "However, if these papers are not available," Smith noted reassuringly, "the man should not hesitate to apply. Such an applicant will be immediately placed under treatment pending the receipt of the necessary papers."[141]

But as time passed, the newspaper provided increasing evidence countering its own declaration that the postwar "machine" for disabled veterans was "gaining in the smoothness of its functioning as the days go by." Peppy cartoons regarding prospective benefits were interspersed with articles detailing the intricate process behind accessing those benefits. Capitalizing on War Risk Insurance, vocational education, and, finally, medical care was more complicated than it may at first have seemed. "Soldiers desiring direct information on government matters are cautioned to be careful to obtain the proper addresses in order to save time and trouble," *The Come-Back* announced in March 1919. The article went on to list a variety of offices where soldiers could write for information about insurance, back pay and personal effects, and liberty bonds.[142] Not only was it complicated to seek assistance, according to *The Come-Back*, but the effort may not bear fruit. A question and answer article about compensation under the War Risk Insurance Act was candid. If an ex-soldier obtained a job, it acknowledged, his disability compensation would be "reduced or discontinued." "Obviously, this is not just. A man with an illness like tuberculosis or Bright's disease might by reason of his necessities be forced to find a job and earn something even in spite of the advice of his doctors." In such a case, "the result would be that the more he earned, the less he would get from the government and the government would profit by that man's industry, even though that man's industry might be one form of committing suicide." However, "such a method of determining the comparison . . . does not take into consideration that most men who had been in the service for any length of time had gained immeasurably by the experience, and probably had improved their earning capacity."[143] Disabled men might have lost their full physical or mental health, *The Come-Back* suggested, but they gained the invaluable experience of service. It was, the paper indelicately implied, a wash.

In its coverage of War Risk Insurance benefits and vocational education, *The Come-Back* sent mixed messages: articles consistently painted a positive picture of opportunities but at the same time acknowledged with increasing frequency that there were limits to and rules about who could access them. Boastful claims that "the United States government intends to put every disabled soldier and sailor into a good job" gave way to warnings that veterans "gotta be real to pass muster."[144] Requests for government-funded college courses from men "with trivial hurts," such as an injured index finger, *The Come-Back* reported in May

1919, would be turned down by a Federal Board for Vocational Education that was scrutinizing cases ever more closely.[145] Straying from its unqualified celebration of government generosity, the newspaper reminded readers that not everyone was entitled to all services.

The Comeback's coverage of post-discharge medical care reflected the larger reality that policies were in constant flux and helped create political awareness among hospital residents. Patients found practical news about meetings among officials of the Public Health Service to address "misunderstandings and delays" in the provision of government insurance and hospital treatment for discharged soldiers.[146] They also learned about a report from a veterans' advocacy group called the American Legion showing that as many as 109,000 soldiers suffering from pulmonary tuberculosis and mental illness had been prematurely discharged from the military "before being properly cured and with no official effort having been made to keep track of them."[147] In March 1921, two weeks before *The Come-Back* ceased publication, it reported a jarring statistic from Ewing Laporte, assistant secretary of the Treasury: the number of ex-soldiers entering civilian hospitals each month was 1,000–1,500 in excess of those leaving them. Furthermore, Laporte estimated, a bed capacity of 30,000 would have to be maintained for World War I veterans "for many years to come."[148] The newspaper of one of the premier military hospitals in the United States was openly acknowledging not only an exponentially increasing demand for services but also the government's desperate, and often unsuccessful, attempts to keep up.

Although *Come-Back* editors, like many army and government officials, subscribed to the belief that the "great need is to guard against hospitalization, that is, [ex-service men] reaching a state of mental and physical inactivity where the thought of initiative or action of any sort takes on the aspects of the impossible," they were faced with the reality that many veterans would seek hospital care for an indefinite period.[149] Patients with tuberculosis and neuropsychiatric diseases posed the biggest societal challenge of all: they would demand institutional care for years to come. As military hospital administrators discharged patients who they argued had reached "maximum improvement," and as men and women who had never been treated in military hospitals—either by choice or because their health maladies arose after service—came forward seeking care, civilian society faced the challenge of answering the needs of a new cadre of wounded veterans.

Army Medical Department officials went to great lengths to fulfill the decree that soldiers would be rehabilitated and prepared for civilian life prior to discharge, growing and diversifying a domestic military medical system in which hospitals served as social, not just medical, environments. During and after World War I, health-related policies assigned great responsibility to the army, but they were also vague enough to be open to interpretation—and cause tension. Army doctors, for example, argued that "maximum improvement" should be defined as the point when a soldier-patient stopped showing signs of physical improvement. After all, they argued, facilities like Walter Reed Hospital were not intended as sites for the provision of long-term medical care; the US military could not spend its time and resources rehabilitating soldiers who would likely never serve again. Meanwhile, injured and ill soldier-patients had a different perspective. Some felt that the government owed them not only the simple courtesy of laundry service but that it should also return them to civilian life only once it was clear that they would need no further care. They resented being discharged physically compromised and therefore with no guaranteed source of a reliable income. While the provision of extended health services went against prewar rehabilitation ideals focused on cure and self-reliance, injured and ill service members viewed it as justice. Expressions of dissatisfaction from men like Samuel Ellis and Arthur Chamberlain gained power as soldiers organized into veterans' advocacy groups.

Indeed, soldiers and caregivers first exposed to government-sponsored care in military hospitals would carry their experiences with them as a veterans' health system took root. For example, George McAdie, who had fought his discharge from the Oteen General Hospital in 1920, continued to struggle with his health throughout the next decade. By 1930, his pulmonary tuberculosis had become, as a medical official put it, "far advanced." That year, he died at Oteen, after it had been reconstituted as a veterans' hospital.[150] His Asheville, North Carolina, tombstone reads simply: "George McAdie, New York, Major 165th Inf., 42 Div., April 23, 1930."[151] Neill MacArten, who was accused of abuse in a Colorado military hospital, later served as medical officer in charge of a Tucson, Arizona, Public Health Service hospital overseeing care for World War veterans.[152] And Paul Bazaar, who wrote of his positive impressions of Walter Reed following the loss of his hands, made his living in the 1920s and 1930s as a manager with the Veterans Bureau in upstate New York.[153] Each of the men was part of an expansive and somewhat haphazard health system that arose as ailing service members reentered society as disabled and ill civilians.

CHAPTER THREE

War Is Hell but after Is "Heller"

An Army Responsibility Becomes a Societal Obligation

In July 1920, Mother Marianne of Jesus was especially worried about two types of patients who occupied the New Jersey convalescent home she managed. First there were the "chronic cases, such as cardiacs, sufferers from sub-acute nervous disorders, &c." Harry Fisher, for example, had "returned home a nervous wreck" after being awarded the Croix de guerre and the Distinguished Service Cross. Anthony Kasswassky, whose entire family was "in that part of Poland now being ravaged by contending armies," had endured three shrapnel wounds to his head and had "the mentality of a boy of ten." Peter Flanagan required "periodic treatment" due to a lung infection resulting from a shrapnel wound but had been "refused further care" by the Bureau of War Risk Insurance. "Quite unable to work," he was forced to support himself on his $80 per month disability compensation.[1]

Mother Marianne also worried about a second group: "those who have not yet developed organic diseases but who are breaking down." Michael Blanche, for example was "told to go back to work" and report to the Bureau of War Risk Insurance if he "became definitely ill." Michael DeLucia was instructed that he "needed six months rest and open air life, but that the Bureau could not give him the care he required . . . In the opinion of our medical attendant, both of these young men could probably be saved from serious organic trouble if they had proper attention now," Mother Marianne noted. "Surely," providing "sympathetic care in congenial surroundings" was "the least we can do for these men who have given for their country all that makes life sweet."[2]

Mother Marianne's case studies highlighted some of the main challenges surrounding the care of recently discharged service members. As it became clear that military hospitals could not handle the ideological and physical problem of thousands of ill and wounded, administrators of existing federal agencies attempted to coordinate care. In response to an unexpectedly high demand, two organizations did the bulk of the work in cobbling together health services: the Bureau of War Risk Insurance (BWRI), the Treasury Department agency created to administer insurance and disability compensation payments to World War I veterans, and the Public Health Service (PHS), which had a widely varied mandate that included protecting US borders from disease, implementing sanitary measures in towns and cities across the United States, and administering a small hospital program. Branches of the military and the Federal Board for Vocational Education were also intimately involved with veterans' aid in these early years, but the BWRI and PHS most directly laid the groundwork for the veterans' health system to come. Neither of those two agencies historically had a mission focused on individualized medical care, let alone the design of a nationwide system that could serve a variety of complex needs like the ones brought forth by Mother Marianne.

In the wake of war, funding consistently increased for the hospitalization of veterans, but government officials found it challenging to coordinate services and determine rules regarding access to and standards of care. In the months immediately following the war, as levels of demand rose sharply, funding and plans for veterans' health programs led the Public Health Service, the Bureau of War Risk Insurance, and federally sponsored Soldiers' Homes to haphazardly enhance their infrastructures. Meanwhile, bureaucrats worked to devise a uniform and objective system for rating veterans' disabilities based on emerging and diverse state workers' compensation programs. Some former service members took issue with their disability ratings and argued forcefully that they deserved to be treated as a class apart from nonveterans who also received government-sponsored care. As former service members complained about neglect in ill-equipped institutions and multiple agencies provided services, no one entity or individual was fully responsible for fixing systemic shortfalls. Bureaucrats, public health professionals, veterans, and advocacy organizations pointed to the inability of existing agencies to fulfill the government's promises as proof that sweeping policy changes were necessary.

Debates about the nature and extent of veterans' health services reflected larger tensions about the purpose, promise, and peril of government intervention in the lives of citizens. While some high-ranking BWRI and PHS officials who came of age during the Progressive Era fought for an expansive system of veterans' entitlements to stave off the twin problems of poverty and ill health, budget-conscious legislators, bureaucrats, and caregivers questioned the personal histories and motivations of patients and argued for conditional and limited benefits. Perspectives about whether and how to provide medical care for individuals like Harry Fisher, Anthony Kasswassky, and Peter Flanagan depended, in essence, on conceptions of the state's responsibility to its citizens.

The Bureau of War Risk Insurance and Public Health Service

In April 1920, Secretary of War Newton D. Baker wrote to Army Chief of Staff Peyton C. March expressing his worry about a policy dictating that all hospitalized wartime emergency officers and soldiers be discharged from army hospitals by the end of June. Focusing on the army's original mandate—that soldiers not be discharged until they were fully rehabilitated—Baker wondered, "Would it not be wise to ask Congress for some sort of legislative authority to retain those who have not at such time achieved the maximum benefit possible from medical and surgical care in Army hospitals?"[3] After all, he argued, "there will be a few officers and maybe a few enlisted men in the hospitals like Walter Reed and Letterman where we have unusual facilities for highly specialized treatment, which can not be expected to be provided with the same degree of efficiency by the Public Health Service." Baker thus implied two things: that the military harbored an obligation to ensure that service members could become productive civilians, and that prospects upon discharge for the sick and injured were relatively dim. "I would not like to have the Army put in the position of turning these men adrift or subjecting them to less favorable conditions for recovery than retention in the Army hospitals would provide.[4]

Baker's ideas about army medical care, which were at odds with those expressed by some officials in contact with patients at institutions like Walter Reed, fit his broader Progressive-minded perspective that the military might shape and help citizens rather than just train them as fighters. When he was appointed by Woodrow Wilson in the spring of 1916, Baker was viewed as a reform-minded pacifist—"the least military figure that it is possible to conceive," as the *Washington Post* put it.[5] A five-foot-six West Virginia–born lawyer, he was a Progressive Democrat who had opposed a 1904 plan to expand the navy and been involved in groups such as the League to Enforce Peace. To many in the military and beyond, his qualifications for the secretary of war vacancy seemed questionable. What could a former mayor of Cleveland, Ohio—who had mandated city control of the local orchestra so the masses could enjoy wholesome entertainment—know about directing an army? But to those who, like Wilson, understood the current conflict as a total war that extended well beyond battlefields, the appointment made perfect sense: a civilian with experience managing relationships between the government, the business community, and the larger public was perfectly suited for the monumental task at hand.[6] As secretary of war, Baker helped shape the Council of National Defense and the Commission on Training Camp Activities, which were based on similar ideological foundations: the state and private industry should cooperate for the greater societal good, using government resources to create a more peaceful world, as well as a healthy, educated populace.[7] Institutional care, in the eyes of Progressives and social reformers like Baker, could serve as a means of helping service members gain a modicum of security and independence.

The army's assistant to the chief of staff, Henry Jervey—a career military officer—was considerably more conservative than Baker in his estimation of military responsibility. The army, he said, "should free itself as soon as practicable of the prolonged care of disabled persons, turning them over to the agencies approved by Congress to provide for their care, thus permitting the Army Medical Department to devote its energies to the normal and proper duties for which it is provided as a part of the military establishment." Those duties included, in Jervey's view, caring for disabled personnel during war, but not afterward. After all, he noted, "Congress has made no provision for the maintenance of the large medical establishment that would be necessary to continue the care and treatment of the large number of disabled persons resulting from the war."[8] Although Jervey recommended against asking permission from Congress to retain disabled men in the army, he tacitly agreed with Baker's point that military hospitals were, in many cases, superior to those of the PHS. Service members, he reassuringly noted, could continue to receive care in some of the finest army hospitals even after discharge—that care would simply be funded by an outside agency.[9]

The Baker-Jervey correspondence demonstrated that a halting transition was under way. In June 1919, the army discontinued the Division of Physical Rehabilitation, created two years earlier. By the end of the next month, it had passed on to the PHS fourteen hospitals containing more than thirteen thousand beds. Around the same time—between June 1919 and September 1919—the number of patients being treated in army general hospitals like Washington, DC's Walter Reed decreased from thirty thousand to slightly less than twenty thousand. By September 1920, there were fewer than three thousand patients in an ever-decreasing number of army general hospitals. In the same period—between May 1919 and October 1920—the number of beds available in army general hospitals decreased from about forty thousand to three thousand.[10]

Some service members went from one bureaucracy to another. When soldiers were discharged from military hospitals, they could turn for assistance to the Bureau of War Risk Insurance, which soon established an uneasy partnership with the Public Health Service in order to provide care. In this moment, one government agency headed by insurance experts (the BWRI) and another focused on sanitation and disease (the PHS) struggled to devise a functional system of hospital care.

Established in September 1914, the BWRI originally had a relatively limited mandate. The agency was intended to oversee insurance policies that covered American ships and freight.[11] But by the outset of war, it was responsible for the difficult task of defining how to implement the exceedingly vague policy contained in the 1917 amendments to the War Risk Insurance Act: "the injured person shall be furnished by the United States . . . reasonable governmental medical, surgical, and hospital services."[12]

Organizing a system of medical care represented only one of many challenges the BWRI faced in the months after the war. The agency's work, as one report put it, was "of appalling magnitude."[13] Its major functions included overseeing allotments and allowances to soldiers' families, adjusting and paying claims resulting from injuries and deaths incurred in the line of duty, and managing insurance policies for "officers and men at cost against death or permanent total disability."[14] In December 1918, BWRI director and former New York insurance broker William C. Delanoy was ousted after the agency endured public and congressional attacks for being inefficient and lax in overseeing the disbursal of compensation checks.[15]

He was replaced by Col. Henry D. Lindsley, a past president of Southwestern Life Insurance Company of Dallas, Texas, and former chief of the War Risk Insurance Section of the American Expeditionary Forces. Lindsley aimed first and foremost to restore faith in the BWRI. He urged Congress not to proceed with a planned investigation of the organization and requested that "a reasonable chance be given to him to satisfy Congress."[16] In March 1919, when a recently dismissed bureau employee charged the organization with "gross inefficiency and wastefulness," Lindsley shot back that the claims were "tissues of falsehoods."[17] In effect, both BWRI leadership and congressional representatives were struggling to prove to veterans that their insurance and compensation payments would be distributed in good faith, that prewar policy promises were not empty and that the government deserved their trust.

Within just five months of his appointment as director of the Bureau of War Risk Insurance, however, Lindsley made a drastic about-face, declaring that the organization he oversaw was "on the verge of breakdown and failure." Lindsley charged that his authority to hire his own staff had been challenged by a Treasury Department that was constantly "suggesting reasons why things cannot be done." Secretary of the Treasury Carter Glass called such claims wholly unwarranted and accused the bureau head of "insufferable personal vanity." In May 1919, Lindsley resigned from the bureau to join the leadership of a newly powerful veterans' social and advocacy organization, the American Legion.[18]

Stepping into the breach in the spring of 1919 was Richard Gilder Cholmeley-Jones, who, according to one reporter, had distinct advantages when it came to both "blood and brains." With a name that "looks, if it doesn't sound, like a freight train," the new BWRI director's wealthy family included poets, artists, archaeologists, soldiers, and explorers. Cholmeley-Jones was born in New York City, grew up in Philadelphia, and graduated from the University of Pennsylvania's Wharton School of Finance. Prior to serving as a colonel in the War Risk Insurance Section in France during the war, he worked in New York's burgeoning insurance industry for the Mutual Life Insurance Company, then independently as a broker.[19] He also served as a member of the business staff of the prominent Progressive journal, the *Review of Reviews*.[20]

Before beginning his wartime government work, Cholmeley-Jones lived in Gramercy Park in Manhattan, where his post as chairman of a neighborhood association "brought him, as he intended, into relations with the poor." That experience helped shape his conception of "Gilder weekly income policies," a form of insurance aimed at helping impoverished families pay for funerals and related expenses by providing them with $75 upon the death of the male breadwinner, as well as weekly payments for one year. "The great object in the mind of Cholmeley-Jones was to give the family of a poor man a little help while it was readjusting itself to meet new conditions," reporter James Morrow wrote in August 1919. "And that is the theory," he perceptively added, "now governing his management of the government's insurance for soldiers and sailors."[21]

As something of a public intellectual, Cholmeley-Jones shared his philosophy on war, life and human nature in essays in the *Review of Reviews* with titles such as "Character," "Perseverance," "Opportunity," "Honor," and "Progress." As the United States mobilized forces, he, like many prominent Progressives, was hopeful that "a military awakening" could present an opportunity for Americans to "respond to the demands which may be put upon us in order that we, of all ages, may successfully take our part in the progress of the world." But it was a piece about "disappointment" that most accurately foreshadowed the difficult road ahead at the Bureau of War Risk Insurance. "Every day brings its disappointments, some of them little ones, and others that seem almost too large to surmount," Cholmeley-Jones wrote. "It is entirely a question of our mental attitude toward disappointments as to how quickly we shall overcome them, and continue our journey towards success."[22]

The spring of 1919, when Cholmeley-Jones was appointed and service members flooded out of the military and its hospitals, was a moment of tremendous growth for the BWRI. There were approximately a hundred employees of the bureau in October 1917. By March 1918, there were three thousand. One year later, the bureau employed more than seventeen thousand workers in its allotment and allowance, insurance, compensation, legal, medical, and other divisions. In June 1920, there were more than seventy-two medical officers reviewing claims in the BWRI central office—double the number from a year prior. At that point, the bureau employed more than 2,400 medical examiners throughout the country.[23]

In the early postwar period, an organization founded primarily to adjudicate financial claims was handling not only a huge increase in administrative work but also the onerous task of arranging for physical exams and extended medical care for millions of prospective beneficiaries. Around March 1919, according to a later BWRI report, "the bureau began to receive claims of disabled soldiers in large numbers."[24] Looking back on this period, a BWRI medical official recalled, "It had not been supposed that the soldiers, sailors and marines would be discharged from the service immediately, as it was understood to be the intention of the government to retain all those suffering from injuries and illnesses incurred in or aggravated by service until the maximum degree of improvement had been obtained." But the bureau "was suddenly confronted with the problem of caring for thousands of disabled ex-service men and women who were presenting their claims daily when no general hospitalization program had been mapped out."[25] The sentiment was repeated almost verbatim in a BWRI annual report: "The Bureau found itself in the position of having thousands of disabled soldiers presenting their claims daily and with no general hospital program mapped out or plans whereby general physical examinations might be conducted throughout the entire United States to determine the immediate nature and extent of the disability from which the disabled soldier, sailor, or marine might be suffering."[26] As early as July 1918, then BWRI director William C. Delanoy had established the principle that his organization would oversee a system of medical care but rely on an outside agency to actually deliver it. "The only 'governmental' hospital services available for this work," Delanoy noted at the time, "are the hospitals and relief stations of the United States Public Health Service."[27]

When President Woodrow Wilson passed an executive order on April 3, 1917, making the Public Health Service part of the military forces of the United States, operating hospitals for the care of merchant marines and a variety of government employees was just one function of the more than century-old organization. It devoted the bulk of its resources to scientific research, the prevention of the spread of epidemic diseases, and the monitoring of state quarantine and immigrant inspection stations.[28] Wilson's April 1917 order meant that "all peacetime activities—investigations of the pollution of the Ohio River, the scientific studies of the laboratories, the rural health demonstrations, programs against trachoma and hookworm disease—had to become a dim background to the more pressing problems of war." High-ranking officials of the PHS were assigned to duty with—essentially, put on loan to—the army, navy, Coast Guard, and, soon enough, the BWRI.[29]

At the outbreak of war, the PHS was focused heavily on battling epidemic diseases and promoting sanitation but was also casting an eye toward the promise and potential of individualized medical care. The agency's leader, Rupert Blue, rose to fame in part by fighting bubonic plague in San Francisco in the 1900s. He then used his perch as surgeon general to bring attention to what he saw as a distinct connection between poverty and health and to advocate for workers' access to medical services. When serving as president of the American Medical Association (AMA)—a post he held in 1916 simultaneously with his PHS surgeon general appointment—he, along with Army Surgeon General William C. Gorgas and many other prominent doctors, supported a system of compulsory health insurance.[30] "Studies of the economic and sanitary conditions affecting the health of the industrial population have shown the urgent need for more effective methods for the relief and prevention of disease among the 30,000,000 of persons who comprise this group," Blue told the AMA in his July 1916 presidential address. "The unskilled, low-paid workers in every community have an excessive morbidity and mortality rate, which is largely accounted for by their economic status and living environment," he said. Most of that population, Blue asserted, "have incomes insufficient to maintain healthful standards of living, much less to provide adequate medical and surgical care."[31] The surgeon general would soon use a similar rationale in arguing for more comprehensive services for recently discharged soldiers.

Blue believed the wartime activities of the PHS were relevant to its general mission. During mobilization, as service members arrived at their US posts from their hometowns and cities, the agency undertook an expansive program of improving sanitation measures in communities surrounding military camps and bases. "If the soldier and the sailor are to be kept well," Blue asserted, "the civilian with whom they come in contact must not be permitted to have a communicable disease, and the civil environment which the fighting man enters must be kept in a clean and wholesome condition."[32] To these ends, the PHS attempted to improve the health of the local populations surrounding cantonment zones, mainly in rural areas such as Petersburg, Virginia; Columbia, South Carolina; and Fort Riley, Kansas, among others. There, agency officers inspected sewer systems, instituted vaccination campaigns, and attempted to ensure a clean water supply and hygienic conditions in local restaurants. According to Blue, the benefits of the PHS efforts went beyond those immediately visible in a few isolated communities. The wartime emergency, he said, was "building permanently for a better public health" and "laying the foundations for an improvement in community conditions which we have every reason to believe will gradually spread throughout the United States."[33]

As BWRI beneficiaries increasingly sought care, the PHS hastily enhanced its medical services, but it still proved difficult to meet the need. In 1917, the agency's 19 hospitals and 119 relief stations offered care for conditions afflicting members of a variety of government agencies including the Merchant Seamen, the Coast Guard, and the Immigration Service. Many sought treatment for tuberculosis, influenza, smallpox, bronchitis, and rheumatism, though sexually transmitted diseases were most prevalent.[34] In the early months of the war, there were 1,500 in-patients in Public Health Service hospitals across the country.[35] By the fall of 1918, ten thousand service members had already been discharged from the army for tuberculosis alone, and Blue worriedly pointed out to the Secretary of the Treasury that his organization had filled many of its hospitals "to over flowing, by placing beds in hallways, on verandas, and even in tents scattered about the reservations." Furthermore, he said, the agency had rented private dwellings and converted them to temporary hospitals, a practice that was "neither satisfactory nor economical."[36] As such, the surgeon general argued that instead of continuing to place an added burden on the limited facilities of the PHS, special arrangements should be made for Bureau of War Risk Insurance patients. "Hospital accommodations," the 1918 PHS annual report said, "should be supplied for the treatment of discharged soldiers and seamen."[37]

The Roots of a Makeshift System

In March 1919, the relationship between the PHS and BWRI was legally formalized when Congress passed Public Law 326. The landmark law signaled that the federal government would attempt to fulfill its promise of providing medical care for veterans by enhancing existing resources. It appropriated $3 million for the takeover of a newly built army hospital in Chicago; $1.5 million to establish a tuberculosis sanatorium at Dawson Springs, Kentucky; $2 million for enlarging a PHS hospital in Stapleton, New York; and $1.4 million for the construction of hospitals for the use of BWRI patients in Washington, DC, and Norfolk, Virginia. It set aside another $1.5 million for an emergency fund that the secretary of the Treasury could use to purchase additional land and buildings, and $785,000 for the PHS to use for hospital operations during the remainder of 1919. In spite of concerns expressed by government officials regarding the "depressing effect" army cantonments could have on BWRI patients, the act also appropriated $750,000 to be used for the remodeling and adaptation of seven army camp hospitals located across the country, which would be transferred to the PHS.[38]

Discussions leading to the passage of PL 326 highlighted some emerging and crucial questions regarding veterans' health care during a time of great transition. First, legislators wondered why such massive appropriations and grand plans were necessary, given the prewar hope of healing soldiers' wounds and ailments before they became civilians: "If they are entirely cured there would be no necessity for discharging them, and they might go back in the service," said a somewhat bewildered Rep. Frank Clark (D-FL) in September 1918. But by that point, bureaucrats working within the system had a firmer grasp on reality. "I do not imagine in time of war it is the business of the Army Medical Corps to try to make healthy civilians but rather to take care of the wounded and injured during active fighting," Charles E. Banks, chief medical adviser of the BWRI said. Once the "time of war" had ceased, he noted, it would be difficult to pursue the prewar policy of treating soldiers within the military health system; all personnel—from conscripted privates to medical officers—were eager for discharge. Plus, he said, it was difficult to justify funding a vast army medical system in peacetime.[39]

More civilian-based services were also necessary, government officials argued, because large numbers of former soldiers were seeking treatment for chronic conditions such as tuberculosis. In many ways, they said, the requirements of such patients were more extensive than those suffering from battlefield injuries. Arguing that tuberculosis was "the great problem" among discharged soldiers and sailors, Banks pointed out that almost one-quarter of those discharged from the army and navy were suffering from the disease. He noted that 14,000 had already been discharged with tuberculosis, and the government was predicting that another 34,000 would be released in 1919; 75 percent of those former soldiers, Banks maintained, were expected to seek treatment in sanatoriums. The demand for care, he argued, necessitated an increase in institutional bed supply, not simply because the government had an obligation to military veterans but because tuberculosis constituted "a great public health and economic problem." "Men who have broken down . . . in a diseased condition," he said, "are a menace to their families and the communities where they reside."[40]

Some legislators could not help but wonder about the appropriateness of offering medical care at the government's expense for a disease that some ex-service members—including those who never saw battle or shipped abroad—likely had long before they enlisted. William A. Ashbrook (D-OH) questioned whether veterans being discharged with tuberculosis had contracted it while serving or, "as a matter of fact, didn't they have it before?"[41] In a separate discussion about disability compensation, John L. Burnett (D-AL) inquired whether veterans who had enlisted with tuberculosis received the same "allowances" as those who had contracted it as soldiers.[42] Banks reported that some service members indeed likely had the disease before serving but that once recruits enlisted they became eligible for BWRI benefits. No one was knowingly accepted to serve who had tuberculosis, he pointed out, though he did concede that draft exams were often "superficial." Furthermore, while some likely had arrested tuberculosis before entering the military, their condition may never have "broken down" if they had not served.[43] The government, Banks suggested, had an inescapable legal and social responsibility.

During debates about PL 326, a cohort of BWRI and PHS experts set an important precedent regarding balancing fiscal considerations with humanitarian concerns. In response to congressional representatives' queries regarding the practicality of opening a 500-bed hospital at Dawson Springs, Kentucky, as opposed to one that might hold 1,000 or more patients, a PHS official remarked that larger hospitals were "more economical" but did not afford the opportunity for families of patients to visit. It was not ideal, he said, to send a man from Maine to Kentucky for treatment.[44] The principle that veterans—even those who had not seen battle—deserved access to institutions close to their homes and families continued to hold throughout the early 1920s and shaped the veterans' hospital system that eventually emerged.

Amid the arguments for more and better veterans' health services, there was some skepticism about the passage of PL 326, and about the general idea of expanding government-sponsored medical services. In January 1919, a bipartisan group of four representatives argued that the war was over and the need for medical care less dire than it once was. In response to earlier claims by BWRI and PHS officials that illnesses like psychoneurosis and tuberculosis required long-term care, the representatives pointed out that the average hospital stay for a tuberculosis patient was just six months—hardly long enough to justify the construction of several permanent institutions. Furthermore, they questioned the worthiness of BWRI patients, some of whom had been in the army no more than a few weeks—accepted by their local draft boards but rejected at their posts or cantonments; just as many of these men had received medical care in local institutions before the war, they could "be cared for better, more promptly, and more economically in civilian institutions now in existence than in any other way."[45] In essence, the report was a statement against prewar legislation guaranteeing that discharged soldiers would have access to publicly sponsored medical care. Although its rationale may have seemed ideologically sound to skeptics, it did little to release the government from its legal obligations.

The House passed the hospital funding bill with 272 yeas and only seven nays. Those who ultimately voted against it were all Republicans, but their ideological backgrounds and reasons for opposition were varied. Montana pacifist Jeanette Rankin and Missouri civil rights activist Leonidas Dyer voted "nay," but so did combat veteran Royal C. Johnson, of South Dakota, who became a staunch advocate for veterans in the 1920s. Fellow veteran and fierce anti-immigration activist Albert Johnson, too, was opposed. Leonidas Dyer expressed one motivation of nay voters: "We ought not to permit the Public Health Service to take over for treatment men who have fought the battles of this Republic," he declared. "It ought to be under the Surgeon General of the Army, who has looked after these men since they left home, who should continue to look after these

men as long as they live, whether they are in the service or have been discharged."
Richard Elliott, of Indiana, had other reasons for opposing the proposal. The
PHS and BWRI, he said, "do not know whether they are traveling afoot or on
horseback," and the current legislation represented a "makeshift measure."
"There will have to be a comprehensive plan adopted," he argued, so that "when
we spend a dollar for the benefit of these boys, they are going to get the benefit
of that dollar."[46] Eventually, more legislators would embrace the call for a broad
systemic overhaul.

Once Congress passed PL 326, the BWRI and PHS attempted to devise a
precise and scientific means of assessing eligibility for benefits and care. The
agencies were guided by practices of state accident commissions administering
emerging workers' compensation laws.[47] State plans were shaped by some of the
same fundamental questions facing BWRI officials: Would rates of compensation for workers be calculated based on their occupation and earning power,
how many dependents they had (in other words, "need"), the nature and degree
of injuries, or a combination of all of those factors? Should medical care be offered as part of an injured person's compensation? How long should beneficiaries wait for services and compensation? Because no consensus existed regarding
these difficult questions, a 1920 Bureau of Labor Statistics report noted, when
it came to states' handling of injured workers, "no two compensation laws [were]
alike."[48]

The BWRI disability rating process, too, involved multiple questions and
multiple steps. Initially, the bureau sent veterans, at government expense, to
be examined by a local PHS doctor. That physician filled out a report regarding
the former service member's condition and sent it back to the central office of the
BWRI, which assessed beneficiaries' percentage of "medical impairment" and
labeled it as "temporary total," "permanent total," "permanent partial," or "temporary partial." A schedule used by the BWRI in 1921, for example, broke down
the diagnosis of dementia praecox into four categories: "complete social inadaptability" after observation of one year received a permanent total rating; "partial
social inadaptability but requiring supervision" received a temporary partial
rating of 50 percent; "partial social inadaptability not requiring supervision"
was rated at 25 percent temporary partial; and "complete social adaptability" was
rated at 10 percent temporary partial.[49] When passing judgments, the BWRI
considered a veterans' social and professional background. As one BWRI official
put it, "the loss of a little finger may be 12 per cent, but on account of the effect
of the loss of his finger upon his vocation as a violinist they may possibly give

him a temporary rating of 40 per cent. We take into consideration his economic handicap as well as his physical handicap."[50] According to one 1920 report, a "leg and thigh with considerable muscle destruction (major disability) does not present a handicap to a man who has an occupation such as Auditor. Yet a stenographer with the loss of . . . any of the fingers (minor disability) would be considered a handicap."[51] Ratings could change over time based on the ex-soldier's progress in vocational training and his ability "to do something else."[52] As per the War Risk Insurance Act, monthly payments were based both on the individual's percentage of disability and on his economic position as breadwinner. A veteran with a disability rating of 12 percent who was married, for example, would receive 12 percent of $100, whereas a veteran with the same rating who had no dependents would receive 12 percent of $80.[53]

As the war became more of a distant memory for many Americans, the PHS consistently took on increasing responsibility for managing its long-term consequences. An ex-soldier who required medical care could report to a PHS hospital, an institution contracted with the Public Health Service (like the convalescent hospital run by Mother Marianne's convent), or, if necessary, a private hospital, which could then be reimbursed by the BWRI.[54] A total of 3,279 BWRI patients were under treatment at PHS hospitals in the summer of 1919.[55] By February 1920, that number had more than tripled, to slightly more than 11,800 patients. Long-term illnesses, rather than battlefield wounds, were the most prevalent among veteran-patients of the PHS. More than 4,200 were being treated for tuberculosis in the winter of 1920, while approximately 3,800 were diagnosed with so-called neuropsychiatric conditions. Another 3,770 were under treatment for general medical conditions (figure 3.1).[56] "Realizing that the existing available Government hospitals were not going to assure sufficient or proper hospital beds for war risk insurance beneficiaries," the PHS opened more facilities and "canvassed civil institutions throughout the country." By June 1920, the agency was operating 52 of its own hospitals containing approximately 11,600 beds, and contracting with more than 1,900 others that offered about 27,000 beds.[57] All told, between June 1919 and June 1920, there were 49,000 admissions to hospitals throughout the country under the auspices of the BWRI.[58]

A November 1919 statement from the bureau about how it was "meeting the herculean problem of examining, rating and returning to physical usefulness minds and bodies wrecked in the Great War" described the organization's challenges and ideals. "No human brain could have foreseen the puzzling maze of intricacies which would follow in the train of [the War Risk Insurance Act]." But,

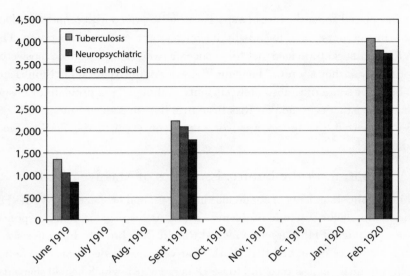

Figure 3.1. Veterans under treatment sponsored by the Bureau of War Risk Insurance, by condition, 1919–20. "Report of the Medical Division for the Quarter Ending September 30, 1919," 6; "Report of Referred Cases and Hospital Standings, Medical Division, for the Week Ending Feb. 26, 1920," 4, both in Records of the Public Health Service 1794–1990, RG 90, Correspondence with War Risk Insurance Bureau and Veterans Bureau 1917–1923, NC-34 23, box 10 and 8, National Archives at College Park, MD

the report said, the BWRI was nobly and efficiently fulfilling its obligations. Take, for example, the case of one man who suffered from shell shock, "having been blown up with high explosives in Belleau Wood," who contacted the Medical Division to report that the noise of plumbers pounding on pipes while his apartment was being remodeled "fair makes me nutty." The BWRI expeditiously had the veteran sent, with an attendant, to a newly opened "psychopathic hospital" at Cape May, New Jersey, "where he received careful attention and accurate scientific treatment." Within a few weeks, the patient was "happy, contented," and "doing splendidly in a business college where he was taking a course at the hands of the Federal Board for Vocational Education." The BWRI also presented the case of a "shy, timid mother" who sought help for her son; he "really isn't crazy . . . he just hears voices," she told a bureau agent. The mother's "aching heart" was somewhat "lightened" when the agency secured a spot for the young man at a Public Health Service hospital in Densville, New York. Then there was a young ex-soldier who had shrapnel lodged in the base of his skull and required special surgery. He was sent, at government expense, to a faraway hospital, placed under the care of a specialist, and provided with round-the-clock attendant and nurse care. Eventually, he underwent a successful operation. The BWRI report acknowledged that "time once was when letters were not answered as promptly as they are now," but "now the work of the Medical Division is and has been for some time absolutely current." Although "the problem of hospitalizing the patients of the War Risk Insurance Bureau is an enormous one," the BWRI reported, the agency was working in concert with the PHS to meet challenges.[59]

A Blueprint for the Future: Estimates of Massive Need

Behind public statements of confidence in a robust and productive BWRI-PHS partnership, major systemic problems existed. As his organization's responsibilities mounted, PHS Surgeon General Rupert Blue brought his concerns to Congress, where he argued that World War veterans needed more and better publicly funded medical care. In House Document 481, which helped shape debates regarding veterans' care during the coming years, he offered data intended to prove that the government faced a great long-term challenge. Blue argued that the resources at hand were insufficient and ill-conceived, and that a total of 30,660 beds—7,200 for general, medical, and surgical conditions; 12,400 for tuberculosis; and 11,060 for neuropsychiatric cases—would be necessary to treat BWRI patients in the near future. In addition, he requested the establishment of two hundred outpatient clinics where state and PHS health officials would work together to organize and offer treatment. At the proposed clinics, medical specialists would see patients before and after hospital visits; ideally, the outpatient centers would cut down on the need for hospitalization. Blue estimated that $85.5 million in government funding would be required to meet the need.[60]

The surgeon general offered various justifications for his request. First, there were the raw numbers: patient load was constantly growing—between April and October 1919, PHS hospitals saw an increase of approximately 140 BWRI patients per week. Blue also noted that Public Law 326 stipulated that the PHS should make use of abandoned military hospitals for treatment of BWRI patients, but bureaucrats who had initially told congressional representatives that beneficiaries would be unwilling to seek treatment at those facilities had, in fact, been proven correct; the PHS had ceased operations at all but two of the military hospitals at which it once admitted patients. Now, Blue said, new facilities were needed to replace those. The surgeon general also pointed out that the request for funding was not spontaneous but instead had been long foreseen by experts. In the lead-up to the passage of Public Law 326, he said, "it was stated many times to many Congressmen that this was only the beginning of what would be the requirements to make adequate provision for the patients of the War Risk Insurance Bureau."[61]

But given that only about 6,300 War Risk Insurance patients were hospitalized when Blue presented his data, the estimated eventual need for more than 30,000 beds necessitated a more extensive explanation.[62] The surgeon general stated that peak patient loads for some neuropsychiatric illnesses would not be reached until the late 1920s, and a need for services would be sustained for decades thereafter. It was preferable, he noted, to treat both neuropsychiatric and tubercular patients in government institutions, as opposed to civil contract institutions, since the latter were "for the most part overcrowded and inadequate to meet the needs of the civilian population, without being forced to care for the large number of cases which have resulted from and have been discovered during the recent war." Although he acknowledged that some regions of the country were overwhelmed with BWRI cases while others had a plethora of empty beds, Blue maintained that institutions serving veterans had to be spread throughout the United States, so that patients could be treated near family and friends.[63]

As he reported that the PHS and BWRI were lacking in resources, the surgeon general also argued for legislation supporting "care for all discharged soldiers and sailors," not just those who had been discharged with a disability rating of at least 10 percent, as the law currently provided. Bringing up an idea embraced by emerging veterans' groups, one that would shape the future veterans' medical system, Blue argued that the burden of proof was on the government concerning those who claimed that their disease was aggravated by or incurred in the service. Furthermore, he said, those who had newly emergent diseases they claimed were connected with their time in service deserved treatment.

Blue offered an economic rationale as justification for providing care to all veterans. Expanding access, he said, will "operate to save the government millions of dollars in preventing or deferring the payment of compensation and insurance claims." It would also, he maintained, foster industrial productivity; it made good business sense to provide "medical supervision for such a large portion of the population at the greatest productive age period."[64]

The surgeon general's assessments of veterans' needs were based in part on an October 1919 report by his confidante and collaborator, William C. Rucker, a long-time PHS officer who was working temporarily as the BWRI's chief medical adviser. As Rucker put it, "the entire problem is one without precedent in history." Although the exact future demand for veterans' medical services was difficult to predict, Rucker argued, "the problem will grow with time rather than diminish, and . . . if mistakes are made they are far more apt to be in the direction of underestimating rather than of overestimating the magnitude of the situation." He offered as partial evidence for his claim the massive increase in numbers of pension requests by Civil War veterans between 1861 and 1897—a parallel prewar policy makers had so adamantly hoped would never be made.[65]

Rucker joined Blue in arguing that all veterans of the war should be eligible for government-sponsored medical care, not just those with disabilities connected to service and rated at 10 percent disability. He noted that claims filed with the BWRI made it clear that military discharge judgments were not always accurate. Sometimes, he said, medical records proved that a service member had a disability upon completion of service but none was recorded. Also, "many service men clamored for their discharges after the Armistice, and were discharged in a disabled condition because they had developed what might be termed 'hospital phobia' and a general dislike for the military service."[66] Despite that many of these former service members had signed away their rights to make future claims on the government, Rucker implied, they should be eligible for medical care.

Rucker's December 1919 testimony was based on his recent experiences fielding complex questions from hospital administrators about veterans' eligibility for treatment. Some PHS officials interpreted a stipulation in PL 326—authorizing the agency "to provide immediate additional hospital and sanatorium facilities for the care and treatment of discharged sick and disabled soldiers, sailors, and marines, army and navy nurses (male and female), patients of the War Risk Insurance Bureau"—to mean that *all* discharged sick and disabled veterans, not only those who had received a disability rating from the Bureau of War Risk Insurance, were eligible to receive medical care. In August 1919, Bert Caldwell, senior surgeon for the PHS in Chicago, wrote to Rucker to ask whether he and his staff were obligated to treat veterans with syphilis or gonorrhea.[67]

Rucker's reply at the time, which cited both the War Risk Insurance Act and Public Law 326, was less than definitive, mainly because those two laws in some senses contradicted one another. According to the War Risk Insurance Act, Rucker explained, a claimant had to be compensable by the Bureau of War Risk Insurance in order to be eligible to receive treatment. Rucker based his argument on the law's statement that "*in addition to the compensation above provided,* the injured person shall be furnished by the United States ... governmental medical, surgical, and hospital services." But, Rucker continued, no compensation was provided for ex-soldiers whose injuries or illnesses resulted from their own "willful misconduct," which, he implied, may bring on bouts of gonorrhea. Rucker also pointed out, however, that Public Law 326 was "far broader in its scope" than the War Risk Insurance Act in its provision for veterans seeking medical care. It was apparently designed, he said, "to care for any person who could show that he had been discharged from the military or naval forces of the United States and was sick or disabled." The entire question, Rucker said, was before the attorney general, who would henceforth notify the PHS of its decision.[68] There, Rucker's letter ended, leaving Caldwell and other PHS officials in the same predicament they had faced since the law was passed five months prior: if they refused to treat patients who were not compensable by the BWRI, they may be acting outside the law. But if they did treat them, it was unclear whether and how the BWRI would offer compensation for services rendered.

A few weeks later, in September 1919, acting attorney general Charles B. Ames reported on his ruling regarding the question at hand. "It was not intended that every soldier who had been discharged and who should afterwards happen to be sick and disabled should be entitled to the benefits of the Act," he stated. Only those who had become sick or disabled in the line of duty were compensable by the BWRI, and only those individuals were eligible for government-sponsored medical treatment.[69]

The debate over the wording of Public Law 326 made it clear that bureaucrats in both the PHS and BWRI were constrained and confused by vague legislation. It also shows that the question of who should have access to publicly sponsored treatment arose soon after ex-soldiers' hospital care was deemed a societal responsibility. The attorney general's ruling did not signal the end of confusion; the point was continually debated throughout the early 1920s. Meanwhile, the seemingly astronomical estimates of need presented via House Document 481—and Rucker and Blue's argument that all veterans should receive care—helped pave the way for future appropriations.

Mounting Challenges

Even as officials at the highest levels advocated for expansive services for veterans, dissatisfaction and frustration grew among patients, the general public, caregivers, and bureaucrats. In January 1920, Walter G. Wilkinson alleged that he had been confined in isolation with no blankets, no food, and no heat at a

Public Health Service hospital in Chicago. Thomas Frymeier said his dressings were rarely changed. Stanley Hyland argued that the institution's food was inedible.[70] In July 1920, A. L. Bender wondered why his tubercular brother had been transferred multiple times, to facilities of varying quality in New York, South Carolina, and Arizona, as his condition worsened.[71] More extreme allegations included those leveled against the PHS hospital in Philadelphia, where veterans and hospital staff testified that patients had endured various types of neglect and abuse in late 1920—hot baths for hours on end, being bound in straitjackets, the mixing of "shell-shocked" veterans with those who had contagious diseases.[72] A 1920 BWRI investigation of Seymour's Sanitarium, a contract institution in Banning, California, documented that nine ex-servicemen and thirty other patients shared one bath and one toilet. The report also noted that "about 70 paces from the main building and 40 paces from the bungalow where an ex-service man with tuberculosis of the intestines and lungs has been placed, is a dumping ground for garbage." One veteran bed patient requested an enema and was told he would have to "buy his own syringe from the drug store." In fact, "all the patients have to buy their own medicine and sputum cups," the BWRI investigation found, "although according to the War Risk Act, everything should be furnished."[73]

On the local level, the BWRI and PHS encountered serious logistical and coordination problems. Throughout the nineteenth and early twentieth centuries, it was common practice—and, in many institutions, seen as a crucial part of treatment—for patients to work on hospital grounds while receiving care, but many BWRI patients felt they should be absolved of such responsibilities. A report on conditions in New York State noted that many BWRI beneficiaries resented the fact that, at some private or semi-private hospitals, they were being requested to perform menial labor because the reimbursement rate of $3 per day was insufficient to cover the institution's costs. Meanwhile, in some New York towns, patients were undergoing surgeries in small hospitals operated by "about six of the local Doctors as a convenience for their own patients, with possibly a bed or two set aside for charity patients." BWRI beneficiaries opted to receive medical care in these community-based facilities in order to remain close to friends and family, but contract services were covered piecemeal: the PHS would pay a set fee of $5 for the use of an operating room and $5 each for anesthetic. Costs for X-rays would also be reimbursed. But "there the [PHS] liability seems to end. No provision at all is made for a surgeon. If the Public Health Doctor happens to be a surgeon well and good . . . although . . . he gets no additional fee." A PHS doctor who had no experience performing surgeries might "decide to make his own attempt . . . seeing even the finest surgeons have to start sometime." Otherwise, a BWRI beneficiary in need of surgical care had "to hustle around to a surgeon and plead with him to operate free of charge." The situation was unsatisfactory not simply because it affected quality of services but also because it was "resented by the local surgeons who feel that under ordinary circumstances the patient would be under their care and that they could charge for their services."[74]

Although Congress had passed legislation intending to make publicly sponsored medical care accessible to former service members, government agencies faced major hurdles when attempting to implement and administer it. The BWRI and PHS had to coordinate staffs and services, determine who was eligible for and worthy of care, and balance concerns about economy with patient demands and complaints. "I have heard some people remark that war was hell, but the after-war effects were 'heller,'" Richard Cholmeley-Jones artfully said during a speech welcoming attendees of a conference between the BWRI and PHS in April 1920. "It is one of the most difficult things to build up an organization, an efficient organization." But, the BWRI director urged his colleagues to rise to the challenge by imagining no "dividing line in the work we are doing" and remembering that "we have one man or woman to serve."[75]

"Dividing lines," however, had plagued the PHS and BWRI from the inception of their bureaucratic relationship. That much was clear when it came to managing the complex process behind examinations and diagnoses. In April 1919, when the BWRI was receiving between three hundred and six hundred claims per day, PHS officials worried that their partner agency was unable to estimate the volume of work to be expected during the following six months, which made it virtually impossible to lay plans for providing hospital care. Meanwhile, a 1919 PHS report noted, no clear guidelines existed regarding how to rate a disability and apply terms such as "total disability, temporary or permanent." The accepted rating of partial disability "undetermined in degree" did little to definitively close cases. In the face of such challenges, PHS officials urged a "systematized and clearly understood plan of cooperation" between the PHS and BWRI.[76] A year later, BWRI officials were complaining that many PHS examination reports were returned to headquarters containing no, or nondescript, diagnoses. One bureau representative was frustrated that the common diagnosis of neurasthenia, which indicated that a patient had symptoms of both nervous exhaustion and epilepsy, "does not mean anything to us. . . . We want to know how many attacks the man is having, what kind, whether day or night. . . . [W]e want a picture of the epileptic. It does not take more than a page of the examination . . . we want a picture of the man's mal-adjustment."[77] In addition, BWRI staff requested that PHS officials be timelier in sending official diagnoses of admitted patients to Washington, DC, so their disability payments could be processed.[78]

Not only was a "system" lacking, but there was also a shortage of ground-level personnel in the face of massive demand. A Red Cross representative, Cora G. Irvine, reported in January 1920 that in Snohomish, Washington, the designated PHS doctor kept patients waiting for hours, sometimes days, before seeing them, then refused to render services until receiving approval for procedures from the regional office. Occasionally, patients were sent to Seattle to see doctors, often at their own expense, Irvine said. The government-approved Snohomish examiner was evidently juggling his veteran-related duties with other professional functions. "For the good of the disabled man," Irvine pleaded, "the suggestion is made that a Public Health Service physician be appointed who would give a specified time exclusively to the Public Health Service."[79]

That may have been easier said than done. The newly appointed PHS surgeon general, Hugh S. Cumming, told legislators in March 1920 that 10 percent of his agency's officers had recently resigned their posts and the PHS was unable to attract medical personnel of any grade—specialists, surgeons, or otherwise—because "the pay offers no inducements."[80] According to the 1920 PHS annual report, in order to meet escalating demand from BWRI patients, even as commissioned medical officers resigned "to accept more lucrative positions in civil life," the PHS recruited reserve medical officers, attending specialists, acting assistant surgeons, and hospital attendants. Some received a "nominal" fee from the agency but served mainly because they were "animated by a desire to render aid to ex-service men." The PHS also created a nursing section in 1919, staffed in cooperation with the American Red Cross. But by 1920, as the PHS struggled to supply new recruits with "adequate and proper quarters," there was "in the discipline of the nursing corps . . . a certain spirit of unrest . . . [and] a very large turnover." Also in 1919, the PHS established a reconstruction section, which by June 1920 consisted of 299 occupational and physiotherapy aids, among others, who offered services at forty-two PHS stations nationwide. In June 1920, the PHS reported that when it came to hiring reconstruction aids, "at no time has a sufficient number of qualified persons been available."[81]

Beneficiaries were directly affected by a lack of bureaucratic coordination between agencies, especially when it came to locating facilities for treatment. Before administrators from particular hospitals transferred or discharged patients, they wired a request to the PHS surgeon general's office in Washington, DC. Officials there then sent a telegram to the central office of the BWRI, advising how to proceed with the case. Then, BWRI headquarters replied to the Washington PHS office, which finally passed on word to the local hospital. The entire process could take a week or more, often leaving both patients and doctors feeling frustrated. Meanwhile, PHS and BWRI officials in Washington and elsewhere exchanged accusations that unnecessary delays were occurring in fulfilling requests for treatment, transfers, and disability payments.[82]

Bureaucratic logistics were complicated by questions about what rights former service members should enjoy as patients. Should they be entitled, for example, to determine where they could access treatment? PHS officials had been informed by BWRI chief medical adviser William C. Rucker in December 1919 that it was "exceedingly improper to issue orders" that a patient be moved to a different hospital, as opposed to "requesting" that he proceed there.[83] When a PHS representative wondered what to do if a patient asked to be transferred in order to be closer to family, BWRI director Cholmeley-Jones likewise urged leniency. The issue "had to be borne with as patiently as possible, and everything must be done to keep the patient satisfied," he said. If the desired institution had an available bed, the patient should have access to it as soon as possible.[84]

The BWRI policy led to great difficulties in administration. In an October 1920 letter to Cholmeley-Jones, intended to answer complaints about a shortage of hospital facilities in Oklahoma, PHS Surgeon General Cumming noted that his organization "had always offered to hospitalize anybody sick in Oklahoma, and up to this time have been successful in doing so, provided they would accept facilities in another state." Cumming argued that it was "impossible . . . for us to guarantee to hospitalize the inhabitants of each state within the boundaries of that state, regardless of the complaint with which they suffer. I do not see," he said incredulously, "how the National Government could undertake to establish hospitals for every type of case in every state in the Union."[85]

The PHS official in charge of the tuberculosis sanatorium in Tucson, Arizona, reported that some patients took advantage of the BWRI policy to locate them according to their desires: "Local patients prefer to live in contract hospitals all account of no discipline." PHS Assistant Surgeon General C. H. Lavinder therefore predicted that, in spite of overcrowding at the Tucson contract institution and the existence of a vast number of empty beds at the PHS facility in the same town, there would be "some difficulty in removing patients from the contract hospitals to the government hospitals." He noted that similar conditions existed in Saranac Lake, New York; Albuquerque, New Mexico; and "scores of health resorts throughout the United States."[86]

Further to this point, PHS, army, and BWRI officials questioned whether bureau beneficiaries should have the rights of soldiers, heroes, or charity cases, and they voiced frustration with the demands and attitudes of their veteran-patients. In February 1920, C. A. Knowles, commanding officer of Army Hospital No. 21 in Denver, Colorado, reported to the army surgeon general that BWRI beneficiaries being treated in military institutions were an especially "difficult class of patients": "Having been petted, made heroes of, on account of their participation in the World War and the disabilities incident thereto . . . there is a feeling among these patients that they are not subject to ordinary discipline and have a perfect right to conduct themselves as they see fit. This condition obviously cannot be permitted to exist."[87] A PHS doctor similarly wondered what to do about the "numerous complaints" regarding ex-soldiers in PHS hospitals who refused to complete the duties required of all patients—making their own beds, for example; "they would say, 'I saved my country from democracy [*sic*] and I will not work.'" Many PHS district supervisors, one doctor noted, had observed "a tendency toward snobbishness in some of the soldiers. Because they were ex-soldiers, they thought they were a little better than other patients, especially the charity ones." To this, the BWRI chief medical adviser could only reply: "This whim should not be encouraged. If allowed to exist, we would create a fine set of parasites."[88]

But veterans and their advocates hardly saw their behavior as "snobbish." To the contrary, they argued, former service members had earned the privilege of being treated apart from general "charity" cases. "Why should our boys be sent to the insane asylums and make no discrimination as to ex-soldiers, no special treatments to try and restore their minds," asked Mayme A. Rock, whose brother, John, was being treated in a state insane asylum in Phoenix, Arizona. "Why," she wanted to know, couldn't "the boys mentally afflicted have special hospitals to care for them properly?"[89]

Cholmeley-Jones gave the benefit of the doubt to veteran-patients and offered little in the way of practical advice for PHS officials. If there were difficulties managing BWRI patients at an institution, he suggested, the PHS should change the commanding officer of the hospital. A better "disciplinarian," he said, may garner better results.[90] The recommendation left unanswered the broad question of deciphering proper expectations for patient behavior.

Such leniency was inappropriate, according to some doctors and officials who questioned whether bureau patients deserved treatment at all. One PHS inspector reported that 80 to 90 percent of patients in hospitals he had recently visited were ambulatory and "seemed to be in excellent physical condition." Suggesting that ex-soldiers should not have unfettered access to government institutions, he argued that PHS doctors should have the authority to discharge such patients in an "unimpeded" manner.[91] Another physician who ran a sanatorium in Fort Dodge, Iowa, reported to Cholmeley-Jones that "many" beneficiaries sent to his institution with diagnoses of tuberculosis did not, in fact, have the disease. In order to remain in institutions like the one in Iowa, however, at least one patient was found to be "borrowing sputum from a man who had tubercle bacilli in his sputum." When such patients were discharged, the doctor argued, they issued complaints with the American Red Cross and veterans' organizations, which did "all they could to discredit our work and the care which we are giving them." Institutions were not only caring for "malingerers," according to the physician, but they were doing so while they waited for six months or more to be reimbursed by the BWRI. The entire system was broken: "many worthy, sick ex-service men" deserved to receive "every care and consideration," but "chicanery and fraud" threatened to undercut the legitimacy of all veterans' claims.[92]

The Fort Dodge official was alluding to the fact that while being treated in a hospital, a service member not only had medical costs covered but also received disability payments equal to a beneficiary with a temporary total disability rating. Cholmeley-Jones explained that policy to skeptical legislators matter-of-factly in May 1920: since patients were "out of employment in the hospital," the bureau took on the responsibility of providing economic support. In the case of the veteran with no dependents who had a 12 percent disability, for example, compensation would increase from $9.60 per month (or 12 percent of $80) while the beneficiary lived at home to $80 while he received hospital treatment.[93] The progressive-minded BWRI director took for granted that the veterans' health system was intended not solely to restore people to self-reliance but also to provide them with financial support in the process—a premise some questioned.

In addition to management and coordination issues there were increasing complaints by 1921 that some institutions where former service members received care were inadequate. In fact, no one—from patients and government personnel (including representatives of the PHS and BWRI) to doctors and emerging veterans' groups—seemed satisfied with the available hospitals. Even though the PHS was charged with inspecting private facilities before approving their use as contract institutions and rejected many, some "inadequate" sanatoriums and hospitals were approved to provide care.[94] In January 1921, Walter L. Treadway, chief of the Neuro-psychiatric Division of the PHS, requested that the BWRI authorize that beneficiaries be "immediately removed" from the Sunnybrook Farm Sanatorium, a PHS contract institution in Illinois that was "poorly administered and poorly equipped"—an apparent adaptation of a previous assessment by veterans' advocates who called the institution, "not fit for a dog."[95] Throughout early 1921, Treadway wrote similar letters about other contract institutions: the Massillon State Hospital in Ohio, he said, was "not sufficiently staffed with medical officers, nurses, and attendants to accord proper treatment to neuro-psychiatric beneficiaries."[96] In June 1921, he expressed some doubt that a doctor at an Augusta, Georgia, facility was "a bona fide graduate in medicine and duly licensed to practice his profession."[97]

"Hundreds of colored people . . . robbed, cheated, deprived of the things rightly due them"

Although BWRI officials attempted to ensure that institutions serving the majority of bureau beneficiaries were of a certain caliber, standards were decidedly lower when it came to providing care for patients of color. In February 1921, Walter Treadway wrote to the Medical Division of the BWRI regarding the Central State Hospital in Nashville, Tennessee. The facility was "not sufficiently equipped or staffed to be considered desirable as a place for the treatment of beneficiaries of the Public Health Service," he said. But he was presumably referring only to white beneficiaries. The hospital, Treadway recommended, might be suitable for the "care of all colored insane residents of District No. 5 and 6," provided that "certain principles in respect to personnel" were observed, including the provision of a minimum number of doctors, nurses, orderlies, and occupational therapists.[98] Clearly, the government was willing to fulfill its legal responsibilities to former service members, but with varying standards. Even so, some institutions did not pass muster for use by any veterans, regardless of color. Soon after he recommended that the Central Tennessee State Hospital be used for African Americans but not for whites, Treadway wrote to the BWRI recommending that "it would not be advisable" to send black war veterans to Maryland's Crownsville State Hospital, which was established in 1910 to serve "the negro insane."[99] These cases suggest that the BWRI sometimes deemed black veterans as being worthy of better care than chronically ill and poor African Americans but not on par with their white counterparts.

As early as 1919, the Wilson administration assigned a black lieutenant, J. Williams Clifford, as the "special representative of the Colored service men in the Bureau of War Risk Insurance."[100] In that capacity, Clifford received telegrams and letters reporting "unjust, discriminating and cruel treatment that is accorded wounded heroes by medical examiners in certain United States government hospitals in the south."[101]

But when Clifford attempted to organize an investigation of one such institution—Camp Logan, in Texas—he said his efforts were "held up, it being claimed that such procedure would get the bureau into trouble." After Clifford was directed "to send my dictated letters down to another office, where a white high school graduate approved and signed them, signing my own signature to my own letters before they were sent out," he resigned in frustration.[102] It had been slightly more than a year since he assumed his federal post.

Following his departure, Clifford shared with the Associated Negro Press excerpts of the letters he received from black soldiers being treated under the auspices of the BWRI, which reflected their unwillingness to accept local customs of segregation. Veteran S. H. Cavitt wrote from Houston to report that, "the doctors and nurses turn deaf ears to (black veterans') pleadings." Another former soldier, Lloyd Bates, wrote from Texarkana, Arkansas, that he was a "cripple . . . unable to walk and work," yet his compensation had been cut: "I want a new rating from some doctor who does not call us Nigger and make us wait two hours until all the whites are waited on." Augustus Stansbury, of Dallas, reported that "it seems that all these white doctors here are giving us a raw deal[;] they will not send in our medical reports so that we can get our compensation." Theodore Roe, of Halley, Arkansas, described a similar problem, adding, "We do know they will write to the Bureau for the white boys but not for us." J. E. Davis, YMCA secretary in Marshall, Texas, suggested that the problem was widespread: "Hundreds of colored people hereabouts in the State of Texas are being robbed, cheated, deprived of the things rightly due them from the Bureau."[103]

In addition to facing bureaucratic challenges, black soldiers and veterans experienced segregation and violence in hospital wards. African American patients at Fort McHenry in Baltimore, for example, reported that they were only allowed to use the Red Cross reading room when white patients were eating dinner.[104] Veterans were segregated not only in the South, but in the North as well. At a PHS hospital in Chicago, a group of black patients complained that when the hospital sponsored a trip for patients to the theater, white patients were escorted in "touring cars and limousines" while black veterans "rode down in an ambulance." The exasperated men wondered, "Haven't we done as much and do we not deserve the same as the whites?[105]

But, in a variety of ways, veteran-patients and their advocates expressed deep resistance to integrated care—just as they had in military hospitals. In February 1922, a riot erupted between black and white veterans at the Edward J. Hines Jr. Memorial Public Health Service Hospital in Mayood, Illinois. The episode began, the *Chicago Defender* reported, when four white ex-soldiers knocked on the door of a room where six black veterans were gathered. "We're going to chase you out of here," one of the white men allegedly declared. "If you were in the South you wouldn't be in any hospital at all," said another. That the white veterans were, in the end, discharged from the hospital proved that there was some limit to the government's tolerance of racially motivated violence, the newspaper claimed. Hospital commander M. J. White told the *Defender* that there were a hundred black veterans and nine hundred white veterans at the facility, and the "whites are the only ones who give the hospital attachés any trouble. The discipline of the Race men is exceptionally good."[106]

The riot at Hines Memorial Hospital was just one clear demonstration that racism would help shape conditions for postwar health care, in spite of African Americans' military service and sacrifices. A San Antonio resident complained that "sick soldiers of both races are mixed indiscriminately in the base hospital at Ft. Sam Houston" and that "irrespective of the record the soldiers made on foreign battlefield . . . the Southern Jim Crow law must be upheld."[107] Representatives of the Disabled American Veterans took up a similar cause when they presented to the Congressional House Committee on Public Buildings and Grounds a report lamenting that white and African American veterans were treated in the same wards at Walter Reed Army General Hospital, where BWRI beneficiaries used some of the facility's beds on a contract basis. On Ward 35, according to the report, there were "26 white men and two negroes," a proportion mirrored closely in several other wards. The suggestion of separate treatment facilities was not meant to be an attack on black former soldiers, argued Frank J. Irwin, national rehabilitation chairman of the Disabled American Veterans. In fact, Irwin felt "they would welcome a change in policy as much as the white patients."[108]

Debating the Utility of Soldiers' Homes

In 1920, BWRI officials attempted to gain control over standards of care and costs by focusing on the goal of locating all patients in government institutions, as opposed to private contract hospitals like Seymour's Sanitarium and Sunny-brook Farm. In addition to relying on federally and state-funded hospitals—which posed their own problems from the standpoint of government officials and beneficiaries—the BWRI turned to Soldiers' Homes as prospective sites of care. But the idea was controversial.

Most of the ten branches of the federally funded National Homes for Disabled Volunteer Soldiers located across the country in 1919 had been founded in the late nineteenth century, after it became clear that private charity efforts could not cover the cost or labor involved in providing for the needs of thousands of aging Civil War veterans. Although hospitals were located on some Soldiers' Home campuses, the primary mission of the institutions was social; homes provided elderly veterans with beds, meals, and the camaraderie of fellow former service members.[109] Because the homes (like PHS hospitals) were government funded, the BWRI could feasibly place beneficiaries in their available beds; as early as 1919, the bureau began to do just that. Even so, as Civil and Spanish-American War veterans died, the total number of sick veterans treated in Soldiers' Homes decreased slightly between 1918 and 1919, but that year, George H. Wood, president of the Soldiers' Homes' board of managers worried about "the great increase in the number of tubercular patients and the lack of proper facilities at the several branch homes for the care of this class of patients."[110]

In addition to the federally run institutions, there were thirty-one state-run Soldiers' Homes in twenty-seven states in 1919.[111] Many of their administrators voiced concerns about admitting veterans of the most recent war, arguing that their facilities were not suitable for the younger population. Some were hesitant to admit World War veterans because they did not wish to work on a contract basis with the Public Health Service.[112] Still, some veterans were placed in the state homes, which BWRI director Richard Cholmeley-Jones argued led to "considerable complaint, because a great many of [them] are not modern in their methods." By way of explanation, Cholmeley-Jones noted, "they are not real hospitals; they are just homes."[113]

It was not just state homes that garnered "considerable complaint." Robert Jones, a World War veteran with tuberculosis who was being treated at the federally sponsored Soldiers' Home in Togus, Maine, reported that conditions there were highly unsatisfactory. Recently discharged soldiers were housed alongside veterans of the Civil and Spanish-American Wars, Jones said: "Not only is there no segregation of men according to ages, neither is there any according to the condition of patients." The hospital surgeon, he added, "frankly admits that he knows nothing about tuberculosis." Residents were offered a steady diet of "steak and eggs—not fresh by any means—milk and potatoes, seven days a week," which Jones maintained was "monotonous and insufficient." The home's lavatories were "not kept clean," and it was "no unusual sight to frighten away all species of water bugs before we wash or take a bath." Because of the conditions, Jones said, he had recently lost weight and "suffered from colds and chest pains."[114]

In July 1919, BWRI chief medical adviser William C. Rucker acknowledged that Jones's sentiments were hardly unique, and he echoed Cholmeley-Jones's distinction between "homes" and "hospitals."[115] "The beneficiaries of this Bureau do not, as a rule, like to go to these homes because they will there mingle with older men," Rucker told Cholmeley-Jones in April 1920. Although a few of the institutions were well located and equipped for the care of specific diseases—Hampton, Virginia, for neuropsychiatric cases; Hot Springs, South Dakota, for tuberculosis—the Soldiers' Homes' hospitals, he said, were "generally not large, and they do not have special facilities, nor the services of specialists for giving treatment."[116]

Nevertheless, bureaucrats and congressional representatives advocated for making better use of thousands of empty beds in federally funded Soldiers' Homes as a means of reining in a disparate system. They were motivated both by economy and ease of management; consolidation in government facilities was preferable to paying per diem rates to thousands of private contract institutions, where conditions and standards were difficult to assess. Cholmeley-Jones noted in April 1920 that it was perfectly legal to send bureau patients to "old soldiers' homes"; his agency simply had to verify that they "in fact, were able to care for them."[117]

Anxious to stave off the critique that "we are doing nothing to help the boys who are so much in need of help," members of Congress supported the use of the government-run facilities. Why, legislators wondered, couldn't administrators "cut the red tape" and get "beds for those boys right away"? The approximately eight thousand beds available at Soldiers' Homes should be put to use for recent veterans, who could be kept "segregated" from veterans of previous wars. Cholmeley-Jones backed the idea. Previous tenants of the homes could be requested to move to alternative buildings or different facilities, he suggested, so that younger veterans could be treated and housed together.[118]

But Rep. Frank Clark (D-FL) found it ironic that one group's needs might be placed above those of another. "I would be loath to fire [veterans of previous wars] out and put them anywhere else that might be available for them," he said, suggesting that all veterans—not just the newest ones—deserved to be treated with dignity. "Would the old soldiers be willing to be segregated in different parts of the homes? Has any investigation been made to ascertain their wishes in the matter?"[119]

While Clark saw a paradox in treating one group of veterans differently, PHS Surgeon General Hugh S. Cumming implied that Civil and Spanish-American War veterans were beyond improvement, as opposed to their younger counterparts, who could still benefit from modern medicine. A great number of World War veterans seeking institutional care were victims of psychoneurosis or tuberculosis, Cumming pointed out; such patients "should not be indiscriminately thrown in among well people." Furthermore, he said, surgical patients of the most recent war required more space and personnel than was typically allotted for Soldiers' Home residents. Therefore, in Cumming's view, the estimate that there was space for approximately ten thousand BWRI patients in just as many Soldiers' Home beds was somewhat optimistic. Unlike most tenants of the homes, who had "nothing particularly the matter" but needed "to be looked over to a certain extent," World War veterans "have to have the best possible treatment."[120] The problem of providing medical care for World War veterans, Cumming suggested, was unique and especially complicated. Existing facilities and agencies would not suffice in the short or the long term.

In spite of the concerns of Cumming and others, and complaints from veterans like Robert Jones, the BWRI continued to make use of beds in Soldiers' Homes in the early 1920s, causing consternation among former service members and their advocates. Older veterans, as Frank Clark had suggested, proved hesitant to leave the homes, and younger veterans resisted inhabiting them. When the BWRI attempted to move World War veterans from a tuberculosis sanatorium in Rutland, Massachusetts, to the Soldiers' Home at Togus, Maine, 200 miles north, more than ninety of the patients signed a petition of protest. In Maine, they said, they would be far from family, exposed to potentially harmful sea air, and given inferior food. "We will go to Hell first," said George A. Bryant, a representative of the group. "We don't propose to go off to some spot to die just to suit them."[121] Standing by his decision to relocate the men, Cholmeley-Jones explained that there was a shortage of hospital beds for veterans in the state and that the move was part of a larger plan to concentrate former service members solely in government-owned hospitals, rather than keeping them scattered in more than a thousand private contract institutions nationwide. The larger intent, Cholmeley-Jones noted, was to "improve the hospitalization program" and "prevent a chaotic condition in the future."[122]

Even as younger veterans resisted being transferred to Soldiers' Homes, their older counterparts resisted leaving. When the board of managers of the National Home for Disabled Volunteer Soldiers requested to remove Civil War veterans from the Northwestern Branch Soldiers' Home in Milwaukee in the summer of 1921 to make room for younger veterans, they had "run across a hornet's nest" and had "practically the entire state, from governor, senators, etc., down, protesting most vehemently." In response, the president of the board of managers of the National Home for Disabled Volunteer Soldiers, George Wood, sent notifications "that for the present . . . no one will be transferred . . . over their individual protest."[123]

"We have assumed this liability"

The frenzy of veteran transfers to and from Soldiers' Homes resulted in part from the June 1920 passage of Public Law 246. The legislation allocated $46 million to the BWRI, to be used for compensation of staff and a variety of beneficiary-related expenses, including "medical, surgical, and hospital services." Some of that money was to be "allotted from time to time" to agencies providing hospital care, including the board of managers of the National Homes for Disabled Volunteer Soldiers, the War and Navy Departments, and the Public Health Service.[124] The law provided mainly for the improvement of existing medical facilities, rather than the building of new ones. It offered millions of dollars for veterans' care but did nothing to alleviate bureaucratic strife.

Although hard-won and seen as a major victory by some veterans' advocates, PL 246 met with hostility from PHS officials who loathed the idea of being forced to seek money and remain subservient to the BWRI. "You give us the hospitals," PHS Assistant Surgeon General Charles H. Lavinder told members of Congress, "but you do not give us any money to operate them."[125] Richard Cholmeley-Jones, of the BWRI, countered that his organization should control funds since "under the War Risk Insurance Act, these men are declared to be patients of the Bureau of War Risk Insurance and we deal with these men and their dependents in several respects."[126]

During debates regarding the passage of Public Law 246, some senators questioned the very idea of earmarking more public funds for the hospitalization of veterans, many of whom they felt were not worthy of such a privilege. James W. Good (R-IA) was disturbed to learn that 22,000 ex-soldiers were classified as "feeble-minded," meaning, according to William C. Rucker of the PHS, they had "never developed to the point of maturity." Why, Good wanted to know, were they accepted into the military in the first place? Rucker explained that entrance exams were brief, so not all cases were detectable. Plus, he pointed out, "a man can 'peel spuds' even if he only has the mentality of a 10-year-old child." Good was aghast. "Here is a person who never did develop mentally, was always feeble-minded, and his service in the war did not make him any more feeble-minded than before, and he is just as healthy and has as much mentality now as he had then," he said. "Why does the government owe that man, because of his service in the war, any greater obligation than any other man who was not injured either mentally or physically because of his service?" Rucker declined to take up the question on an ideological level but instead made a legal argument. By virtue of previous legislation, he said, it was assumed "that the men who are accepted shall be accepted as of sound condition." And it was mandated that the government would provide necessary medical services for all those who served.[127] In a sense, Rucker was saying, even if the system was flawed, the government was legally obliged to ensure that it remained functional.

Francis E. Warren (R-WY) focused less on the question of preexisting health maladies and more on whether individuals were consciously besting the system. Were veterans, he wondered, remaining in hospitals or on the disability rolls not because they had legitimate needs but simply to garner monthly payments? Warren, like some PHS officials who lamented that patients sometimes feigned illness to remain in institutions, worried that Congress was "setting up a premium upon shirks and slackers by paying them a good deal more than they can get in wages." At some point, "somebody somewhere has to say 'No' and stop the flood leading to indolence."[128] Concerns voiced by Good and Warren were typical of those who questioned the effectiveness of legislation granting expanded rights and services to veterans throughout the early 1920s.

The contrast between some legislators' and bureaucrats' perspectives represented tensions about the larger purpose of veterans' health services. Lawmakers like Good and Warren asserted that former service members should receive entitlements because they earned them. But for some officials from the Public Health Service and the Bureau of War Risk Insurance, veterans' benefits held the larger potential of alleviating poverty and bolstering public health.

Advocates of Public Law 246 overpowered the opposition, in part by arguing that Congress had an obligation to approve the request for funding because of guarantees contained in 1917 amendments to the War Risk Insurance Act regarding war-related illnesses and injuries. According to a June 1920 congressional report regarding new hospital facilities for war veterans, 155,000 veterans were entitled to treatment from the BWRI: "We have assumed this liability," the report said. "Under the law, we are obliged to meet it . . . we must make adequate provision."[129]

In spite of the passage of PL 246 and funding increases, systemic problems continued to plague the PHS and the BWRI throughout 1920 and 1921. The question at hand had evolved from whether the system was working to who was to blame for, and what was to be done about, its sundry problems. By the fall of 1920, PHS and BWRI officials were accusing each other of active malfeasance. In a letter that he asked be considered "confidential in the extreme," PHS senior surgeon William S. Terriberry explained to a colleague that he had obtained a copy of a letter from a BWRI official requesting that the Red Cross visit PHS facilities and "make certain investigations as to the satisfaction of the patients with their treatment," including their feelings about their doctors, food, and living conditions. Red Cross personnel, Terriberry reported, replied that they were unwilling to use their organization to "spy" on the PHS. A frustrated PHS officer shared news of the accusations with a Boston reporter, who duly noted in a newspaper article that the organizations were sparring, Terriberry said. Now, Cholmeley-Jones had complained to the secretary of the Treasury that PHS officers were "engaged in political propaganda."[130] The tension was evident on the ground level, too. At a Public Health Service facility in Louisville, Kentucky, a BWRI inspector was greeted by a hospital official who would not allow him to distribute questionnaires to patients in spite of his reassurances that he was "not sent for the purpose of inviting criticisms . . . but merely for the purpose of cooperating with the U.S.P.H.S. . . . . to create a pleasing impression with the ex-service men themselves."[131]

Terriberry's suspicion that the BWRI had asked Red Cross officials to visit PHS facilities was, in fact, correct, but bureau officials represented the endeavor as wholly innocuous. In July 1920, BWRI representative J. H. Widerman wrote

to a Red Cross worker in Camp Sevier, South Carolina, requesting a "confidential report" regarding how patients were being "treated by our . . . surgeons . . . ,
with what degree of sympathy," and, in general, "how they are being cared for."[132]
Approximately one month later, Grover F. Sexton, the head of the BWRI's Investigation Field Services, took things a step further and sent a memorandum to
his agency's representatives throughout the United States requesting "a general
clean-up of all delayed cases." He asked that BWRI employees visit PHS hospitals, "preferably in company with representatives of the American Legion or the
American Red Cross," to assess patients' opinions "of how service is being rendered" and physicians' thoughts on patients' conditions. "The Director desires
that he shall be able to say that a representative of the Bureau has called on every
man in every hospital, ready to render every service possible," Sexton reported.
He asked BWRI representatives to "search" PHS office files "to see if there are
any delayed cases" but advised them to do so "in conjunction with" PHS officers,
and noted that there was "to be nothing of criticism . . . only a most energetic
effort to serve every disabled man and woman that we can reach."[133]

The heads of the BWRI and the PHS each backed the accounts of their representatives. Cholmeley-Jones wrote directly to Surgeon General Cumming asking that he advise local hospital commanding officers to allow BWRI representatives to question patients. The visits were meant to serve less as "inspections"
than as a means to make the work of the two organizations "more effective."[134]
But Cumming demurred: "the investigations," he believed, were meant to "discredit the work of the Public Health Service." Sexton's original letter regarding
a "clean-up" campaign was not so innocent, he argued, and had prompted BWRI
field representatives to "find something of which a complaint could be made."[135]

The 1920 correspondence between the two government agencies signaled
the dawn of a new era in veterans' medical care, wherein the impressions and
opinions of former service members held great import. In each of their letters
regarding the investigation and standards of hospitals, Sexton and Terriberry
hinted at the impetus for their actions: the emergence of a new and powerful
organization called the American Legion. According to Terriberry, the PHS and
BWRI should sort out their problems before the annual meeting of the Legion,
or else damaging charges of infighting were "apt to be thrown about."[136] Eager
to uphold the congressional mandates set out for them, yet frustrated by limited
resources, disparate government agencies were unable to maintain appearances
of harmony once veterans' groups arrived on the scene, raising demands and
expectations. Throughout 1920 and 1921, advocacy organizations helped bring

to a close the era of PHS-BWRI joint authority over veterans' medical care and played an integral role in the successful fight for the August 1921 establishment of the Veterans Bureau.

By March 1921, the PHS was treating 26,000 hospital patients, and the tide showed now signs of ebbing; an average of 2,000 BWRI beneficiaries were being admitted for care each week, while only 1,700 were being discharged, leaving a net increase of approximately 1,200 patients per month. In all, by the summer of 1921, the PHS had overseen treatment for 150,000 BWRI patients in a multitude of public and private medical facilities.[137]

Around that time, bureaucrats involved with the system took to defending their agencies. Surgeon General Cumming's sentiments regarding the Public Health Service's performance were reminiscent of those expressed by Army Medical Department officials earlier in the war effort. His agency had been forced to put into operation various hospitals "in haste" in 1919, Cumming said, and "with a full realization that many . . . were not satisfactory for the purpose." Still, the organization fulfilled its responsibility to answer an "urgent need . . . pending the adoption of some program which would more adequately and more permanently meet the needs of the situation."[138] Representatives of the PHS, Cumming pointed out, had repeatedly argued in Congress and beyond that more facilities and funding were necessary. Their early predictions, he said, which were initially criticized as "pretentious," had, in fact, proven prescient, as demand increased over time. "I know that we have sincerely attempted to render . . . the best service possible under the circumstances," Cumming said in July 1921. "I realize that we may have fallen short of our ideals in a great many respects, yet I feel under the circumstances that disabled veterans who have come under the care of the Public Health Service have received sympathetic consideration as well as good professional care and treatment."[139]

Other PHS officials expressed similar perspectives. The agency had been "improperly organized to take care of the disabled men of an army of 4,650,000 soldiers," senior PHS surgeon B. W. Brown, told a gathering of veterans in June 1921. Still, he maintained, "We did not utter a complaint. We jumped into the breach, and with our 22 hospitals, 700 doctors, we did the best we could do for you."[140]

BWRI director Cholmeley-Jones, too, had adopted the attitude of a concerned realist by the early 1920s. The hospitalization situation, he said, was "manifestly unsatisfactory to the disabled ex-service men and women and to the government alike." Federal agencies had not had time to acquire "adequate hospital facilities," and it had thus become necessary for them to conceive of a revamped plan to provide medical care to veterans.[141]

In June 1920, Cholmeley-Jones made several recommendations to repair—and expand—a broken health system. First, he said, all veterans—not just those rated with disabilities of 10 percent or more—should be able to access free medical care. Also, he suggested, although the War Risk Insurance Act stipulated that the BWRI provide medical treatment along with compensation, it should be amended to allow the agency to offer short-term services—the extraction of a tooth, for example—without providing payments to patients.[142] Furthermore, it was "impracticable" for the government to treat a patient for a service-related disability or illness and "to ignore other new injuries or diseases which in themselves affect very materially the patient's progress in the recovery from the injury or disease contracted in or aggravated by military service." The War Risk Insurance Act, the BWRI director said, should be amended to allow the government to provide medical care for such "new" health conditions. Finally, joining a chorus of bureaucrats and veterans' advocates, Cholmeley-Jones recommended that "Congress . . . consolidate all Federal agencies dealing with ex-service men and women, centralizing responsibility, authority, appropriations, and disbursements."[143]

Soon after Cholmeley-Jones put forth those recommendations, he died of heart disease. He was 38 years old. The illness, his friends believed, "was superinduced [*sic*] by the hard work he performed in connection with the war." Cholmeley-Jones had served as director of the embattled Bureau of War Risk Insurance for two tumultuous years, from May 1919 through March 1921. By the end of his tenure, the *New York Times* reported, "most of the pending cases [were] cleared up and every bit of the official machinery [was] working in coordination." Upon his death, the American Legion referred to Cholmeley-Jones as the "staunchest supporter in the fight for justice to disabled men."[144]

"Colonel R. G.," as his friends called him, built that legacy in part by maintaining a relatively liberal interpretation of the purpose and potential of veterans' benefits.[145] Like Rupert Blue and other bureaucrats who found their professional footing during the Progressive Era, he saw government sponsorship of veterans' health services not just as a tool for displaying gratitude to valiant citizen-soldiers but also as a means of alleviating poverty and bettering society. As such, he believed, they should be widely accessible. But bureaucrats had to turn an eye toward economic efficiency and mind the sentiments of legislators, who sometimes expressed hostility to the idea of providing entitlements to individuals who had questionable service or health histories. Congressional representatives found themselves torn between enhancing benefits for former service members and demonstrating economy by questioning the veracity of claims that more hospital services were necessary.

Meanwhile, even as memories of the war faded in the public eye, veterans' demands and expectations of their government grew. Savvy advocacy groups were able to win expansive health entitlements for constituents in part by pointing out how dysfunctional the system was as it stood. Veterans, they argued, had been shortchanged, and they deserved better.

CHAPTER FOUR

The Debt We Owe Them

Advocating, Funding, and Planning for Veterans' Health Care

On a fair spring day in March 1920, members of the American Legion's National Executive Committee gathered for a closed-door meeting in the nation's capital. They had come from all over the country to testify in Congress about the necessity for more government benefits for veterans of the recent war. Thomas Miller, chairman of the American Legion Legislative Committee, urged those present to take the afternoon to visit their state representatives and senators in advance of the hearing. "Mention generally our legislation covering the disabled men," Miller said, referring to a variety of bills authored by Legion leaders intended to enhance hospital and medical care. "We have been criticized by the statement that we have not looked out for the disabled man." James G. Scrugham, of Nevada, added a note of urgency: "Every one of you here," he pleaded, should take "a personal interest" and feel "a personal responsibility in putting the thing through. When you go to see your Congressmen and Senators, let them know we have a good hard kick behind us. It is no child's play," he said. "You have to go to it and go to it hard and persistently and continuously."[1]

The next morning Scrugham rose to his own challenge. During congressional testimony, he spoke forcefully about the necessity to distribute cash and land allotments to those who had served. Offering generous federal entitlements, he argued, would combat a "dangerous unrest that is spreading through the country."[2]

The story of soldiers' and veterans' medical care in the World War I years is, in part, a story about veterans' activism. The advocacy organizations of the Great War built on the achievements of their nineteenth-century predecessors—groups that helped ensure the creation of a massive veterans' pension system—by arguing that former service members deserved special privileges from their government as repayment for their economic and physical sacrifices. But veterans' advocates of the World War I–era also capitalized on the widely held view that cash pensions were no longer considered an ideal form of recompense. They fought not only for monetary payments but focused as well on securing other lasting and extensive rights: among them, special access to jobs, land, and institutions such as hospitals. The American Legion, Disabled American Veterans (DAV), and other organizations founded following the Great War helped shaped veterans' policies and benefits for the remainder of the twentieth century, in part by legitimizing the idea that the federal government bore a responsibility to offer care for a wide variety of health conditions.

As veterans' hospital care remained in disarray under the auspices of the Bureau of War Risk Insurance (BWRI) and Public Health Service (PHS), advocacy groups made it clear that the idea of enhancing health services for veterans was ideologically adaptable. DAV national commander Robert Marx, like PHS Surgeon General Rupert Blue and BWRI director Richard G. Cholmeley-Jones, argued that offering medical care to former service members could better society, help alleviate some of the most dire consequences of poverty, and foster self-reliance and self-improvement. But as social and fiscal conservatism gained favor among both Republicans and Democrats, political operatives in the American Legion and beyond offered an additional justification for expanding benefits: more extensive entitlements for injured and ill veterans, they argued, might stave off political radicalism. In order to maintain a love of country, they claimed, veterans needed certain things from their government, including good medical care. Veterans' advocates thus provided legislators of a variety of political stripes with diverse reasons to support increased funding for veterans' hospital care, even though some questioned whether all eligible former service members deserved it.

The American Legion and DAV served both political and social purposes. Many who joined the groups following World War I did so primarily to become part of a larger veteran social community rather than to satisfy a hunger for government benefits. Thousands likely became members with no knowledge of—or, indeed, in spite of—the organizations' efforts on Capitol Hill.[3] In fact, as the American Legion waged successful battles in the early to mid-1920s for the establishment of the Veterans Bureau and increased access to veterans' hospitals, the group actually saw membership rolls fall from a high of approximately 795,800 in 1920 to 609,000 in 1926. Only after veterans had won increased rights, and especially with the onset of the depression of the 1930s, did the organization's numbers increase.[4] While they did not necessarily lead to direct gains in membership, battles for government entitlements were an important pillar of veterans' organizations' general agendas. In the early 1920s, the American Legion and DAV served as crucial partners for bureaucrats who argued for more and better hospitals for former soldiers. By putting a human face on the problem and bringing it to public attention in the context of conservative social values, they played an integral role in the establishment of a nationwide veterans' health system.

The American Legion and the Fight for Disabled Veterans

The officers who conceptualized the American Legion in Paris in January 1919 aimed to create a new veterans' organization that would provide US soldiers of all ranks with a forum for mutual aid and friendship but also counterbalance the supposed gathering threat of Bolshevism. Those founding principles helped shape two intertwined legacies for the Legion of the interwar years. The organization was sometimes unabashedly anti-immigration, anti-egalitarian, chauvinistic, racist, and antiradical. But it was also instrumental in securing long-lasting and extensive rights for many former service members and putting in place a framework on which all US veterans—regardless of race, ethnicity, or sex—could eventually lobby for their own enhanced rights. The group's leaders advocated tirelessly for injured and ill veterans because of humanitarian concerns, but they also hoped to foster a certain brand of patriotism and stave off political radicalism among seemingly vulnerable veterans.

During the Legion's earliest meetings, members argued that disabled and ill veterans had unique concerns and represented an important constituency. In May 1919, at the group's first stateside caucus in St. Louis, Missouri, Harry Mock, an Illinois surgeon who had served in the Army Medical Corps, noted that there would be hundreds of thousands of soldiers, sailors, and marines released from the military with a disease or disability, who would not only be "discouraged" because of their handicaps but would also resist joining the Legion unless "stimulated to do so." In order to tackle the latter challenge, Mock suggested creating a division of disabled soldiers of the American Legion. Fellow representatives opposed the idea, suggesting that organizational unity, based on the virtue of having served, and not one's post-service condition, was paramount.[5]

Although Mock's idea was rejected, the Legion was determined to make the rights of disabled and ill veterans part of its organizational mission. At the group's first national convention, in November 1919, members agreed to a resolution stating that legislation should be passed "making sufficient appropriation to provide adequate hospital and sanitarium facilities for the care and treatment of all persons discharged from the military and naval service." Additionally, the government should pay for "surgical treatment . . . irrespective of the service origin or aggravation of their disability." Iterations of the resolution were passed each year throughout the early 1920s.[6] Such measures became the blueprint for the Legion's proactive Legislative Committee, which lobbied on Capitol Hill in the hopes of ensuring that federal policies paid heed to the interests of the organization.

Within one year of the Armistice, the American Legion was using its growing national network to gather firsthand evidence of shortfalls in the provision of medical care to soldiers and veterans. In November 1919, its National Executive Committee received a visit from an official of Battle Mountain Sanitarium in Hot Springs, South Dakota, one of the Soldiers' Homes where discharged soldiers with tuberculosis were treated courtesy of the BWRI. Post adjutant Ranson, who before working at the sanatorium had been a patient there, described a dire situation. The institution, he said, not only lacked adequate space and food but was also intended primarily to treat "stomach and rheumatism troubles." The sanatorium doctor was a "wonderful surgeon, but not a T.B. man." Ranson assured Legion leaders that he and his fellow ex-servicemen were not looking for a handout; he, for one, had sought care from a public facility because he did not "want to stay around home and run the risk of giving the disease to some of my relatives." But he came forward because conditions were so bad at the institution that cure seemed impossible. For example, wages at Battle Mountain were so low that only former patients were willing to work there, many of them still "spitting bugs—as we call it—or spitting T.B. germs." One patient was so miserable that he wrote to the Public Health Service asking to be transferred to a private sanatorium. The PHS sent him to a facility in St. Paul, Minnesota, that was full to capacity and turned him away.[7]

Some members of the National Executive Committee were more sympathetic to Ranson's cause than others. A representative from South Carolina voiced his concern that more facilities and services may not necessarily be better for soldiers and veterans. He had served as a medical examiner for the BWRI, he said, and as such was authorized to provide any treatment necessary to patients who visited him. "It is their own fault," he said of ex-soldiers who failed to get proper treatment for their ailments. But a representative from South Dakota disagreed; he argued that the Legislative Committee should lobby vigorously for legislation to provide for more extensive hospital facilities.[8] The latter, more sympathetic, perspective prevailed in the American Legion in 1919 and the early 1920s.

By teaming with government officials and people with special knowledge of the system, Legion representatives compiled a body of evidence that indicated that the medical care problem was systemic and not the product of irresponsible or irrational demands from former service members. One Legion report cited evidence shared by doctors and bureaucrats that demonstrated that soldiers remaining in military hospitals were "quite unhappy and dissatisfied" and "tired of hospital life," which featured subpar food and a corps of social service agencies, nurses, and doctors whose ranks had been depleted since the Armistice. These ailing soldiers often insisted on being discharged "before being cured in the hope of receiving better treatment" as ex-servicemen. But the report maintained that as veterans they continued to encounter problems—especially if they sought treatment for neuropsychiatric illness. Presenting the perspectives of a judge who had encountered mentally ill veterans in his Chicago probate court, the Legion report maintained: "The gravest problem throughout the country at the present time is the proper hospitalization and care of nervous and mental cases. Neither the men nor their families liked the idea of being sent to State Institutions, or to be rendered inaccessible by distance." Furthermore, the Legion pointed out, "The parents of insane or neurotic ex-service men resent the attitude of the Government and the local authorities in putting men through the ordinary routine of a court and detention station."[9]

As the Legion relied on experts for data and opinions, doctors and government officials eager to see improved health facilities turned to the organization to advocate for their causes. Thomas Salmon, chief executive officer of the National Committee for Mental Hygiene and chief consultant in psychiatry for the American Expeditionary Forces (AEF), expressed his faith in the potential of the American Legion to serve as liaison between veterans and the government. "Believe Legion has great opportunity in securing treatment needed by Comrades in greatest distress," he wrote in a telegram to the organization's hospitalization committee. "Future lies in your aid now."[10] Salmon realized that a group advocating for the rights of disabled and ill veterans could be a powerful ally as he continued to pursue his long-term professional mission to modernize psychiatric care. Indeed, the Legion's willing cooperation with his efforts "helped to alter public perceptions of mental illness" and "advance psychiatry from the confines of the insane asylum and into the public eye."[11]

Many Legion leaders believed that fighting for rights for veterans with disabilities was not only worthy in itself but could also serve as a powerful means of earning public support and political legitimacy for the organization. The Legion needed to "emphasize two things," Chaplain John Inzer told the executive committee in June 1919. "Pure democracy and unpolluted Americanism, and that we are going to take care of the discharged and disabled soldiers. With that kind of a program the whole country is back of us."[12]

Legion members and official reports repeatedly noted that those who were disabled in service had sacrificed the most and should be the top priority of the organization. "The Congress of the United States and the responsible people have been so derelict in their duty to these men that it is fitting at this time to call public attention to it and take some affirmative action," said Legion representative Foreman of Illinois, at the March 1920 executive committee meeting.[13] He went on to describe a dire situation in his home state, where there were not enough beds in government institutions and mentally ill ex-soldiers were being sent to charity facilities against the will of their families. Foreman's appeal for the Legion to support an emergency appropriation for the construction of facilities was met with applause. Representative Emery of Michigan seconded the sentiment, adding that tubercular ex-soldiers were "walking the streets and they ought to be hospitalized." In Michigan, he said, the problem was not a dearth of funds but a lack of organizational power on behalf of the Public Health Service, which was charged with caring for the ex-soldiers. The PHS had funding, but it was "a hard thing" to find the buildings, doctors, and nurses that would constitute a proper hospital. Representative Hoffman of Oklahoma concurred, saying there were three thousand tubercular ex-soldiers in his state with nowhere to turn. "They simply send them down to New Mexico or Texas but the conditions have been investigated there and are not satisfactory and these men . . . want to stay in their own home and among their own friends."[14]

Hoffman also expressed frustration with the idea that the American Legion should assist the PHS in locating viable facilities, which he saw as "passing the buck." "We weren't asked for any conditions when we were called into the Service," he said, "nor told that if we became injured you had to hunt out a place and lie down in it." The American Legion, he argued, was becoming the "catch basin" for doing the complicated work of a variety of government agencies.[15]

But Delaware Legion representative Thomas Miller, chairman of the organization's Legislative Committee, pointed out that the group was much more than a thankless government workhorse. Leaders were working vigorously on Capitol Hill for a variety of measures, including the Wasson Bill, which was intended, among other things, to establish fourteen district offices throughout the country, in addition to unlimited suboffices, for handling the claims of BWRI patients.

Legion Legislative Committee members were also advocating for passage of the Darrow Bill, which would provide $100 per month for all ex-soldiers enrolled in government-sponsored vocational training, and the Rogers Bill, which would consolidate veterans' services overseen by the PHS, the BWRI, and the Vocational Training Boards Rehabilitation under one cabinet officer. Finally, in addition to helping ensure that ex-soldiers were not discharged prematurely from military hospitals, the Legion was also actively attempting, through its local chapters, to assist the government in locating more than thirty thousand beds needed by War Risk Insurance patients. "Your Committee and your National Organization," Miller noted, "have not been recreant to your resolutions . . . saying that the duty of The American Legion first was to the disabled men and the families of the fallen."[16]

The Disabled American Veterans and Robert Marx

At the first convention of the Disabled American Veterans in June 1921 in Detroit, Michigan, the organization's national commander addressed a packed house, and explained the group's ideological origins and basis. "During the long years to come, while the paths of the able-bodied service men may tend to diverge," Robert Marx said, "the life paths of the disabled men will run closer together." Although a disabled service member may receive public sympathy and medical treatment to heal his wounds, when "he leaves the hospital . . . his disability continues. He loses the protection of the institution, the friendly and the helping hand. He is still disabled but in the public imagination, he is now one of them and must shift for himself." Marx explained that "through an association such as ours, the needs of this man are met, the comradeship, the friendly advice and the helping hand continued."[17] DAV membership was initially limited to those who were "wounded, injured, or disabled by reason of such service during the period of the Great War of 1917–1918."[18] The organization, Marx said, would not only offer social support but also help veterans work through a "tangle of red tape" to secure medical treatment, compensation, and vocational training.[19] An increasing number of veterans were attracted to the cause in the early 1920s. Between 1921 and 1924, DAV membership grew from approximately 17,400 to more than 44,000.[20]

A barometer of major causes and lesser-known eccentricities of his time, Robert Marx was a fortuitous choice as the DAV's first spokesman. He was a successful lawyer and judge, a proud ex-serviceman, and an articulate and instrumental Democratic Party standard-bearer. Indeed, Marx's political connections helped the DAV find its national footing in the early 1920s. From the DAV, Marx gained visibility as a prominent war-wounded veteran, which proved to be a professional and political asset. A pillar in the Midwest legal community, he was involved in some landmark cases of his time; in one of the most famous libel lawsuits in US history, he helped Aaron Sapiro, who was briefly his law partner in the mid-1920s, elicit an apology from auto tycoon Henry Ford for making anti-Semitic remarks in his *Dearborn Independent* newspaper. He was also instrumental in establishing a compulsory auto insurance law.[21] Of German-Jewish descent, Marx was secular but spoke publicly about the contribution of American Jews to the war effort. At the same time, he declared himself American before Jewish; he was outwardly opposed to the idea of Zionism and a Jewish state.[22] Marx was a loyal subscriber to fitness magazines and spent his spare time pursuing wrestling, mountain climbing, "hand-balancing"—the practice of holding his own or another man's body weight while posed in a physically challenging position—and other hobbies that promoted health and well-being.[23] While Marx was a firm believer in the power of exercise and other forms of what could be construed as self-help, as the DAV's first national commander he also tirelessly argued that the US government had an obligation to provide material support for wounded veterans. A bachelor until his death, in 1969, Marx lived well—he traveled widely and had multiple vacation homes—but he also created a rich legacy. In his will, he left substantial portions of his fortune to universities, libraries, and the veterans' organization he helped launch to national prominence.[24]

Robert Marx's passions were rooted in his upbringing. Within a year of his birth, in 1889, his parents, William and Rose, relocated from an apartment above a shop in downtown Cincinnati to the upscale suburb of Avondale. William Marx, a successful shoe salesman, had connections and ambitions in the Democratic Party. In 1906, his friend and frequent lunch date, Cincinnati mayor Edward J. Dempsey, appointed him president of the Board of Public Service. William Marx's assignment ended abruptly when he accused his fellow board members of "prejudice." But he was remembered, upon his death from cancer in 1915, as boasting a "kindly genial disposition, a quick, active mind, and a splendid executive ability."[25]

Young Robert Marx possessed similar qualities. The 1906 Walnut High School yearbook noted that he was a member of the debate club and the football team and that he had "oratorical qualities which fill the rest of his classmates with pride." He also possessed "that power of winning the audience to his side."[26] In 1910, Marx was admitted to the Ohio bar and began making a place for himself as a prominent member of his community. He became involved in various civic organizations and helped establish an Americanization program meant to encourage immigrants to assimilate.[27]

Not quite thirty years old when the United States declared war, Marx eagerly answered the call. In the winter of 1916–17, he served as chairman of a local enrollment committee, which aimed to enlist Cincinnatians to train at US military camps. Marx himself completed a naval training cruise aboard the battleship *Illinois* in the summer of 1916 and was sworn in as a second lieutenant in August 1917. Assigned to the 357th Infantry, 179th Brigade, at Camp Travis in Texas, he was appointed senior instructor in physical training and the regimental athletic officer.[28] Marx was shipped overseas in July 1918 as a captain with the 357th, which participated in some of the most intense battles of the US war effort.[29] All the while, Marx exercised strict discipline with his soldiers. In between frenzied frontline battles, he proudly recalled after the war, "I required every man to shave himself every day, as nothing does so much to increase morale as a clean shaven company of men." He also mandated that trenches be "kept clean." "Clean shaven faces and clean trenches are bound to promote clean rifles and clean ammunition," Marx declared. "Added together, the whole creates pride, confidence, and spirit."[30]

Like other officers of the professional middle class, Marx expressed reverence for service members stationed near the front.[31] "The mere private, the insignificant doughboy is the one man who should be worshiped by every American at home or abroad in or out of the army," Marx wrote to his mother in October 1918. "Nothing is too good—nothing ever can be to good for the boy who has fought in the front line infantry in France." Still, Marx believed it was important not to "pity" the soldier. He "eats well—he has three blankets—he gets his mail —his daily newspaper—splendid hospital and first aid service when wounded— everything that can be done for him . . . is done."[32]

Marx soon experienced that splendid hospital and first aid service firsthand. In the closing hours of the war, he was stationed with his battalion in the small village of Baalon in northeastern France when a barrage of German shells began dropping "with alarming accuracy." He never heard the one that eventually struck him; he only knew he was hit in the head. Fighting the urge to faint, Marx attempted to walk toward medical assistance but found he was unable. Years after, he recalled, "I sat down and ten minutes later, men came with the stretchers. The only thing I know of the trip back is that it was equally as dangerous as the advance had been. Every foot of the way was through a shell swept area. The number of gas shells used was so large that the stretcher-bearers had to put my gas mask on in spite of all my head wounds." But Marx recalled that he did not dwell on his own injuries: "I did not suffer so much, but that I could not help marveling even in that state, at the courage of the men who persisted in carrying me back three long kilometers without regard to the peril or danger to them."[33] Alfred Segal, a columnist for the *Cincinnati Post*, saw Marx soon after his injury, and described his legs and arms as being "peppered with high explosives," and generally, "quite a wreck." He had fourteen wounds, Segal reported, including a skull fracture and "a gaping hole in his shoulder and one in his neck."[34]

As a result of his injuries, Marx was exposed to a variety of the medical care facilities available to US soldiers. His first stop was at a regimental first aid station for an anti-tetanus serum. From there, he was transported by ambulance to the 90th Division triage station at Sun-Sur-Meuse and finally to a mud-floored mobile hospital at Verannes, where he received an operation and "hovered between life and death."[35] "When I became conscious, it was November twelfth," the day after the Armistice, Marx later recalled. "I asked how soon I could go back to my outfit; the doctor answered: 'no hurry boy, the war is over.'" Soon after the injury, Marx reported to his mother that his wounds were "all from shell fragments but no vital parts are affected. I have some flesh wounds in my shoulder and in my arms which are rapidly healing and some scalp wounds which are steadily improving."[36] By the time Marx was finally discharged six months later, he had experienced "delightful" American Red Cross hospitals and "most unpleasant and unsatisfactory" base hospitals in France, as well as "comfortable" convalescent hospitals in New York and New Jersey.[37] As Marx recovered, his fellow patients made a powerful impression on him: "the legless, the armless, the lungless, the sightless," he later reflected. "To them the war was barely begun, for their suffering and sacrifice were just commencing."[38]

Before Marx was discharged from the army, in May 1919, Cincinnati's local newspapers heralded his service and endorsed him for election as a judge in the city's superior court. His victory as a Democrat in an otherwise Republican-dominated race in November 1919 was a testament not only to his personal and professional qualifications but also to the political power of a battle injury overcome and a "gallant military record," as a *Cincinnati Post* editorial put it.[39] In the lead-up to the election, Marx's proponents regarded him as a "most excellent soldier" whose efforts as a captain "contributed no little to the glory of the brigade . . . and the ultimate victory of our army."[40] His "fearlessness," they said, had "been tested" and he had "proved himself of the courageous stuff public officials, especially judges, should be made of."[41] "This is your first chance to honor a service man with your vote," a newspaper advertisement by the local Soldiers and Sailors Committee charged. "He fought for us over there; let's vote for him over here!"[42] In the end, Marx's slim margin of victory was attributed to the unflagging support of fellow veterans. His election made it clear that when former soldiers stood by their "comrade," their power was immense.[43]

The DAV Finds Its Voice

Robert Marx played a central role in the founding of the DAV, though there are differing accounts of the particulars of the organization's origin. According to Marx, a group of disabled veterans gathered at the American Legion National Convention in 1919 and "discussed the need for an organization to represent the disabled veterans, and concentrate on their particular needs." Following that meeting, Marx "invited a hundred men for dinner and discussion," then, within a few weeks, "asked that a committee be formed to work with him in charting the organization's beginning."[44]

An alternative, more detailed, account of the organization's formation located its roots in a government-sponsored vocational education program. Veteran and Ohio native Charles C. Quitman, who enlisted in 1916 and served as a stretcher-bearer, recalled in a sworn affidavit in 1926 that he approached Robert Marx in the locker room of the Cincinnati Gym and Athletic Club, where both men were members. He and other students from a University of Cincinnati vocational class, he said, were organizing a meeting of disabled veterans, and they hoped the newly elected judge would be willing to address the group. Marx agreed, according to Quitman, and spoke about the necessity of an organization whose sole focus would be to represent the needs of disabled veterans. By May 1920, the group had met three times to discuss possibilities and goals, eventually drawing more than two hundred disabled veterans from Ohio and neighboring states. As support for the cause mounted, Marx helped draft a constitution and bylaws for an organization that would henceforth be called the Disabled American Veterans of the World War.[45]

Marx helped spread the word about the growing Midwest-centered organization during an August 1920 cross-country train trip with the Democratic presidential candidate, Ohio governor James M. Cox, and his running mate, Franklin D. Roosevelt. While Marx's main focus on the trip was to help the Democrats gain veteran backing, he also used the thirty-two-state tour as an opportunity to address local groups of disabled veterans and encourage them to join a growing national organization. In the process, he successfully solicited an endorsement from Governor Cox, who referred to the DAV as "the right kind" of organization.[46]

Marx also received support from Franklin D. Roosevelt, who offered "a telegram of greeting and good wishes" to the 1921 DAV convention. "I hope," FDR wrote, "you will keep together and work together until the debt of gratitude has been paid to the lowliest among you."[47] In his correspondence with Roosevelt, Marx represented himself as a temporary head of the DAV—more of a fellow political operative than an advocate. "For the moment I am the national president of this association, known as the Disabled American Veterans of the World War," Marx wrote in 1921. "May I suggest that the delegates would sincerely appreciate a telegram of greeting and good wishes from you to be read at the convention."[48] Marx's correspondence with Roosevelt—the two remained in touch at least through the early 1930s—is especially notable given FDR's efforts in his early presidency to scale back veterans' benefits.[49]

As the Disabled American Veterans of the World War gained members and garnered publicity, its leaders identified several key goals, including more and better hospitals, quality vocational training, an adequate employment program, just compensation, and social services for disabled veterans.[50] In so doing, they trumpeted sentiments of entitlement and anti-dependence, echoing and validating the fundamental ideals of military reconstruction efforts even as they argued that the latter had fallen short of expectations. In September 1920, about a hundred disabled veterans from Ohio, Kentucky, and Indiana nominated the DAV's officers and proclaimed their determination to "assist disabled soldiers and suppress efforts to exploit public sympathy."[51]

Marx, the organization's now popularly elected chairman, was candid about his belief that veterans should aim for self-improvement and self-reliance. His sentiments correlated with his interests in strength training and his reverence for bodybuilder Bernarr MacFadden, who deplored "weakness."[52] Veterans' advocacy, in the eyes of Marx and many others, was a means of fostering independence and strength. The main goal of the DAV, he told the gathering, was "to inspire in its members a determination to come back and to take their place in the nation as self-supporting and independent citizens."[53]

The young organization took as a cornerstone edict the idea that disabled veterans were entitled to certain medical and educational benefits. Instead of having other groups plead their case, DAV officials said, disabled veterans should band together in a group and "determine for themselves what they want."[54] The group prided itself on holding the government accountable for making good on its promises. "The community," Marx said at the DAV's first annual convention, needed to "pay its obligations" to wounded soldiers.[55]

At the same meeting, DAV chaplain Rabbi Michael Aaronsohn, who had been blinded in battle, voiced a related yet somewhat rare sentiment: disabled veterans should see themselves as part of a larger group of civilians with disabilities. "The war wounded have been peculiarly favored with the care of a generous and wealthy government," he told the convention. "However, we must not overlook those about us who are similarly crippled or handicapped by the loss of some member or organ of the human body."[56] In a later memoir, Aaronsohn shared poignant impressions of being wounded and his subsequent experiences living with a disability. And he voiced beliefs that may have been held, but were rarely shared publicly, by other war-wounded ex-soldiers. Why, he wondered, did public sentiment favor disabled soldiers and veterans over those who served without enduring injuries? Aaronsohn expressed gratitude for the care offered him in military and other publicly funded institutions following his injury, but he also argued that the U.S. government should work to ensure that all people with disabilities (veterans or otherwise) were integrated into society. He wondered, for example, why blind veterans should be educated separately from others when they would have to work with sighted people for the rest of their lives.[57] Aaronsohn's perspectives demonstrated that, in more ways than one, not all disabled veterans saw themselves, or people with disabilities, as a class apart.

But the DAV's ability to bring together ailing ex-soldiers en masse drove home the point that wounded veterans had unique and common experiences, needs, and desires, and it allowed the organization to have a wide-ranging public impact. The group—and the publicity surrounding its formation and events— introduced the general public to the stories of individual ex-soldiers. In a time of demilitarization and growing weariness with war-related funding, it helped bring attention to the plight and demands of disabled veterans. As *Stars and Stripes*, the military's newspaper of record, put it soon after the establishment of the DAV: "So many organizations have undertaken to aid the wounded and disabled in various ways that an expression from these men . . . would be watched with great interest."[58] In an article previewing the DAV's 1922 San Francisco convention, The *Vallejo Chronicle* conveyed a similar idea: "Such a convention in every city of the land would bring home to the citizenry of the country the debt we owe them."[59] Newspaper articles about the San Francisco convention featured inspirational stories of individual attendees and the cause of the organization. A

Tucson Arizona Star headline read: "Vets will try to unravel red tape in federal bureau's work when they hold meeting." The "army of broken boys" gathering in San Francisco, the article said, "look to the government as a worthy son looks to a father."[60] The *Tacoma Washington Ledger* reported that four local veterans would attend the DAV meeting; Merwin Stewart, who had lost both his legs, would drive the car.[61] The *Santa Barbara News* noted that a veteran named Charles G. Galloway, who had his leg amputated below the knee following an injury during the Battle of Belleau Wood—a "badge of honor," the story said—was passing through town as he made his way from San Antonio, Texas, to the convention in San Francisco. "Galloway is a merry-appearing youth," the *News* reported, "who even though he is minus a leg, appears to know how to get lots of real joy out of life." Earlier in the week five disabled veterans—two who had legs amputated and three with "severe scars"—had passed through Santa Barbara on their way to San Francisco from New York.[62] The *San Francisco Examiner* urged readers to "listen carefully" to the veterans gathering in their city. "They are a race apart," the paper reported, "these men who have gone half the distance that separates the living from the dead, but returned."[63] Likewise, the *San Francisco Bulletin* argued, "the most American thing in America is an American war veteran with a wound. . . . He is the true American aristocrat."[64] Headlines in newspapers from Utah to California echoed the sentiment: "City Honors Heroes of Struggle"; "Heroes of War Modest Men"; "Vets Will Further Peace"; "Toll of War Shown as Veterans Meet"; "Cut Red Tape in Caring for War Heroes Demands Disabled Vet Chief."[65]

Even though the DAV was attracting increasing attention, members of Congress from both parties, when asked to approve a federal charter for the organization in the early 1920s, wondered whether the group might be redundant. John Newton Tillman (D-AR) and Earl C. Michener (R-MI) maintained that too many organizations were appealing for federal recognition. As a case in point, they noted that a group of women had attempted to obtain a charter for a national business and professional women's league. "There is no end to applications," Tillman said. However, given the nature of the DAV's mission, both acknowledged, "from a sentimental standpoint, it would be rather difficult to deny these crippled boys this privilege if they feel they should be put in a class by themselves."[66] Other congressmen voiced concerns about whether recognizing another veterans' organization could make it more difficult to legislate. After all, they wondered, wasn't the recently incorporated American Legion the mouthpiece of veterans nationwide? Wasn't that group already "covering the issues"?

Why was a "separate and distinct organization to take care of the disabled . . . necessary"?[67]

It was a testament to the power of the American Legion that Robert Marx and others justified the incorporation of the DAV, in part by noting that Legion leaders supported it. Robert Marx, in fact, served on the Legion's hospitalization committee when he initially began directing the DAV, and he assured legislators that the two groups would not take contrary political stances. There was "no possibility for duplication" of work between the two organizations, Marx said, pointing to "numerous instances showing [their] cooperation." Making a powerful argument, Marx proclaimed that the granting of a charter was a matter of lending dignity to those disabled in war, who were "distinct and apart" from their "able-bodied" counterparts: "There is only one man who can instill in his own heart the will to win out, and that is the disabled man himself."[68]

For some, disenchantment with the American Legion served as a motivating factor to support the DAV. Rabbi Michael Aaronsohn, the DAV chaplain, recalled in the early 1940s that soon after World War I, the Legion represented to him a "grand monopolization of patriotism." "The arbitrary classification of men according to war service was," Aaronsohn believed, "an affront to the loyalty and devotion of those who were not 'privileged' to bear arms." He was an admirer of Col. Frederick Galbraith, the Legion's national commander in 1920 and 1921, who was widely viewed as a great advocate for the disabled. But after Galbraith was killed in a car crash in June 1921, Aaronsohn said, "it seemed that those who came after . . . only promised whole-hearted devotion to the cause of the needy and afflicted at opportune occasions."[69]

Aaronsohn was not alone in his skepticism. A representative of officers hospitalized at Walter Reed in Washington, DC, Lt. Graham, told Legion leaders in May 1920 that "the officers and men in the various different hospitals are very much disgruntled and very much dissatisfied with the attitude of the American Legion." Their "spirit" was "getting lower and lower all the time," and they felt that the Legion should use "at least as much effort for the disabled men as you are using for the bonus." It was clear that the organization had "not been on the job regarding the disabled men."[70]

Apparently, Graham and Walter Reed patients were swayed by arguments of budget-conscious government officials who argued in 1920 and 1921 that disabled veterans had to choose between pursuing their own rights and services and supporting a cash payment—sometimes called a bonus or adjusted compensation —for all former service members. There was not enough money, the officials maintained, for the government to provide both. According to former secretary of war Henry T. Stimson, "the real bonus issue, now as in the past is whether more than $2,000,000,000 in gratuities shall be disbursed among the able-bodied veterans or whether several hundred million dollars shall be available annually for the care of the tubercular and mentally disabled, the crippled and handicapped veterans." Secretary of the Treasury David F. Houston made a similar point: "The country must pay a tremendous price for the present and future care of the disabled, and the ability of the country to pay cannot be jeopardized by the distribution of several billions of dollars to their more fortunate comrades."[71]

The coverage of Walter Reed Army General Hospital's newspaper, *The Come-Back*, reported a rising hostility to both the American Legion and legislation for a bonus payment in the spring of 1920. The Legion started off on solid footing at Walter Reed, but over time some disabled soldiers became increasingly focused on their own concerns and identities as distinct from those of nonwounded ex-soldiers. When American Legion national commander Franklin D'Olier visited Walter Reed Hospital in December 1919, "men crowded into the Red Cross hut . . . though it was chow time." D'Olier was met with "a burst of applause" when he guaranteed that the Legion would not "appear before the American people as asking for a specific sum of money as payment for service" but would focus on obtaining a "square deal" for all veterans and prioritize fighting for improved treatment of the wounded.[72] At Walter Reed, patients established a Legion post, which held regular, well-attended meetings. But over time, as dissatisfaction with available services inside and outside military hospitals mounted, patients started groups of their own, focusing on obtaining access to better medical care and other benefits.[73] By early 1920, Legion meetings at Walter Reed were less popular and the organization was "bending every effort to secure larger attendances."[74] In March 1920, the Legion's district commander felt it necessary to "exhort the Reed men to be punctual in their attendance." For its part, *The Come-Back* reprinted the preamble to the organization's constitution, "owing to a misunderstanding on the part of many men as to what the American Legion stands for."[75]

"The prey of the I.W.W."

Some Legion leaders worried that the rising sense of skepticism was indicative of a dangerous ideological defection. Veterans' advocacy efforts were shaped not only by firmly held beliefs that the nation had obligations to the war-wounded but also by deep-seated fears about the prospect of veterans' dissent. As early as 1917, Joel E. Goldthwait, director of the army's Division of Orthopedic Surgery, expressed concern about political radicalism based on what he had seen in England. "At least half a dozen times," Goldthwait later recalled, "persons in high authority" reported that each of the more than 600,000 "mutilated" men "represented a center of unrest, and that unless something could be done to improve their condition, or at least to have them feel that the Government had done its best for them, these individuals would become centers of revolution, and . . . no Empire or Nation could survive that."[76] In the early 1920s, advocates and government officials alike argued that offering veterans generous benefits represented a viable means of staving off a potential political catastrophe.

The sentiment was problematic for Legion officials who believed that fighting for government entitlements contradicted the organization's central principles. The Legion, after all, was founded to "be a great, American, unselfish organization, that would devote itself to the problems of Americanism and patriotism and not to the obtaining of material benefit for its members," a representative from Arkansas argued at a March 1920 meeting. It was intended to put "something into the Government, not take something out of it."[77]

But others maintained that post-service benefits were assets in an ongoing battle for the malleable hearts and minds of former service members. "We cannot put anything finer into our Government than to do something to save those men from the doctrines of the radical agitator," said a Washington representative. "We must take some action or urge the Government to take some action which will make it impossible for the agitator to say to him, 'what has your Government done for you? They have been unsympathetic when you have asked about your War Risk Insurance. . . . They have been unsympathetic if you have been a wounded man. You have been underrated in many instances as to your disability. The Government has nothing for you whatever.' "[78]

The Legionnaire's ideas were rooted in the larger social climate. In the first decades of the twentieth century, labor organizers had been gaining sympathizers and enemies by demanding humane working conditions and a more equitable economic system. One of the more radical groups born in the "western timber and mine lands" in this period, the Industrial Workers of the World, or IWW, distinguished itself from the growing trade union behemoth, the American Federation of Labor, by advocating worker control of industry. Class revolution would come, the IWW maintained, only if unskilled workers from a variety of trades could band together in true solidarity.[79] By January 1917, the IWW consisted of six industrial unions, as well as their hundreds of affiliates. The organization had a total of 60,000 dues-paying members, though it counted in its ranks 300,000 "workers . . . in good and bad standing." Between 1905 and 1917, the IWW organized strikes across the country, from Maine, Connecticut, and Massachusetts to Ohio, Washington, and Louisiana, earning a reputation among business owners and many members of Congress as a threatening menace.[80] Washington state was a center of labor unrest and tension between conservative veterans and radicals. Drafted soldiers, many of whom were illiterate, said a Legion representative who hailed from there, "are the prey of the I.W.W.," and they were to be "pitied not blamed" if they succumbed to pressure from leftists. "Remember when a man wants sympathy and does not get it, that he is a good, fit subject for the radical agitator."[81]

Others agreed that veterans' benefits could tame a volatile political climate. John Edward Holden, state adjutant of the Utah branch of the American Legion, had a litany of injuries from his time in the military: "wounded in both legs, both arms, lost my left eye, and my teeth have been wired." Holden told legislators during congressional hearings that he was approached at a train station by "a beautiful young woman who presented to me a paper entitled 'What the Government is doing for the ex-soldier.'" Initially "real enthusiastic to read something that was going to benefit me directly," he soon realized the document "condemned the form of Government, and at the bottom of it it said, 'To remedy this join the I.W.W. organization.'"[82] Holden implied that the distribution of such literature was endemic in hospitals housing soldiers and veterans. Noting that he would "rather lose the other eye and lose my arm than have that presented to me over again," he testified that he was approached in a similar fashion while being treated at Fort McHenry in Baltimore. "A woman came there with some fruit and some candy and dropped me a note, and in this note there was more I.W.W. literature, condemning the form of Government and the way the ex-service man was being treated." Holden said he had "no complaint, as a wounded man," and that he was "being well taken care of" in government hospitals and vocational education programs. But, he added, many ex-soldiers who were "voicing the opinion that the Government [was] not doing justice to them" were joining the ranks of the IWW, "whose purpose is to overthrow the Government."[83]

Walter Reed's newspaper, *The Come-Back*, reported a similar incident on the hospital campus. "An effort to distribute anti-government propaganda among the patients of this institution last winter met with dismal failure when the man who sought to spread the radical ravings was guyed down in an attempt to talk to a group of the veterans in the post exchange," the newspaper reported in April 1920. "The hospital men simply would not have the paper around."[84]

Some legislators were skeptical about using monetary rewards as a means of enhancing patriotism. "I think the American people have great hopes that these 4,500,000 men [who served during World War I] will be a safety valve in the Americanization problems of this country, and I believe they will myself," John Nance Garner (D-TX) said during hearings regarding the cash bonus in 1920. "I have intense confidence in it, but I doubt sir, whether the payment of three or four hundred dollars to two or three million of these men will tend to make them better citizens, or increase their patriotism or their Americanism."[85]

Skepticism dissipated somewhat when conversations centered on veterans who were wounded or ill. During legislative debates in 1921 focused on providing millions of dollars worth of funding for veterans' medical care, Rep. Clarence J. McLeod, veteran and Republican from Michigan, bolstered the idea that veterans were especially ideologically vulnerable. "Let us of America take warning against the danger of neglecting our disabled heroes," McLeod said forebodingly. "The surest investment we can make for the national safety, for the perpetuation of American ideals, the Declaration of Independence, and the Constitution is now to decently and gratefully mete out justice to the men who carried the flag virtuously through the Nation's latest and gravest peril. It is well to remember that even as republics have been ungrateful so have they gone down into dust and oblivion."[86]

Other legislators similarly linked soldiers' complaints about compensation rates and medical care to what Iowa Republican Burton Sweet called "a universal unrest throughout the country."[87] Sweet offered his commentary at a December 1919 dinner reception in the dining hall of the House of Representatives, where the American Legion had invited legislators and Walter Reed Hospital patients for a meeting. One of the patients, Corporal Butte, who had a leg amputated, said that hospital patients were "fighting all of the possible handicaps that can be thrown in their way." In spite of having "placed every confidence in the men whom this government had placed in charge of the things that were vital to them," Butte said, "it seems at the present time that the only guarantees we were blessed with was that we might be allowed a discharge." Butte's frustration and anger were palpable.

> Would any of you gentlemen be willing to trade places with one of these cases now at this hospital, living on a liquid diet? Now, by liquid diet, I mean mashed potatoes, raw eggs whipped up to a liquid, some times forced through a tube in the mouth, other times through the diaphragm into the stomach. . . . Then, maybe, you will be told that your chances of getting well will never be good, or perhaps you will go through fourteen operations, both minor and major, suffering the pangs of a super-hell, and then be told you will outgrow your disability in time . . . these men are not professional soldiers in any sense but were called by the draft into this war, and . . . the idea was conveyed to them that they would be taken care of in every way possible.[88]

Royal C. Johnson, a fellow South Dakota Republican, decorated war veteran, and Legion member, was hopeful that Butte and other patients would "realize the American Legion [was] willing to present their case" and come into the fold of the organization. "Unless we are going to have the Ugly Head of Bolshevism rise up in our midst, some of the things that we have listened to are absolutely true, and they are the kind of things we can't let go in this country," Johnson said. "The only way to keep them below the surface is to meet the honest, fair, demands of these men."[89] Johnson and Sweet would become two of the staunchest advocates for veterans' entitlements in the months to come.

For the American Legion and its supporters, the fight for government benefits was central not only to a larger mission of saving former service members from the menace of antigovernment sentiments but also to its attempt to gain credibility as an advocate of the rank and file. A Michigan representative reported, "the I.W.W., the labor agitators, got busy early last summer and fall, saying in open meeting and through their labor paper, mind you, that the Legion represented big business, that the Legion never would represent the service man, the rank and file, that the Legion was composed of officers, and tried to put us on the defensive." At the state Legion convention soon after, the organization "went unanimously on record" in favor of offering ex-soldiers "adjusted compensation" or cash payments for their time in service.[90] A fellow Montana representative also characterized the organization's support of a bonus as being directly related to an attempt to undercut that state's IWW "agitators." "We have got our problems out there that you fellows back east here haven't got," he said. "Near the home and the habitat of the industrial worker of the world," the

Legion could combat its reputation as "a wolf in sheep's clothes" by supporting veterans' entitlements. A counterpart from Washington was most explicit:

> We have, in the state of Washington, like my friend from Montana, a hotbed of I.W.W. and reds of the various classes and they are making a great play to the ex-service man in our state to secure them in their ranks and they make this plea that the government has done nothing for the ex-service men and they say to them that "you can't get Congress to do anything to help you now, you join our ranks and we are going to bring about the reform and get those things to which you are entitled." Now, there are a few of the illiterate, uneducated men falling for that propaganda. There are a lot more in the balances, who are subject to being taken and converted into the ranks of the radical or of being stabilized by the American Legion. Lots of them haven't joined the American Legion for the reason that they say they want to see what we can do.[91]

Although some Legion members were ideologically opposed to the idea of expansive government benefits, they eventually favored them, in part to ensure that the organization could appeal to the masses.

Even as the American Legion was influenced by the potential appeal of the ideals expounded by groups like the IWW, it helped inspire the missions of veterans' organizations that embraced socialistic, pro-labor, antimilitary ideals. Such groups claimed that veterans should fight for material rewards from their government based on the conviction that they had been unjustly exploited and thanklessly discarded. The Private Soldiers and Sailors Legion, for example, lambasted the American Legion for proposing a universal military training bill, arguing that "war is the greatest curse of the world."[92] The organization demanded jobs, land, and cash payments on the basis that the government should be obliged to "let down the bars of monopoly" and "let people have access to opportunity." But according to the Private Soldiers' Declaration of Principles, veterans did not intend "to be used as crow bars to pry some other man or woman out of a job. Nor do we intend to be . . . used as a lever to force down the wages of other citizens."[93] Similarly, the World War Veterans of America, which described itself as having "somewhat of a radical slant," was in 1920 "endeavoring to recruit now members from the ranks of those enlisted men who joined the American Legion."[94] Its aims included the formation of "one great fraternal organization for the mutual protection of our rights, advancements of interests, promotion of our welfare . . . to secure forever the blessings of liberty, equality, justice and peace to ourselves and all of our fellow citizens."[95]

Some DAV members, too, sometimes wrapped arguments for veterans' benefits in political language. The organization's spokesman, Ralph A. Horr, argued that antiradicalism should be a priority of the organization, and he justified the claim that veterans deserved publicly funded medical services by juxtaposing their sacrifices against leftists' supposed anti-Americanism. At the 1921 DAV convention, Horr told the crowd of approximately one thousand that he had visited a hospital in Chicago and met a disabled veteran who was showing signs of infection following the amputation of his arm. There were soldiers like him throughout the country, Horr reported to applause; they had problems the DAV had to "attend to," problems that were "almost political." Immediately following his discussion of the Chicago hospital, Horr described other lingering threats: "German-speaking societies" in the United States and supposed radicals who were "in communication with the Soviet of Russia. . . . We have problems to solve as disabled veterans of this great war that are national and international in their scope."[96] Fighting for enhanced rights for disabled veterans and taking a stand against radicals, Horr implied, were complementary missions. At hearings regarding the granting of a federal charter for the DAV, Horr said that the organization aimed, among other things, to keep members "out of other organizations that would amount purely and simply to the exploitation of the disabled men and result in embarrassment to the government."[97]

Horr and fellow DAV members who favored a greater emphasis on surveillance of immigrants and suspected communist agitators gained enough support within the ranks of the organization to spur conflicts between attendees of the DAV's meetings and members of the comparatively left-leaning Disabled Soldiers' and Sailors' League.[98] When a representative from the latter group, Mr. Bodine, visited a DAV meeting in May 1921 and fiercely criticized Robert Marx for praising the government, he and his comrades were shouted out of the room, accused of being radicals, Bolshevists, and troublemakers. One newspaper reported that as Bodine exited the meeting, he yelled back: "We are proud to be called Bolshevists. Although we have not so many members as this association we will start a drive tonight to enlist all the 'radicals' we can find among the disabled veterans who want a square deal."[99] About a month later, Horr led a contingent of DAV members into a socialist convention in Detroit and announced that "the Americans who fought against a foreign enemy would fight as hard against enemies at home if the need should arise."[100] At its June 1921 annual convention, the DAV passed a resolution stating that socialist "utterances not only are unpatriotic and un-American, but disloyal and treasonable" and that "ways and means should be evolved by the national and State governments for the suppression of those persons guilty of using the same."[101]

There were members of both the American Legion and the DAV—Robert Marx and Michael Aaronsohn, for example—who did not support the inflammatory tactics bolstered by leaders like Ralph Horr.[102] But the groups' conflicts with the IWW and so-called socialists, which were widely reported in newspapers, helped them gain notoriety as protectors of conservative American values. That impression helped ensure that their requests for extensions of government entitlements seemed justified and rational, not radical.

The conflict between mainstream veterans' groups and radical organizations was part of a sweeping and largely effective effort on the part of conservative lawmakers and advocates to rein in the power of leftist groups in the World War I era. Spurred by the fear that workers' rights movements would lead to economic instability, and gaining momentum from the perceived threat represented by the 1917 Bolshevik Revolution, business elites (some of them members of groups like the American Legion) endeavored to mobilize public opinion against organizations like the IWW. In order to convince military veterans to reject ideas that could be construed as socialistic, they came to believe, they had to offer something tangible in return. It was hardly a unique approach. Proponents of pathbreaking welfare reforms in Germany in the late nineteenth century, for example, had "strategic and cooptative motives vis-à-vis the labor movement . . . although economic and altruistic motives predominated in their public justifications." In general, advocacy groups and elected leaders have sometimes supported and adopted entitlement programs in part to "exclude radical voices from policy discussions."[103]

Advocacy in Action: The Langley Bill and Funding for Hospitals

In the closing hours of Woodrow Wilson's presidency, advocates and bureaucrats pushing for a more expansive hospital system won a major legislative victory. As Wilson "waited upon Congress in its final hour in his room off the Senate Chamber," one of the bills he signed into law was an $18.6 million appropriation intended for the improvement, expansion, or building of hospital facilities and dispensaries for BWRI patients.[104] Public Law 384—known as the Langley Bill—stipulated that $6.1 million could be used for the improvement of existing institutions and the remainder for the construction of new facilities.[105]

The Langley Bill's journey to passage demonstrated the potential political power of veterans' advocacy groups. The Legion appeared before the Committee on Public Buildings and Grounds four times urging a favorable report on the bill, which, in its original form, provided $10 million for hospitals to be used for BWRI patients. Just before the House adjourned in June 1920, the committee finally placed it on the calendar, then voted unanimously for the appointment of a subcommittee to secure a special rule to allow the bill to be brought to a vote. The special rule was granted on January 11, 1921.[106] One of the landmark pieces of veterans' health entitlement legislation thus received a hearing and became a reality in large part because of a mighty effort on the part of the American Legion.

The Langley Bill marked a turning point for two reasons. First, it was a *hospital* bill above all else, based largely on the requests of the Public Health Service rather than those of the director of the Bureau of the War Risk Insurance. Although both the BWRI and PHS were part of the Treasury Department, previous legislation concerned with veterans' medical care left the BWRI in control of funds, engendering complaints from PHS officials about a lack of access. It was impossible to plan a hospital program, they argued, when approval and funding for every project or idea had to be sought from an outside agency.[107] The passage of PL 384 indicated legislative acceptance of the claim that hospitals should be funded apart from other benefits.

Second, the new law allowed medical experts, rather than elected officials, to decide where hospitals should be built. In its original form, the bill proposed that the recommendations of a "commission composed of congressmen" recommend locations for new hospitals. According to Wesley L. Jones (R-WA), the involvement of legislators in the selection of sites would "save the government a good deal of money." But a few of Jones's colleagues spoke against such a provision. James W. Wadsworth (R-NY) argued that a commission ruled by congressmen and senators would "take months to bring about any decision." Almost as a case in point, the Senate hearings soon devolved into a series of senators' calls for the Langley Bill to include funding for the enhancement of specific facilities in their own states. "If we want to save time, if we want to do this thing effectively," Wadsworth suggested, sites for new institutions should be chosen by the Public Health Service, subject to the approval of the president.[108]

Democrats in both the House and Senate concurred with Wadsworth's suggestion that representatives of the PHS and other medical experts had the best knowledge of which facilities were needed where, and that they should be left to autonomously decide the matter. Would a senator with "a sick friend or, unfortunately, an ill relative, consult a physician or four politicians?," asked Henry F. Ashurst (D-AZ).[109] Ladislas Lazaro, a Democratic representative from Louisiana and a doctor, made a similar argument in the House. Health professionals, Lazaro said, "who know how to treat those cases" should say "where they should be treated." The "medical authorities who have charge of this money," he suggested, "could select a commission composed of experts, especially in these tuberculosis cases, who would make a rapid survey and then decide where this money should be spent and where these boys should be treated."[110] Lazaro's idea bolstered the precedent that hospitalization was a wholly medical problem, rather than a social or political one. It was greeted with applause.

Debates over the passage of the Langley Bill featured a fair amount of partisan bickering but demonstrated that many had come to accept the general principle that hospitals—regardless of where they were located—constituted a persistent need. Democrats were eager to write "broad" legislation that would, as Otis Wingo (D-AR) put it, "adequately take care of the hospitalization of our soldiers in every section of the country." Likewise, the bill's sponsor, John W. Langley (R-KY), maintained that the legislation marked "merely the beginning of a great hospital-building project, which may ultimately cost many times the amount authorized by this bill."[111]

Langley, who was elected to Congress a decade before the war and chaired the influential Committee on Buildings and Grounds in the early 1920s, earned a reputation in that post as one of many "rollers of the pork barrel" who chased patronage via expensive legislation. In 1923, when he proposed spending $1 million to erect post offices and other federal buildings, the *New York Times* suggested that he and like-minded colleagues had forgotten "that attempts [were] being made to run the United States on a budget basis."[112]

But hospitals for veterans were different from post offices. In fact, many maintained that Langley's 1920 bill was insufficient given the extent of need. In the Senate, as in the House, legislators argued that the bill represented only the beginning of much more expansive provisions, though members of opposing parties differed as to what that meant for policy in the short term. Joseph T. Robinson (D-AR) noted that the surgeon general of the PHS had requested $35 million, much more than the $18.6 million allotted in the legislation. "If we only authorize the amount carried by the committee's provision [the amount that could be spent within one year] we will never catch up with the requirements of the service or even approximate that accomplishment," Robinson said. "The construction of permanent, suitable institutions" could not be accomplished within the confines of fiscal year appropriations. He estimated that it took five to six months to locate a site for a hospital, and even longer to secure contracts and devise building plans. "If we wait and only make the authorizations now of such sums as will be actually expended during the coming fiscal year we will be no nearer up with the requirements of the service at the end that time than we are now," Robinson said. Reed Smoot (R-UT) attempted to quell his colleague's concerns. "I am positive that at the end of the year, when the next appropriation bills come up, or, if necessary, a bill carrying the amount outside of a regular appropriation bill before the appropriation bills pass . . . whatever is necessary to take care of hospitalization for the ex soldiers will be granted by Congress at any time."[113]

House representatives passed the bill in a landslide: 239 voted in favor, and none voted against it. Even though some believed the legislation fell well short of providing what was necessary, they went on the record with a "vote to provide hospitalization for the soldiers."[114] Like so many pieces of veteran-related legislation before and to come, congressional representatives voted based on the generally understood principle behind the law—that former soldiers should have access to better hospital facilities—and not on their judgments regarding its specific contents and logic.[115]

Public Law 384 was a relic of Wilson's administration, but it would be implemented under a new Republican president, Warren G. Harding. Throughout his campaign, Harding sharply distinguished himself from his Progressive Democrat predecessor, guaranteeing Americans he would usher in a "return to normalcy," approve lower taxes, and lessen government intervention. He won the accolades of veterans' groups early on. In December 1920, the president-elect made time to meet at his home with a fellow Ohioan, DAV leader Robert Marx. Although Marx had campaigned eagerly for Harding's Democratic opponent, once the returns were in he offered qualified praise for the president-elect. Harding, he said, was "simple and democratic" and "as plain as an old shoe." He also had "a very keen understanding of the problems facing the disabled soldiers and sailors; a very sincere and heartfelt sympathy for them and a firm determination that they shall be the first charge and first duty of the nation as soon as he becomes president."[116] Two weeks before he assumed office, Harding attempted to affirm this belief with a public statement: "I shall make it one of the first items of important business to see that the conditions affecting the government's care of our disabled veterans are rendered more efficient."[117]

To those ends, in the days immediately following the passage of the Langley

Bill, Harding's new secretary of the Treasury, Andrew W. Mellon, appointed a board of medical experts to decide how to disburse the money allocated by the legislation. The Consultants on Hospitalization, referred to as the White Committee after its director, William Charles White, was tasked with conceiving a building program for hospitals that would serve veterans.

The committee took as its point of origin not only the recently passed Langley Bill but also Public Law 326, which in 1919 authorized the Treasury Department, and by extension the PHS, to take over a Chicago army hospital; establish a tuberculosis sanatorium at Dawson Springs, Kentucky; enlarge a Marine hospital in Stapleton, New York; and build new hospitals in Washington, DC, and Norfolk, Virginia—all for the use of World War veterans. According to the White Committee, PL 326 "did not take into consideration at all the question of a consistent program for the complete hospitalization of the veterans of the world war; nor did it make any attempt to provide a hospital system in relation to centers of military population."[118] The White Committee intended to right such previous wrongs and offer professional advice that was untainted by politics or greed as, it was understood, previous parties had been when proposing isolated hospital projects in particular districts.

The committee consisted mainly of nationally renowned and public-minded experts who personified the Progressive Era's wide-ranging health reform efforts. They came to the project with long-held commitments to the idea that a rationally administered, scientifically based system of medical care could promote better health. Most specialized in care for people with mental illness or tuberculosis, two of the primary health threats facing ill and disabled veterans. Prior to the war, committee chair William C. White had worked with the Public Health Service and helped lead the National Association for the Study and Prevention of Tuberculosis, which prioritized the scientific study of the disease and the construction of adequate facilities where patients could receive care. White's public health work earned him national notice, and during the war he headed the tuberculosis unit of the American Red Cross in France. Fellow White Committee member Frank Billings, who served during the war as head of the rehabilitation program of the army surgeon general and chairman of an American Red Cross mission to Russia, had also previously been involved with the National Association for the Study and Prevention of Tuberculosis. Another committee member, John G. Bowman, had served as codirector of the American College of Surgeons from 1915 to 1921 and was a leader in the emerging field of hospital standardization. In 1919, after visiting hospitals across the country and encountering "horrifying conditions," he published the first volume of the formative *Minimum Standards for Hospitals*.[119] In 1921, Bowman helped lead meetings of the American Conference on Hospital Service, which brought together representatives of fifteen health organizations, including the American Medical Association, the American Nurses Association, the Medical Department of the US Army, the Public Health Service, and the National Tuberculosis Association.[120] White Committee adviser Thomas W. Salmon had a varied career as a country doctor, a bacteriologist with New York State mental hospitals, a Public Health Service immigrant inspector at Ellis Island, and chief consultant in psychiatry for the AEF. He had long been a harsh critic of contemporary practices in diagnosing and treating mental illness and helped bring attention to the shortfalls of local systems of asylum-based care.[121]

The White Committee undertook detailed studies of available government-owned hospital beds, creating copious charts, reports, and maps describing its findings. Its members not only visited institutions but also interviewed the foremost experts on hospital and medical care for veterans and the greater population. In a preliminary report released soon after the committee's establishment, an advisory group laid out a "comprehensive plan of hospitalization" for veterans with tuberculosis and mental and nervous diseases. (A separate report on the needs of general medical patients would be submitted in the near future.) The report maintained that the recent $18.6 million appropriation was hardly enough to solve the problem at hand and offered concrete suggestions for providing enough hospital beds for veteran-patients. In order to organize treatment of patients with mental diseases, for example, Thomas Salmon suggested that the White Committee plan for three distinct stages: a "relatively slow ascent," a "rather long level phase," and finally a "slow descent." He recommended additions and improvements to four PHS hospitals in Pennsylvania, Maryland, Georgia, and Iowa, along with the construction of several new institutions in the districts with the most limited resources and the highest ex-soldier populations, including California, Illinois, Minnesota, and Colorado. In a report to the President, the White Committee also emphasized cost-consciousness: "with few exceptions," the group pointed out, many of the six thousand beds to be added to government facilities for the use of ex-soldiers would be "enlargements of government-owned properties."[122]

The $18.6 million allocated by the Langley Bill was granted to the Department of the Treasury and it was clear that the White Committee envisioned a hospital system that would serve veterans in the relatively short term but benefit a larger population—in Treasury Department facilities such as Public Health Service hospitals—at a later date. "In locating these hospitals your consultants have had in mind the permanent value to the Government of its investment in these institutions," noted one committee report. "It will rest with the Government to determine their final use."[123] A "crisis expansion" of veterans' hospitals, the group maintained, would be short lived; most of the resources provided would be useful later for purposes other than providing medical care for former service members.[124]

"So far as treating them in separate institutions, it is almost a necessity"

Among other issues, the White Committee debated how to provide for African American veterans, some of whom had sacrificed their health while serving but were still deemed unworthy of the privileges of full citizenship. Veterans of color attempted to establish a place for themselves in the American Legion and Disabled American Veterans, but the groups' leaders—in some cases hesitantly—erected barriers to full membership and prioritized the loyalty of white constituents. Minority veterans remained fiercely engaged in their own right, but few organizations had the political clout—or the ear of as many members of Congress—as the Legion and DAV. It followed that the veterans' hospital system, which was shaped in part by the largely segregated American Legion and DAV, would be less accessible to minorities than it was to white men.

Drawn by the social appeal and political power of the DAV and the American Legion, African Americans challenged the groups' national leaders to address contradictions between the organizations' practices and the stated egalitarian policies of their national constitutions. Austin T. Walden, a former captain in the 365th Infantry, and Charles A. Shaw, a former lieutenant with the 92nd Division, wrote to Legion headquarters on letterhead from Walden's Atlanta law office in September 1919. They, along with "several other Colored officers and soldiers who served in the late War," had applied for membership in the organization, but the Georgia Division had rejected their request, telling them that only white veterans were allowed to join. Walden and Shaw therefore applied on behalf of "thousands of colored soldiers in Atlanta and Georgia" for permission to establish a separate state organization "composed exclusively of colored men, with representation in the National Convention as provided by the National Constitution of the American Legion."[125] Similar requests streamed in to the Georgia Legion throughout 1919, according to the state secretary, C. Baxter Jones: "We did not anticipate that . . . there would be as many requests for Charters as there have been," Jones reported to the organization's national headquarters.[126] In Louisiana, black soldiers from various regions banded together and referred to themselves as "delegations." In July 1919, representatives from New Orleans, Alexandria, and Shreveport attempted to gain entry to the state convention in Alexandria but were told that "as colored men" they would not be granted charters from the Louisiana Division. "This information," they said, came to us "like a thunderbolt from a clear sky." After being turned away from the state convention they wrote to national headquarters for "advice."[127]

As Legion leaders worked to grow the organization and attract members, they faced dueling perspectives from white members regarding what they commonly referred to as "the negro question." Some argued that the decision by individual states to reject black ex-soldiers as members "was not in any way a satisfactory solution." According to a member of the National Executive Committee from Georgia, it was imperative for the American Legion to accept African Americans as members. "We in the black belt of the South are sitting on the edge of a powder keg as far as the race problem is concerned, and are very anxious that all opportunity be given for a smooth adjustment of the situation," he said. Most white members of the Atlanta Legion chapter, he added, were "embarrassed" by the vote at Georgia's state convention to reject all black veterans from the organization.[128] One Louisiana delegate said he would resign from the Legion if black veterans were forbidden to join. The organization, he argued, was in a position to act as a "stabilizer" in the region if it adopted egalitarian policies.[129]

Those perspectives contrasted sharply with other southern Legion members who saw the prospective acceptance of African Americans as a means of guaranteeing turmoil, not promoting progress. The state adjutant of South Carolina ominously predicted that if black veterans were admitted to the organization in that state, "no more white people would care to join, and probably those already members would withdraw." He argued that officials at the Legion national headquarters—located in New York—should not dictate to state leaders how to handle "the negro problem." Southerners, he argued, were "peculiarly qualified" to deal with it themselves, and the idea of white and black individuals associating —even if they were all veterans—was unthinkable.[130] "There will be no colored brethren" in the Virginia American Legion, declared the department commander of that state. The organization was to be "100 percent white."[131]

The Legion's national leaders recognized the paradoxes and fragility of the situation. Chairman Henry D. Lindsley answered a letter from a Georgia representative who opposed membership for African American veterans by noting that the matter would have to be discussed at the annual convention. "I am, myself, from the South . . . and I, of course, understand the situation in a general way that pertains to your state relative to this matter," he noted delicately.[132] At the June 1919 national Executive Committee meeting, in the midst of a debate about the issue, representative Miller of Delaware asked, "Does the tentative constitution as adopted recognize the absolute equality of every member of the A.E.F.?" Indeed, it did, he was told by Chairman Lindsley. "Then," Miller asked, "can this committee approve a scheme which would tend to inequality?"[133]

But the only viable solution was to leave the question to the states, even if some inequality should result, according to Legion chaplain John Inzer. "We must do something for the negroes. We must give them their rights, because those that had the opportunity to do were good soldiers." But, Inzer worried that African American veterans were "coming home to assert themselves" and that in many towns in Alabama, Georgia, and Mississippi, black men and women outnumbered whites. "If we were to throw down the barriers and make anything like equality in the membership of the American Legion, it would stimulate those negroes down there to almost an uprising in lots of places."[134]

In the end, in spite of the perspectives of Lindsley, Miller, and others, the Legion adopted the policy of local control. Rather than risk losing support among segregationist whites, national Legion leaders allowed each state to reach its own conclusion about extending membership privileges. Segregated posts were established throughout the country. The largest black post was in Louisville, Kentucky, with 110 members. The Legion's failure to restrain the exclusionary impulses of its Southern constituents had serious implications for growing the organization's membership: in some regions of the South, more than half of AEF soldiers were black.[135]

Like the American Legion, the DAV was challenged by the matter of whether to welcome into its ranks black veterans. Many of the organization's officials from the Northeast and Midwest felt strongly that the group should include all former service members regardless of race. Rabbi Michael Aaronsohn's account of the first annual DAV convention painted a picture of a highly egalitarian organization, which promoted "the friendship of Christian and Jew, of nonbeliever and priest, of Republican and Democrat, of Indian and immigrant, of Negro and Caucasian" and united them in "brotherhood."[136] At the same meeting, however, members shared laughs and applause after one delegate opened his speech about the necessity of land grants for veterans with a joke about a "darkey." Like their American Legion counterparts, attendees also passed a resolution urging that "foreign-born Japanese shall be forever barred from American citizenship" in spite of opposition from a member named O'Boyle, who felt it went beyond the DAV's "sole object . . . to work for the welfare of the disabled, and nothing else."[137]

Indeed, members like O'Boyle and Aaronsohn faced strong ideological opposition from their counterparts—many from the South and West—who were not only strongly anti-immigrant and antiradical but also staunchly segregationist. The proposed policies of the latter group prevailed at the June 1922 annual convention in San Francisco when three black veterans from Fairview, Texas, were denied seats after traveling across half the country in order to attend. The incident prompted National Commander Marx to announce that like the American Legion the DAV's official policy would be to allow state departments to determine whether black veterans would be recognized as members. Marx noted that DAV headquarters had granted the Fairview men a chapter charter before the Texas state department was functioning, but due to that office's recent passage of a whites-only policy, the charter would be revoked.[138] The organizational constitution, adopted at the 1921 Detroit convention, explicitly said that state departments and local chapters could "admit or reject any applicant for reasons satisfactory to such State department or local chapter."[139]

The segregation condoned in policies of veterans' groups was mirrored in government-supported health institutions. In the spring of 1921, according to a White Committee report, African American veterans with neuropsychiatric illnesses were treated apart from their white counterparts in institutions in Mississippi and Louisiana, and in separate facilities entirely in Georgia, Alabama, and Texas. One of the largest of those facilities, in Marshallville, Georgia, housed more than four thousand patients. White Committee adviser Thomas Salmon referred to the hospital as "very unsatisfactory."[140]

One of the major disadvantages of treating white and black patients in the same institutions, Salmon said, was that white patients "will not work where the negroes are working." So in southern hospitals, "all the [white] patients sit on the porch and the negro does the work, which is fine for the negroes but bad for the white patients, because there is no occupation for these agricultural people except farm labor." Since white veterans could not receive proper work training when housed and treated among their black peers, Salmon suggested, "I do not think there is any question but that they should be in separate institutions."[141]

Salmon further reported that African Americans were seeking hospital care at a much lower rate than white veterans. In southern districts, the BWRI and PHS admitted 4.4 white veterans per thousand for tuberculosis treatment, compared with 2.1 per thousand black veterans. The difference was even greater when it came to neuropsychiatric disorders: 5.1 of every thousand white veterans was admitted, as opposed to 1.5 of every thousand black veterans. The discrepancies between treated conditions of whites and African Americans could have been due to several factors, including black newspapers' reports of hospital riots and unequal treatment or stigma regarding mental illness. Motivations aside, the low admission rates among black veterans presented a major problem, according to Salmon—though not only for prospective black patients: "If they did not need hospitalization, that would not make any difference but somewhere the negro insane are a danger and they are much more liable to be a danger to white than to negro."[142]

In order to solve the "emergency problem," committee members discussed the possibility of establishing a world premier "negro scientific institution" in Tuskegee, Alabama. It would be in the vicinity of the highest concentration of black veterans and the famous Tuskegee Institute, an industrial and agricultural school run by and for African Americans. Thomas Salmon noted that a hospital for black veterans should also be close to training facilities for black doctors and nurses, including "a negro medical school." While the future location of such a facility remained, for the time being, undetermined by the White Committee, the general idea met with universal approval. "I think it would be extremely unwise to put white and colored in one institution," psychiatrist George H. Kirby maintained. "It seems to me that so far as treating them in separate institutions, it is almost a necessity," agreed C. H. Lavinder of the Public Health Service.[143]

For their part, a rising generation of activists and health professionals, who spearheaded efforts at the turn of the century to found new hospitals solely for African Americans, viewed all-black health institutions as potential bastions for professional development and havens of protection from discriminatory treatment. "It may be objected and is frequently a source of controversy that separate hospitals are non-essential," the educator Alice Dunbar Nelson wrote in 1919. But she argued that such reasoning was "idle and fallacious." Hospitals for African Americans "are needed in some places as schools, churches and social organizations are needed."[144]

But representatives of the National Association for the Advancement of Colored People (NAACP) and others who viewed segregation as unconditionally "wrong in principle as well as practice" initially balked at the Tuskegee proposal, especially the idea that the hospital be located in the Deep South city of Tuskegee, Alabama.[145] "One needs only read both white and colored newspaper [*sic*] to find out how welcome the colored soldiers will be in that hell-ridden section," one World War veteran wrote to the *Chicago Defender*. "Our newspapers and race organizations owe it to the Colored soldiers who were shot and gassed in France and maltreated on their return to America to take steps to see that this outrage is not consummated."[146] The National Committee on Negro Veterans Relief and other organizations agreed, reiterating the argument made by Thomas Salmon in a May 1921 White Committee meeting: a hospital for black veterans, committee members said, should be located "near some recognized medical center," such as Howard University, a premier institute of higher learning for African Americans. "We do not believe Alabama, or that general vicinity offers such a strategic location." The committee argued that the "bulk of the probable cases" were actually not located near Tuskegee and that "the men generally would prefer to dispense with medical treatment altogether than to receive it at an institution in the proposed environment."[147]

African American advocates became even more hostile to the idea of locating a veterans' hospital in the Deep South when federal officials mandated in 1923 that although Tuskegee would be staffed by black professionals, whites would occupy the highest posts at the hospital. The move led to calls of injustice and black doctors' refusal to work there. Only after President Harding guaranteed that African Americans would wholly control the hospital did the NAACP and other groups lend their support.[148]

As veterans' groups gained backing and made the fight for the rights of ill and disabled former service members a central mission of their organizations, they served as willing allies for medical professionals and bureaucrats attempting to set the terms of the debate regarding veterans' hospital care. Political change took compromise, and in some cases contradictory action. In many ways, veterans' activism in this era showcased democracy at its finest. Working- and middle-class Americans banded together to have their demands met. But veterans' groups won the fight for access to hospitals and other benefits for their constituents in part by cloaking their demands in rhetoric of "100 percent Americanism" and antiradicalism. As such, they argued that only some citizens—indeed, only some veterans—were worthy of special privileges. Officials of the DAV and American Legion heeded the requests of zealous members, and initially denied minority

veterans access to the group's conferences and existing posts, and condoned segregation in both military and veterans' hospitals.

Although their efforts were steeped in the predominantly anti-egalitarian
ideology of the times, advocacy groups founded in the years following the Great
War were instrumental in securing long-lasting and extensive rights for former
service members. The political victories of the Legion and DAV, among others,
helped bring about not only a federal hospital system for veterans but also the
1944 GI Bill and a flurry of government benefits for former service members in
the following decades. They also provided a framework on which minority former service members could lobby for their own enhanced rights.

In the short term, veterans' organizations and bureaucrats gained support
among legislators attracted to ideals of self-reliance and antiradicalism and
among health professionals who had long advocated for a better, more organized, health system. Members of the White Committee intended to use public
funds to establish a vast and comprehensive system of care for some of the
neediest Americans, but the group's autonomy in creating a network of hospitals
to alleviate a temporary, emergency situation was soon to be challenged. Within
less than two years, its building program would be subsumed by a brand new and
increasingly powerful government agency called the Veterans Bureau.

CHAPTER FIVE

Administrative Geometry

Creating and Growing the Veterans Bureau and Its Hospitals

It was paradoxical. Warren G. Harding and his underlings blazed into office guaranteeing they would streamline the federal bureaucracy. But they simultaneously promised that theirs would "go down in history as an administration that did not forget its sick and wounded soldiers, and brought peace and contentment to every fireside where assistance on the part of the government was requested and was due."[1]

While Progressives viewed the consolidation of veterans' health services as a means of alleviating illness and poverty, and some social conservatives represented it as a means of staving off radicalism, the new presidential administration of Warren Harding perceived it as a way to decrease government wastefulness. In the early 1920s, advocacy efforts surrounding medical care for veterans shifted from focusing primarily on short-term needs for additional and better facilities to the merits of more permanent and far-reaching legislation. The Veterans Bureau (VB) was approved in August 1921 because politically powerful groups like the American Legion and knowledgeable bureaucrats were able to represent it not as a revolutionary agency that would oversee an array of new entitlements for a select group of citizens but instead as the most cost-effective, efficient, and politically expedient means of alleviating a dire, emergency situation. That was an appealing argument at a time when a Republican president and legislators were drawn to "more efficient business in Government administration," as Harding had put it in his March 1921 inaugural address.[2] In an attempt to sidestep what they viewed as federal malaise, legislators ensured that the Veterans Bureau would be an independent agency rather than part of any existing department.

In its original form, the new Veterans Bureau had few vested powers when it came to structuring a national system of veterans' hospitals, but it had great potential for expansion. Charles R. Forbes, the bureau's first director, is most commonly remembered as a corrupt figure who bilked the government and the country's former service members out of millions of dollars. But his aggressive drive to expand the powers of his agency helped ensure that the Veterans Bureau would gain control of all hospitals treating veterans, and that the system would be both highly autonomous and in place for many years to come. Within approximately one year of its establishment, the VB went from overseeing the care of its beneficiaries in a variety of government and private institutions to managing forty-seven of its own hospitals. It also won funding to undertake its own hospital-building program. By the early 1920s, advocates joined forces with VB bureaucrats to argue that veterans' hospitals should be open to all former members of the military, not just those whose injuries could be connected to service, in part because there was a surplus of beds after a frenzied expansion.

Their requests were answered with the 1924 passage of the World War Veterans' Act, which helped ensure that demand for newly planned facilities would continue, and likely increase, for years. The act granted former service members a distinct entitlement as a reward for their membership in a powerful interest group of citizen-veterans, not solely by virtue of having incurred an injury or illness in the line of duty. While the precedent for universal veterans' benefits and a "citizen-veteran" class had been set by the liberal pension laws of the nineteenth century (the laws that policy makers had railed against while laying plans for the War Risk Insurance Act in 1917), the establishment of the privilege of access to hospital care had unique and enduring consequences. It granted veterans a highly visible and increasingly valuable institutionally oriented connection with their government, and it paved the way for a veterans' health system that would remain intact throughout the following century.

Pushing for Systemic Change: The Rogers Bill and Political Challenges

Before Harding's inauguration, opinions among bureaucrats were virtually unanimous: "Beyond all question," as the Bureau of War Risk Insurance 1920 annual report put it, "it would be to the mutual advantage of the government and its beneficiaries if Congress would consolidate all federal agencies dealing with ex-service men and women, centralizing responsibility, authority, appropriations, and disbursements."[3] The Public Health Service similarly declared that one "administrative head" should oversee the major agencies involved in veterans' care.[4]

American Legion officials took it upon themselves to make those ideas a reality. John Jacob Rogers, a veteran, Legionnaire, and Republican representative from Massachusetts, put forth the earliest legislative iteration of the Veterans Bureau in December 1920. Rogers, born to "one of the leading families" in the industrial town of Lowell, Massachusetts, graduated from Harvard University and practiced law before being elected to the House in 1913. During the war, he took a hiatus from his post to serve in a field artillery unit.[5] His wife, Edith Nourse Rogers, the daughter of a prominent Lowell mill agent, also traveled to the battlefields of Europe, where she "gave much attention to hospital conditions in England and France."[6] Upon her return to Washington, she volunteered among other "society women" as a Red Cross nurse at Walter Reed Hospital, where patients referred to her as "natural and unaffected" and "the angel of Walter Reed."[7] Edith Rogers prioritized the rights of disabled and ill veterans in the 1920s and long thereafter. Presidents Harding and Calvin Coolidge each appointed her as their unpaid personal representative to investigate conditions in government hospitals, and in 1925, she replaced her recently deceased husband in Congress, where she vigorously fought for veterans' entitlements through the following three decades.[8]

A result of a three-day meeting of "high Legion officials with the chiefs of various government bureaus," the bill introduced by John Jacob Rogers contained a wish list of requests from the powerful advocacy group.[9] The main function of the legislation was "consolidation at the top and decentralization in the field," as Rogers put it.[10] It would establish a "Bureau of Veteran Reestablishment," in Washington, DC, with one director who would oversee fourteen or more regional offices. The agency would be charged with "treating all the necessities of the disabled man, whether that be hospitalization, compensation, or vocational training." The bill's contents, said Abel Davis, head of the Legion's newly created hospitalization committee, were based not on "any theoretical discussions with experts as to what is the way of handling problems of this sort" but instead on "practical knowledge" of veterans' needs.[11]

Debates over the Rogers Bill showcased some of the core issues connected with—and the primary arguments for and against—establishing a special government bureau solely intended to oversee the needs of veterans. Supporters of the bill cited various justifications for its passage. Although Congress had been generous with funding for ex-soldiers during the past three years, Davis argued, it was relying on disparate entities to handle treatment, compensation, and rehabilitation, which resulted in conflict and "passing the buck." In other words, no one was wholly responsible for fulfilling veterans' needs, and therefore no one was fully culpable for systemic shortfalls. The current bill, Rogers said, ensured that there would be "some one whom we can hold individually responsible if things go wrong."[12]

Veterans' advocates also made economic arguments. Although the government might be overspending, Legion officials maintained, many veterans were not getting their due. If beneficiaries enrolled in vocational training programs, for example, they were eligible for compensation from the Federal Board for Vocational Education and therefore should have been taken off the rolls of the Bureau of War Risk Insurance. But in some cases paperwork was delayed or bungled, and the government was paying double compensation.[13] According to one 1920 estimate, the BWRI had made more than $11,000,000 worth of overpayments to veterans due to faulty communication between the BWRI, army, and Federal Board for Vocational Education.[14] Drawing on the latter point, Robert Marx, testifying both as a representative of the Legion's Hospitalization Committee and the Disabled American Veterans, emphasized that consolidation would, in fact, save the government money.[15]

Centering authority in one bureau, advocates suggested, could not only enhance economic efficiency but also lead to more uniform treatment of beneficiaries. Frederick W. Galbraith, the newly elected national commander of the American Legion, argued that awards were unpredictable. He said he had recently visited a hospital where two men with the same disease were receiving different monthly payments—one $8 and the other $80. The latter had been rated when his tuberculosis was at full force while the former had been rated when it was arrested.[16]

In addition to alleviating such discrepancies, Galbraith argued that passing the Rogers Bill would fulfill a duty rather than constitute an expensive and ideologically questionable expansion of government. He reminded representatives that men were subject to the draft, "without regard to their desire" and "accepted the obligation willingly." The government, he argued, "said to these men, when you are disabled . . . we pledge our national wealth and our sacred honor that you should be cared for." Galbraith hinted at the next frontier of the Legion's advocacy work for disabled soldiers, which was intimately connected with the current bill: the building of new hospitals solely for the use of veterans. Before the war, Congress had failed to mandate a hospital-building program, and now "men are still suffering."[17] The Legion's John H. Sherburne concurred. The veteran who was in need of hospital care "absolutely throws his hands up," he told legislators. Instead of getting into a "terrific tangle of red tape" by attempting to access care at a government hospital, men were going to local charities for help. Sherburne dramatically conveyed the gravity of the situation as he saw it, and the possible benefits of passing the bill: "The government today has the chance to salvage more human wreckage than they have ever had in a similar situation before."[18]

Thomas Salmon, who had served as the chief consultant in psychiatry for the American Expeditionary Forces and visited asylums, jails, and hospitals in twenty-six states to assess conditions, seconded the opinion that only a small percentage of soldiers who needed treatment had come forward to get it. He also reiterated Galbraith's point that veterans and their families loathed the idea of charity and state institutions and that more hospitals intended specifically for former service members were necessary. If institutions were built "for young men in full vigor," Salmon said, veterans would not be in the embarrassing situation of having to receive care alongside the elderly and the poor, and they would "come in numbers that will surprise you all."[19] The statements of dire need found willing support among some congressional representatives. "I, for one," said John G. Cooper (R-OH), "think it is about time that our Government established institutions to take care of these patients."[20]

But government officials from the Federal Board for Vocational Education (FBVE), the Public Health Service, and the Bureau of War Risk Insurance—the three agencies that would be affected most directly by the legislation—cited problems with various portions of the Rogers Bill. Secretary of the Treasury David F. Houston acknowledged that the Legion's wish to eliminate delays was "very commendable," but he called the notion of creating a new bureau, the head of which could be held fully responsible for veterans' welfare "inadvisable and impractical." First, he noted the breadth of the work of the Public Health Service, arguing that consolidating it with the Bureau of Veteran Reestablishment would "impair the efficiency of a governmental agency concerned in matters affecting vitally the entire population solely for the purpose of rendering service to . . . one group of people." He hypothesized that such an organization "would not function satisfactorily" and would fail to effectively serve both veterans and nonveterans.[21]

Other government officials agreed that the legislation was too broad and sweeping. Before reassigning the job of veterans' welfare to a new agency, argued the secretary of the interior, Congress should investigate and address systemic problems.[22] James P. Munroe, of the FBVE, maintained, "No facts have thus far been produced to show that any greater efficiency would be achieved, any more sympathetic consideration would be given to the disabled soldiers, or any more economical administration would result from combining the rehabilitation service with the other bureaus." Munroe joined the secretary of the Treasury in his skepticism regarding whether current administrative problems could be solved by the "mere expedient of consolidation under a single officer." The FBVE's work was temporary in nature and "through experience, more efficient every day"; to reassign its duties to "new and untried hands" would be both costly and "injurious to the disabled soldiers."[23]

Hugh S. Cumming, the surgeon general of the PHS, agreed; far from serving to coordinate the workings of the three bureaus, the measure "absolutely disrupts the Public Health Service and its personnel, serves to destroy its carefully constructed corps of medical men, professional nurses, and other trained personnel. . . . Confusion," Cumming said, would be the only result if the "ill-considered" and "radical" Rogers Bill became law. Like the secretary of the Treasury, Cumming said he believed that veteran-related work of the three bureaus should be overseen by one individual, but he argued that no one director could be, as he put it, a "Poo Bah." It was impossible "to gather together in one individual a doctor, a financier, and an educator." Division of authority, he implied, was wholly necessary.[24]

At the center of debates over the Bureau of Veteran Reestablishment (and later, the Veterans Bureau) was the question of whether the legislation would lead to the creation of a long-term federal hospital system for veterans. The "ultimate hope," according to Abel Davis of the Legion, was that the PHS would cede control over hospitals where veterans were treated to the new bureau. But even as they advocated for the creation of a distinct veterans' health system, Legion officials attempted to assuage the fears of cost-conscious politicians. One congressman wondered whether a PHS "general" hospital system would eventually exist and another system "exclusively for the service of ex-service men." That was not a "necessary conclusion" of the legislation, according to John Jacob Rogers, but "in the main, and rightly, it would be the rule."[25] The Legion's assertion that the new Bureau of Veteran Reestablishment, not the PHS, should have authority over hospital facilities and care represented more than just a stance on semantics and administration. The group was laying the groundwork for the argument that veterans should have access to an autonomous federally sponsored hospital system. Advocates and government officials agreed that the system was broken, but the Rogers Bill stalled because they had not reached a consensus regarding how to fix it.[26]

Continuing the Drive for Consolidation

Approximately one month after his inauguration, President Harding, determined to show that he was fulfilling his campaign promises to veterans, convened a group of experts to recommend ways of dealing with the general administrative problems facing disabled ex-soldiers seeking government benefits. "I should like you to make . . . an effort to find out just where the Government agencies are in any way lacking in authority, neglectful, or failing to carry out what is the un-questioned intent of the Congress," Harding wrote in his letter establishing the "Committee to investigate the administration of the law in caring for the crip-pled and impaired soldiers of the late war." It was unquestionable, Harding claimed, that the government aimed to provide the best possible care for former service members, but he urged the group to help establish a "firm foundation" for the rational management of veterans' benefits by examining past "abuses" and "regulations." After all, "the policies adopted at this time are very likely to be in effect for a full half century to come."[27]

In April 1921, during three days of meetings, representatives from a variety of groups, including the American Legion and the Red Cross, questioned officials from the BWRI, PHS, and FBVE, repeating many of the concerns expressed in hearings regarding the failed Rogers Bill. Charles G. Dawes, the banker and long-time Republican loyalist who oversaw the discussions, expressed his deter-mination to remain focused on solutions, not problems.[28] "We know the condi-tions, and they are deplorable," he said. "The thing is to find a remedy." Dawes encouraged his committee to act like "officers of a big corporation" instead of members of congressional investigative committees.[29] While Dawes maintained a tone of urgency that helped keep committee members focused, and ensured that discussions extended through meal times, and late into the evening, he re-scinded control of the proceedings to Frederick W. Galbraith, national com-mander of the American Legion.

The Dawes Committee broached a series of difficult questions. How, for example, should a prospective veterans' bureau be organized? Would each state have a district office, or would the agency follow the structure of the FBVE and the PHS, which had fourteen regional offices? There was also the issue of salary limits. BWRI, FBVE, and PHS representatives all reported that it was difficult to recruit qualified personnel given restrictions on how much they could pay them. How could this new organization get around that matter? Another press-ing concern was what to do with the estimated 20 percent of veterans who remained in institutions even though they were well enough to be discharged. Uniform rules and regulations had to be adopted to ensure that patients were not spending an unnecessarily long time in hospitals, but who would conceive of and enforce them?

The committee also addressed questions about the provision of facilities. Charles Sawyer, who was President Harding's personal doctor and was detailed to the committee as his "special representative," wanted to know why more than ten thousand available beds at army and navy hospitals could not be used for veteran-patients in need. "Our house is on fire," Sawyer said, arguing that patients needed to be put in any institution that had space. Doctors familiar with the situation took issue with that rationale. Hospitals, Thomas Salmon argued, were not like "stables or garages." They had limited numbers of beds for specific types of cases. Patients with mental illness and tuberculosis—patients who may be threatening suicide, for example—could not be placed in just any ward. Not to mention that, as Army Surgeon General Merritte Ireland noted, "a man can not be grabbed up and taken to a hospital." Unless facilities were relatively advanced and close to former service members' homes, they would likely resist seeking treatment.[30] William C. White articulated a related point: "The only way to get beds for mental or tubercular cases is to build them at the government expense."[31] The point met with the approval of American Legion representatives, who repeatedly argued that the $18 million allotted in the March 1921 Langley Bill was not nearly enough to accomplish all that was needed. The government could immediately place ex-soldiers in available empty beds in the short term, they said, but many millions of dollars more would be necessary to undertake a "permanent building program."[32]

Charles Sawyer became a powerful force as Warren Harding increasingly relied on him to coordinate federal health-related activities. His focus on economy above all else was only one quality that drew skepticism from veterans' advocates and bureaucrats. Sawyer ran multiple lucrative sanatoriums in Ohio and had earned the Harding family's trust by defending the future president's mother and fellow homeopath, Phoebe Harding, against claims that her prescribed treatment played a part in the death of a young boy in 1897. Soon after the episode, Sawyer began managing the treatment of Florence Harding's floating kidney condition; she came to believe that "Doc" (as the Hardings called Sawyer) "was the one man who could keep her alive." By the time Harding ran for president, in 1920, Sawyer had become a close personal friend, and he served as an invaluable local booster during the campaign.[33]

But government officials and veterans' advocates were skeptical. According to Joel T. Boone, a navy doctor who also cared for the Hardings during the administration, Sawyer was commissioned as a brigadier general in the reserves mainly because "President Harding realized that unless he paid him himself, Doctor Sawyer would have to have some military status." The action, Boone said, "brought forth much public criticism."[34] Indeed, scholars have called Sawyer "the suddenest brigadier general in history."[35] But members of Congress felt they could not justify opposing his nomination, given that they had approved a similar request by President Wilson for his physician to be appointed a rear admiral in the Navy Medical Corps.[36] Still, Sawyer's willingness to wear a uniform in spite of his lack of military experience gave "offense to real soldiers and sailors," including some of the veterans' activists who came to strenuously disagree with his stance on policies.[37]

Sawyer's focus on economy at the April 1921 Dawes Committee meetings corresponded with his general outlook on minimizing government spending and largesse. Similar ideals guided him as he advocated for a consolidated Department of Public Welfare in May 1921. Part of President Harding's plan to reorganize the executive branch into ten concentrated departments, the new entity was intended to oversee "affairs relating to public welfare," including public health and "social justice," which the president felt were "vital to the nation's perpetuity."[38] Inspired by the finding that two-thirds of those eligible for the draft during the recent war had been rejected because of "lack of physical capacity" and "mental inability," as Sawyer put it, the Department of Public Welfare would allow the US government to proactively aid in the production of "the biggest, best and strongest citizen."[39]

The proposed department, which would contain four branches—education, public health, social service, and veterans' services—also represented an effort by the Harding administration to respond in one fell swoop to various factions that had been lobbying for federal funding and power. "If cabinet officers were allowed to each one who is asking for it," Sawyer contended during hearings regarding the Department of Public Welfare, "it would result in a very unwieldy body as a cabinet of the United States." Specifically, education advocates were fighting for their own department, as well as a law that would provide social and health services for impoverished women and children, and veterans' advocates were lobbying for the Veterans Bureau. The Public Health Service cost nearly $50 million annually, and the "social service" problems of vocational accidents and "children's well-being" were costing the government more time and money each year. In all,

Sawyer estimated, the PHS, Bureau of War Risk Insurance, Children's Bureau, National Home for Disabled Volunteer Soldiers, Employees Commission, Pension Bureau, Federal Board of Vocational Education, Bureau of Education, and other related departments were allotted more than $701 million annually. The proposed Department of Public Welfare, he suggested, would "bring them all into one united family" with the dual goals of "economy" and "efficiency."[40]

Sawyer's tendency toward thrift was evident in his proposals for the department's veterans' branch. Disregarding previous controversies that had erupted following the transfer of Great War veterans to Soldiers' Homes and prior discussions regarding the necessity of specialized beds for tuberculosis and mentally ill patients, he consistently argued that existing institutions should be used to house injured and ill veterans of the recent war.[41] He understood that veterans' advocates wanted former service members treated close to their homes in up-to-date facilities. But, he noted, the Soldiers' Homes scattered throughout the nation were "wonderful properties." Their population was "decreasing very rapidly," and the government had "no other apparent use for them." Since most of the homes boasted extensive grounds, buildings could be erected, expanded, and improved according to need. World War veterans—who the Legion and other activists argued were too young to be confined to institutions with aged Civil War veterans—could bring the latter "joy and satisfaction." At the same time, Great War veterans could "take lessons" from their older counterparts. "It will redound to the good of both." Sawyer maintained.[42]

Not surprisingly, many legislators and advocates felt their agendas were threatened by Sawyer's attempt to include their causes in his Department of Public Welfare "united family." Horace Mann Towner (R-IA), a tireless advocate for federal allotments for local education and a primary sponsor of legislation intended to create health care and education programs for poor women and children, told Sawyer in no uncertain terms that he believed his constituents' priorities "would be subordinated" in the department.[43]

Just months after the Department of Public Welfare was proposed and languished in Congress, the Sheppard-Towner Act and Veterans Bureau legislation were both passed. Although the two laws served different constituencies—Sheppard-Towner was largely intended to provide education and health services for women and children—each was based on the ideal that targeted populations should have access to government assistance. Both were landmarks in the history of federal entitlements to citizens.[44]

As the Department of Public Welfare debates demonstrate, when the Dawes

Committee met in the spring of 1921, the future of veterans' health care was unknown. That much was clear when late on the first night of meetings the Legion's Frederick Galbraith posed a crucial question: if the government forged ahead with its plan to put in place a permanent hospital system, which government entity would operate the facilities—the new veterans' agency, the PHS, the military? While the American Legion clearly aimed to demonstrate the need for institutions that would be used indefinitely and solely for veterans, William C. White's response revealed that civilian medical professionals intended to create a temporary fix, then arrange for facilities to be turned over for the general use of the public. The hospitals, White told Galbraith, would be run not by the proposed Bureau for Veterans Affairs but instead "by the departments for which they are built," such as the Public Health Service and the National Home for Disabled Volunteer Soldiers.[45] In a later memo to President Harding, White laid out a plan for increasing veterans' hospital facilities across the country and noted that he and his colleagues were "considering your interest in fitting these needs in a general welfare program."[46]

Apart from some significant areas of disagreement and difficulty, the Dawes Committee was able to reach a consensus regarding three important matters. First, the government had to deal with the emergency situation and get soldiers who needed care into hospitals immediately. Second, it would have to fund a large-scale building program to meet current and future patient loads, which experts predicted would peak in the late 1920s. Third, one government agency should oversee the administration of rehabilitation, medical, social, and vocational services for veterans. What that agency would look like and who would lead it was unclear, but committee members concurred that it should assume control over the BWRI and any activities of the FBVE and PHS that pertained to former service members. They also agreed that whoever was chosen as the director of the new entity should be seen as having "one of the greatest honors that the president can bestow" and have a tremendous amount of freedom and autonomy.[47]

Thanks in part to Dawes's ability to consistently bring his committee members back to what he called the "bird's-eye view" and emphasize points of harmony, after three days of meetings, the group was able to compile seven recommendations for President Harding. Among other things, the list included the suggestions that a veterans' service administration be established encompassing the BWRI and sections of the FBVE and PHS; that "inconsistencies" in past legislation be eliminated and the director of the new agency be allowed to determine employees' salaries; that all government hospital facilities be made available for the use of the new agency; and that a "continuing hospital building program to provide satisfactory care for the disabled veterans of the world war be entered upon at once." The latter, according to the recommendations, should be overseen by the White Committee, the group of doctors and public health experts that had been placed in charge of deciphering a hospital improvement and expansion program in March 1921.[48] Bold, but short on detail, the committee's final recommendations served as a foundation for what would become the Veterans Bureau, and for the building of a nationwide hospital system for former service members.

The Establishment of the Veterans Bureau, and the Seeds of a National Health System

Less than two months after the Dawes Committee meetings, in May 1921, Rep. Burton Sweet (R-IA) laid out his plan for a Veterans Bureau. The Sweet Bill's twenty-nine sections put in place almost all of the committee's recommendations, and then some. Like the Rogers Bill, it was based on suggestions from government officials involved in the system, as well as representatives of advocacy groups. Unlike the Rogers Bill, it garnered enough support to become law.

Sweet, like other elected officials, was committed to veteran causes for personal and political reasons. Although he had never served, he visited Château-Thierry with fellow members of Congress in the summer of 1918 and "saw boys torn by shot and shell." Americans, he said, had an obligation to make those service members "as contented and as comfortable as possible."[49] Sweet also doubtless saw the benefit of courting the soldier vote in a state where Progressive Republicans and Democrats were appealing to farmers and laborers and threatening to unseat him and fellow conservatives. Sweet authored three bills while serving in Congress from 1915 through 1923, all of them concerned with expanding veterans' benefits.[50]

In the summer of 1921, legislators agreed about the necessity for a new agency to oversee veterans' welfare, but they debated where in the federal bureaucracy it should be based. During hearings on the Rogers Bill, both Robert Marx of the DAV and Col. Frederick Galbraith of the American Legion had argued that the Department of the Interior would be a suitable home. Treasury, as Galbraith put it, was "fiscal," whereas Interior, which housed the Bureau of Pensions, national parks, and schools for American Indians, was "educational and physical." Similarly, John Jacob Rogers argued that the Department of the Interior was a "natural repository" for the Bureau of Veteran Reestablishment.[51] But during Dawes Committee meetings and later legislative hearings, advocates and government officials had proposed that the new agency should be part of the Department of the Treasury, not least of all because two of the main agencies involved in veterans' welfare work (the PHS and BWRI) were located there.[52]

Amid debates regarding a home for the new agency, officials from the Bureau of Pensions voiced concern about whether it was redundant. According to a Bureau report, the words "compensation" (used to describe disability payments authorized under the War Risk Insurance Act) and "pension" (generally used to describe outlays to war veterans of the Civil and Spanish-American Wars), meant essentially the same thing. The Pension Bureau, the report said, should handle all Bureau of War Risk Insurance business related to disability ratings and payments, since it had been undertaking such work "since the foundation of the Republic."[53] Like officials of the Public Health Service and Federal Board for Vocational Education, Bureau of Pensions personnel questioned why a new agency should handle tasks that might fall under the auspices of an existing organization.

But some elected officials eager to please veteran constituents looked at the issue from a different perspective. Instead of combining it with a federal agency like the Pension Bureau, which had a decidedly mixed reputation among both veterans and fiscal conservatives, or place it in a larger department, they argued, a new bureau for veterans' affairs should be autonomous. In fact, Senator Reed Smoot (R-UT) proposed "taking [the bureau] from under the Treasury Department entirely." The new agency's director could then "report directly to the president of the United States." Noting that when members of Congress wrote to the BWRI, their correspondence often traveled up and down the Treasury Department's chain of command, Smoot argued that establishing an independent entity would help accomplish a primary goal: "I want to wipe out all the 'red tape' that is possible." "That," said David I. Walsh (D-MA) is a very happy thought."[54] By making the new Veterans Bureau an independent entity, policy makers hoped to increase efficiency and avoid assigning it an identity as a primarily fiscal insurance program (in the Department of the Treasury) or one centered on social assistance and welfare (in the Department of the Interior).

Another sticking point during hearings on the Sweet Bill was the question of expansiveness and longevity. Edwin Bettelheim Jr., chairman of the Veterans of Foreign Wars (VFW) Legislative Committee, requested that PHS hospitals be immediately turned over to the new bureau. He also asked for the removal of a clause in the bill stipulating that all the agency's regional offices would be terminated by June 30, 1926. "There is not a man in this country who can tell when those offices should terminate," Bettelheim said. The director of the new bureau, he argued, should have the power to eliminate the offices only after it was clear that they were no longer needed. Senators Smoot and Walsh both retorted that as the number of patients decreased during the next five years, the law should provide that the number of administrative offices would also decrease. Smoot argued that including a termination date was beside the point, since the legislation would likely be amended well before 1926.[55]

Smoot also relayed his concern with a section of the bill stipulating that benefits would cover not only veterans whose injuries or illnesses could be conclusively proven to be "upon service origin" but also ex-soldiers whose ailments had been "aggravated" in service. For example, according to the proposed legislation, if a soldier's military intake forms indicated that he had arrested tuberculosis, he would be eligible for medical and disability benefits for that condition within two years of his discharge.[56] The government had already set the precedent that benefits could be granted for injuries or illnesses aggravated in service, most recently via June 1919 amendments to the Vocational Rehabilitation Act. But when it came to hospital care, such a guarantee, Smoot said, would "work havoc." If an injury was of service origin, it should be "taken care of," but he contended that "this thing is wide open … every soldier thinks his case is an aggravated one. There will be no end to the examinations; there will be no end to the dissatisfaction; there will be no end to the demands for the next 50 years."[57]

In spite of their concerns regarding some details of the bill, Smoot and Walsh eventually supported its passage and even worked to expand its provisions. They, along with a great majority of their congressional colleagues, believed that the Veterans Bureau represented a viable solution to the economic, moral, health, and public relations problem posed by underserved veterans. "Further continuation of the present system of separate bureaus handling the problems which are so closely interrelated," a 1921 Senate report said, "would be not only unfavorable from the viewpoint of our incapacitated war veterans, but would be a pitiable reflection on Congressional inability to bring about quick beneficial changes in the present laws."[58]

While finalizing legislation that shaped the US veterans' health system, lawmakers prioritized the concerns and complaints of veterans rather than medical expertise, which they occasionally deemed questionable. In the lead-up to a Senate vote on the bill on July 20, 1921, David I. Walsh urged an amendment that would absolve veterans with tuberculosis or "neuropsychiatric disease" from having to prove that their conditions were contracted in military service. He justified his proposal by citing the dissatisfaction of BWRI beneficiaries: "The men who have been most disappointed, the wave of protest, I might say, against these bureaus and the Government have come from these men who have these diseases, know they have them, have had it demonstrated by doctors that they have them, and then have the Government say to them, 'Prove it, prove it, prove that you have the disease as a result of your service.'" The rule resulted in veterans having to "go about looking for affidavits and looking for evidence," leading to "much trouble and inconvenience." Walsh looked for approval from Smoot, who responded that he had "no objection" to the amendment. Soon after, the bill was passed.[59] Legislation to establish the Veterans Bureau also found strong support in the House. There, not one representative voted against it.[60] Finally, the bill went to conference, where a bipartisan group of eight senators and representatives discussed points of contention. On August 1, 1921, Smoot presented their report in the Senate, which brought about a discussion about presumption of service origin of tuberculosis. "The medical authorities have almost the power of lawyers," Senator Walsh said with derision. "A great many of the hardships about which Senators have received complaints have been due to medical opinion relating to the length of time when diseases traceable to service should develop."[61] As such, Walsh advocated for extending presumption of service origin to two years following discharge, rather than one year. In the late stage of formulating the bill, members of Congress, not medical doctors, made rules about access to care.

Ultimately signed into law on August 9, 1921, an Act to Establish a Veterans' Bureau granted extensive power to the organization's director and laid the groundwork for the most far-reaching system of federally sponsored hospital care in the United States. The new agency—"an independent bureau under the president," as the legislation read—would replace the BWRI and assume responsibility for all the veteran-related functions the FBVE and PHS had performed. Each of those three agencies would transfer records and personnel to the Veterans Bureau. Although the new director would determine details regarding the bureau's structure, the legislation stated that there would be a central office in Washington, DC, 14 regional offices, and up to 140 "suboffices" scattered throughout the country.[62] Concerns mentioned by Bettelheim of the VFW regarding the inclusion of a termination date for the regional offices went unheeded; by legislating that the offices would close on or before June 30, 1926, members of Congress demonstrated their initial conviction that the VB should be a temporary, or at least shrinking, bureaucracy.[63]

Other aspects of the legislation, however, ensured that the new organization would be—as veterans' groups had hoped—a lasting institution. In addition to overseeing the disbursal of insurance benefits and vocational education, the bureau would be responsible for providing examinations, hospital, dispensary, and convalescent care not only for veterans who had incurred injuries or illnesses in the line of duty but also for those whose preexisting conditions had been aggravated in service. The latter clause, as Senator Smoot predicted when he questioned it during congressional hearings, helped pave the way for a subsequent extension of access to *all* veterans. The law also included the proposed amendment to extend presumption of service origin for tuberculosis and neuropsychiatric diseases to two years following discharge, a major boon for veterans' advocates, who wanted VB hospitals to be fully accessible to veterans suffering from common chronic conditions.

Two other measures included in the VB legislation, regarding institutional expansion and control, helped ensure that the agency would grow over time. The law provided that PHS hospitals housing veterans could be transferred to the VB at the president's discretion. It also stipulated that if proper facilities were not available to provide care for veterans through the PHS, army, navy, and Soldiers' Homes, the director of the new bureau could "acquire additional facilities." These could then be placed under the direct control of the VB, as opposed to being handed over to other agencies, as William C. White and fellow White Committee members suggested should be done. The head of the new bureau was thus given license to grow a veterans' hospital system however he deemed fit.

"My job deals with the rehabilitation of men"

Initially, the creation of the Veterans Bureau led to more, not fewer, bureaucratic challenges. The task of transferring paperwork, office space, facilities, and personnel from the BWRI to the new agency proved onerous.[64] Furthermore, VB staff, officials from federal agencies already involved in veterans' care, and members of the White Committee had questions regarding how they would divide and share responsibilities. Would the PHS and White Committee serve the VB or be overtaken by it? There was also the crucial issue of leadership: who would take the helm of the new bureau?

In March 1921, Warren G. Harding had barely served a day in office when R. G. Cholmeley-Jones, considered by veterans' advocates to be a great friend of disabled and ill veterans, stepped down from his post as director of the Bureau of War Risk Insurance to return to work at a financial services firm in New York City.[65] Harding chose as his replacement Charles R. Forbes, who, after emigrating from Scotland as a child, had made his living as an engineer in the construction industry. Forbes served in the army during the Spanish-American War and then as a sergeant in the Signal Corps. Prior to World War I, he was working on various federal committees in Hawaii, where he met and became fast friends with a traveling Harding.[66] Forbes's apparent lack of specifically relevant experience for the task at hand was highlighted by a *New York Tribune* article noting that up until the day before his appointment, the president was debating whether to appoint him the governor of Alaska or head of the BWRI.[67]

With the establishment of the Veterans Bureau imminent, the recently appointed BWRI director became the prime candidate to lead it. "The new bureau needed someone of impeccable status, a rock-hard reputation, first-rate professional credentials, and superb people-skills," one scholar notes. "Forbes had none of these attributes."[68] Veterans' groups registered their early reservations with the new appointment. Edwin S. Bettelheim Jr. of the Veterans of Foreign Wars testified at a Senate hearing that although "Colonel Forbes [was] a very good man," he should not automatically be appointed the head of the Veterans Bureau.[69] In spite of such reservations, Forbes got the job; he was one of many who found himself in his Harding administration position less because of his professional skills and credentials than because of a history of friendship with the new president.

By the August 1921 founding of the Veterans Bureau, the bulk of veteran-patients were in Public Health Service hospitals, though many were scattered in other federal, state, and private contract institutions. Meanwhile, the White Committee forged ahead with plans to systematically improve medical facilities serving veterans across the country. By the time Forbes assumed his position as head of the VB, that group had released a comprehensive plan regarding hospital needs and received approval to build, expand, or improve thirteen facilities across the country.[70]

Forbes's effort to gain control over the hospital program was emblematic of his convictions that the VB could serve as a shining example of the Harding administration's efforts to streamline government operations. The Treasury Department and the White Committee, he believed, were the epitome of federal malaise. About a month after the establishment of the Veterans Bureau, Forbes and his staff met with White and members of his committee and indelicately implied that the medical group had been inefficient and lackadaisical. As each party shared impressions of prospective facilities throughout the country, Forbes grew increasingly frustrated with statements about the necessity to go through the time-consuming processes of seeking approvals, inspecting properties, and, generally, working within "the Government machine." "If any of these new projects are handled in such a way as to prolong the work," he told some of the foremost public health and medical men in the country, "I am going to ask the President and [secretary of the Treasury] Mr. Mellon to stop the cause of delay." When White suggested that his committee was simply following rules dictated by the Treasury Department, Col. Robert U. Patterson, a career Army Medical Department doctor who was newly detailed as the assistant director of the Veterans Bureau, chimed in: "Write a letter to the Secretary of the Treasury saying you are not satisfied with the method; that you would like to have the places and specifications made out in a more expeditious way."[71] Two weeks prior to the meeting, Patterson had written to William White and advised him that "the greatest emergency for the hospitalization of beneficiaries of the U.S. Veterans' Bureau *exists now*."[72] The distinguished doctors volunteering their services and following occasionally time-consuming governmental procedures, it would soon become clear, resented being chastised by newly assigned federal appointees.

About a month after his tense meeting with the White Committee, Forbes approached the newly formed Federal Board of Hospitalization (FBH) with the idea of soliciting public funds to be used for a building program overseen and controlled by the VB. Established by Harding in November 1921—three months after the Veterans Bureau—the FBH was intended to "consider all questions relative to the coordination of hospitalization" overseen by federal entities: the new VB, the army, navy, Public Health Service, National Home for Disabled Volunteer Soldiers, Department of Indian Affairs, and the Government Hospital for the Insane, St. Elizabeths in Washington, DC. Growing in part out of a larger contemporary movement to ensure that hospitals across the country met particular criteria, the board aimed to "standardize requirements" so that facilities, supplies, and buildings could be shared between government departments. It was also intended to "formulate plans designed to knit together in proper coordination the activities of the several departments" in the interest of improving efficiency.[73] During early meetings of the FBH, the issue of veterans' medical care commanded much attention.

Soon after the board's 1921 founding, Forbes drafted a letter asking its members to support the "second Langley Bill," which would allocate $17 million to the VB to oversee eight new hospital projects. The institutions, Forbes said, would be pursued separate from the projects already under the auspices of the White Committee, which had control over the $18.6 million allocated in 1921— before the establishment of the VB—under the "first Langley Bill."[74] "It is felt that the recommendation of your board . . . in the matter of hospitalization will be a source of strength to this Bureau in making its wants known to Congress," Forbes wrote.[75]

Shortly afterward, during Senate hearings on the second Langley Bill in December 1921, Forbes not only argued that the $17 million appropriation was necessary but also touted the judgment from the FBH that "the money provided" should be "disbursed under the direction of the Director of the United States Veterans' Bureau." VB assistant director Robert Patterson reinforced the point: "The board expressed the opinion that [the funds] should be disbursed as the director [of the VB] sees best, in his judgment, and not by the Secretary of the Treasury."[76] Forbes and Patterson were guided by their belief that the intention of the Sweet Bill establishing the Veterans Bureau was that the director of the new agency could "deal directly with the Surgeon Generals of the Army, Navy, and Public Health Service, without being obliged to go through any Secretary or Assistant Secretary of a Department."[77]

When senators questioned the status of previous allocations, and hospital projects being overseen by the White Committee, Forbes dismissed the group's efforts: "None of the hospitals that were to be constructed from this $18,600,000 are completed. There are some of them that are not started." The Treasury Department, Forbes maintained, was slow to take action, and wasteful in the way it assigned contracts.[78] In later hearings, Forbes detailed the "crying demand" for more hospitals in populous districts like New York, improved facilities in the South, and more dispensaries nationwide. Expansions and additions provided for under the White Committee, he maintained, were insufficient.[79]

Thanks in part to Forbes's lobbying, the spring of 1922 saw a great expansion in VB powers. An April 29, 1922, executive order referred to previous legislation that had established the VB, which stated that its director could request additional facilities if they were deemed necessary, and went even further. Although the White Committee would continue to exist and pursue projects approved under the first Langley Bill, the order stipulated that the VB would take charge of those facilities once they were completed. It also gave the VB control of fifty-seven Public Health Service facilities primarily serving former soldiers, sailors, and marines.[80] Forbes's agency gained further power and autonomy with the

May 1922 approval of the second Langley Bill, or Public Law 216, which granted $17 million directly to the VB to "provide for the construction of additional hospital facilities and . . . medical, surgical, and hospital services and supplies" for veterans.[81]

Another, related act—a response to claims that there was "clear discrimination against" those who served in previous conflicts who were "not getting an equal show with the veterans of the late war"—significantly enlarged the VB's pool of potential claimants.[82] It stipulated that the bureau would sponsor medical care for aged veterans, not just ex-soldiers of the World War. Congressional representatives claimed that a law passed in March 1919, which opened Public Health Service facilities to all "discharged sick and disabled soldiers, sailors, and marines," meant that all veterans were already guaranteed access to government hospitals. Yet representatives of Spanish-American War veterans claimed they were being denied treatment. By naming in legislation the groups of veterans that would have access to hospitals, advocates argued, the confusion could be avoided. As William L. Mattocks, editor of the *United Spanish-American War Veterans National Tribune* put it, "We, of course, feel that the veterans of the Spanish War are entitled to the same medical attention" as those of the World War. Thanks to the efforts of the older veterans, Public Law 194 ensured that hospitals and other medical provisions of the VB would be available to "persons who served in the World War, the Spanish-American War, the Philippine Insurrection, and the Boxer Rebellion."[83] Gradually, the government was expanding benefits and growing the purview of the health service arm of the Veterans Bureau.

By June 1922, less than a year after its establishment, the VB was overseeing care for more than eighteen thousand patients in ninety-six government hospitals. It owned and operated forty-seven of the institutions. Those "veterans' hospitals" provided treatment for almost twelve thousand patients. In addition to working with existing facilities, the VB pursued its own hospital projects, adding 3,650 beds to 13 institutions in 1922, all but one of them intended to serve neuropsychiatric and tuberculosis patients—individuals whose illnesses were long-term and chronic.[84] At the same time, the White Committee was overseeing the construction or expansion of eleven veterans' hospitals; once completed, the VB would assume control over them.[85]

Under Forbes's watch, the goal of ensuring that all injured and ill former service members would receive care in *government* hospitals gradually gave way to the ideal that they would be treated in *veterans'* hospitals—facilities intended solely for them. After the spring of 1922, the Treasury Department became increasingly removed from the administration of veterans' hospital care as the Veterans Bureau gained ever more autonomy. The June 1922 VB annual report referred to the establishment of the agency as "one of the great epochs of veteran relief."[86]

Scandal, Bureaucratic Growth, and the Legacy of Charles R. Forbes

In the winter of 1922–23, frustration with—and eventually suspicions of—the seemingly autocratic VB director began to grow. While fighting to ensure that his agency gained control over a veterans' hospital program, Charles Forbes drew the ire of veterans' groups, White Committee members, and fellow Harding appointees. They began to suspect that he was, at worst, embezzling or, at best, placing bureaucratic and financial concerns above the needs of veteran-patients.

Tensions mounted in the spring of 1922, when the transfer of facilities from the Treasury Department to the Veterans Bureau allowed for plenty of federal spending and a vast expansion in the capacity of the VB, but few newly available beds. A White Committee report blamed Forbes, arguing that he had hampered the group's efforts to provide fully functioning hospitals. Once President Harding transferred PHS supplies to the VB in April 1922, the report said, the bureau "refused the use of surplus supplies, and for weeks it was impossible to draw on supplies for equipment." The committee was therefore forced to purchase equipment to complete Treasury hospitals before transferring them to the VB.[87]

Forbes's haggling over funding may have been interpreted as proof of a disregard for veterans' welfare. "I had no way of foreseeing what shortcomings would result by reason of the hospitals constructed by the White Committee," the VB director wrote in August 1922 to Albert A. Sprague, chairman of the National Rehabilitation Committee of the American Legion. "They made their own plans and specifications and constructed their own hospitals." Furthermore, Forbes unapologetically noted, "it was not my intention nor would I under any consideration use any money of the second Langley Bill to complete and equip the hospitals that were turned over by the White Committee from the first Langley Bill."[88]

Sprague was perturbed by Forbes's apparent lack of concern that throughout the time of political wrangling, none of the institutions would be ready to receive patients. "Out of this new quicksand of difficulties, we must take another step at once and go all the way to solid ground," Sprague told Forbes in September 1922. If the funds allotted for hospitals were insufficient, he maintained, the director of the Veterans Bureau should "not . . . delay the presentation of actual needs to Congress. . . . The American Legion will back you to the limit, and so will the American public when they know the facts."[89]

The correspondence between Forbes and Sprague reveals two things. First, Forbes could not win. Advocates were disappointed that more and better hospital beds did not exist within a relatively short time. In many ways, Forbes (like officials of the BWRI and PHS before him) was being blamed for problems arising from prewar plans gone awry and expanding expectations of government responsibilities. The correspondence also demonstrates that suspicions of the VB director were growing. Veterans' groups and others questioned how and why the government was spending millions of dollars on veterans' health services yet facilities remained insufficient. Increasingly, they suggested that Forbes's own impropriety was to blame.

Within the Harding administration, many had heard reports of Forbes taking cross-country "junkets," during which he and his traveling companions enjoyed "a constant flow of liquor, movie stars as party guests, and occasional swims in full evening dress." Beyond the fun, there were accusations of outright graft. In August 1922, Forbes allegedly sold government hospital supplies from a storage site at Perryville, Maryland, to associates for a fraction of their actual cost and simultaneously restocked Perryville with merchandise he purchased new with government funds. The transaction drew the suspicion of Charles Sawyer, among others, who alleged that the VB director received kickbacks on both ends of the deal. Forbes maintained that he was merely replacing damaged supplies with new ones. As rumors flew about embezzlement and corruption, Florence Harding, who hoped to keep intact her reputation as an advocate for disabled veterans, asked friends who worked for the VB to keep her informed about interorganizational activities.[90]

Throughout the summer and fall of 1922, Harding's physician and Federal Board of Hospitalization head Charles Sawyer trained a close eye on Forbes. On one occasion, a Veterans Bureau executive officer, T. Hugh Scott, transmitted to Sawyer a copy of an FBH report marked with question marks and notes that had been "found in Colonel Forbes' desk."[91] A few months after forwarding the report, the VB transferred Scott from his post in Washington, DC, to a veterans' hospital in Muskogee, Oklahoma. One journal reported a suspicion that Forbes orchestrated the transfer as punishment for Scott's reconnaissance work: "Perhaps T. Hugh Scott of Oklahoma, who took straight to the White House some accounts of things done and left undone, will tell how he was shifted overnight from high authority in Washington to exile at a distant hospital."[92]

By mid-1922, Forbes's frequent absences from FBH meetings were causing his colleagues continued frustration, but his notes from visits to hospitals during that time reveal that he was spending days talking with beneficiaries. Indeed, Forbes was more tolerant of Veterans Bureau patients than he was of fellow government officials. "Boys complain of claims being held back by bureau," he jotted down in a notepad during a visit to New York's Sea View Hospital in April 1922. "Is this fault of individuals in bureau? Also complain bureau is 'down on them.'" Patient Manuel R. Trupillo, Forbes noted, was "awarded permanent total. Says he hasn't received insurance. Why?" And from the Naval Hospital in Brooklyn: "Frank N. Hillinghby . . . operated on for ulcer by outside physicians, said he didn't know anything about the Public Health Service or U.S Veterans' Bureau except in a very vague way. . . . Morale of patients who aren't under USVB excellent. USVB patients feel they're not as well treated as Navy patients." At a Marine Hospital in New York City, Forbes wrote, "No complaints, advise sending lots of patients here."[93] Getting into the field was one way (in addition to ceaselessly pursuing funds) that Forbes attempted to get around bureaucratic malaise and live up to a declaration he had made to members of the White Committee in the fall of 1921: "My job deals with the rehabilitation of men."[94]

As tensions escalated among federal officials, Forbes became somewhat defiant. When the matter of the Perryville sales came up at an FBH meeting in December 1922, Charles Sawyer stated his belief that it had been a great mistake to sell the supplies instead of keeping them on hand for future use. Forbes responded that if he was to continue as the head of the VB, it was necessary for all parties to understand that "the internal management of the bureau was his responsibility only."[95]

Within just a few months, however, the suspicions of the Legion and others led Congress to open an investigation into Forbes's agency.[96] As news of the probe trickled out of Washington, he finally resigned from his post. "There is little understanding of the magnitude of this task, and there is little appreciation of the splendid service of its employes [*sic*] in the interest of the disabled men," he said in a statement immediately following his resignation in February 1923. Inefficiencies in his bureau, he maintained, were due to attempts by unnamed parties to "inject politics."[97]

In the short term, it seemed that designating an all-powerful director for the Veterans Bureau had backfired. In 1924 and 1925, a congressional investigation and a subsequent grand jury trial found that Charles Forbes had cheated the government—and, by extension, the veterans he was meant to serve—out of millions of dollars. The legal episode, which included gripping accounts of Forbes's fondness for parties and liquor, as well as an affair with the wife of one of his accusers, were widely reported in newspapers. Among other things, Forbes allegedly sold government property at well below cost to personal friends and reaped his own financial rewards in the process. His denial of all charges and his claim that Charles Sawyer and other witnesses who testified against him were undertaking a politically motivated conspiracy came to naught: he was sentenced to serve two years at the Leavenworth Federal Penitentiary.[98]

In the spring of 1923, around the time Congress undertook its investigation of Forbes, the White Committee submitted its final report and exited the field of veterans' hospital policy and planning. In spite of facing challenges during its twenty-month existence pertaining to relations with the VB and interdepartmental transfers of power, the committee had forged ahead with its mission to recommend a comprehensive national building program for veterans' hospitals. By 1923, based on the suggestions of the consultants, work was mostly complete on nineteen hospital projects designed to provide approximately six thousand beds for veterans. Four new hospitals had been constructed, three purchased and later remodeled, and twelve transferred from the PHS or War Department. An additional three projects consisted of additions to existing National Home for Disabled Volunteer Soldiers.[99]

In a November 1923 report, the White Committee recorded its frustration with what it viewed as separatism and redundancies on the part of the Veterans Bureau. In response to Charles Forbes's repeated claims that the group had been inefficient and wasteful, committee members pointed out that eighteen months after the April 1922 passage of the second Langley Bill, the Veterans Bureau had provided only two hundred new beds for occupancy, and those were "at a hospital in Memphis, Tennessee, which was purchased completely equipped, and ready to operate." Furthermore, the VB only had completed an average of 68 percent of the thirteen hospital projects it had started. At the same time, the efforts of the White Committee had allowed for the provision to the VB of more than 2,900 beds (many of them, the report neglected to mention, also in previously existing institutions) and completed 84 percent of its "total program." By May 1924, the White Committee noted, the VB would receive more than 5,800 new beds, thanks to the efforts of the Treasury Department.[100]

But amid statements of productivity, the White Committee brought up a thorny question: had the government fostered "overhospitalization"? Since 1917, $316 million had been used for hospital construction, "a great deal" of which was "spent for temporary hospitals established during the war which had to be abandoned." Getting to the supposed root of the problem, the committee noted: "If the United States Government had had a Federal plan for its hospital work, probably much that was otherwise wasted could have been preserved as permanent institutions for use in the situation that confronts the country to-day."[101] Following the release of the final White Committee report, newspapers echoed the sentiment: "Charge Huge Waste in Hospitalization," screamed a *Washington Post* headline. "Medical Experts Find U.S. Built Many Institutions That Will Not Be Needed."[102]

It was politically expedient—and, in part, accurate—to cite previous policy oversights as the culprit, but efforts to guard against bureaucratic growth and redundancies were unsuccessful for at least four complex reasons. First, because of the unpredictable and chronic nature of two pervasive conditions—tuberculosis and mental illness—it was, according to the White Committee, "impossible . . . to give accurately the numbers of [veteran] beneficiaries."[103] Over time, the problem only became more acute. It was difficult to definitively limit access to care as patients with chronic diseases that were vaguely defined and understood placed heavy demands on the system.

But haphazard growth also occurred because it was difficult to assess how many beds were actually in existence and useful at any given time. For example, in January 1922 the White Committee recommended that a total of twenty thousand beds be made available for veterans: eight thousand for patients with tuberculosis, eight thousand for patients with neuropsychiatric disease, and another four thousand for general medical or surgical cases.[104] According to the 1922 annual report of the Veterans Bureau, there were 27,985 government beds available.[105] On the surface, it seemed simple enough to conclude that meant a surplus of more than seven thousand beds. But health professionals joined veterans' advocates in pointing out that beds had to be of a certain quality and type, and in locations relatively close to veterans' homes. Also, they argued, tuberculosis and neuropsychiatric patients needed to be housed in buildings specially suited to their conditions; not just any empty bed would do. Neuropsychiatric patients posed a particularly vexing problem, and resources were especially scarce for their care. While the VB had successfully located more than 70 percent of both tuberculosis and general medical patients in government hospitals by June

1922, only 50 percent of neuropsychiatric patients were in government facilities by that time. Most of the new facilities proposed in 1921 and 1922 by Treasury Department and VB officials were aimed at alleviating that specific problem, even as other (unsuitable) government beds sat empty.[106] For members of Congress, it was challenging to understand the actual numbers—of patients or necessary beds—involved. Eager to avoid reputations as anti-veteran, many reacted by simply granting more funding when it was requested.

The third reason why the number of hospitals increased was because government committees and organizations were operating at cross-purposes and competing for resources. The White Committee moved forward on conceptualizing a national system of veterans' hospitals even as the new VB director undertook a separate building program and strove for control over all facilities and services. Both parties were propelled by veterans' groups, which argued that former service members needed access to more and better facilities.

Finally, a veterans' hospital system grew in the 1920s because of the structure of the bureaucracy. Forbes's true motivations for doggedly pursuing the mission of expanding the purview of the VB, which he publicly attributed to a desire to decrease wastefulness and increase quality of care, are, perhaps unknowable. But more important than understanding his individual psychology is to reckon with how and why it was possible for a bureaucrat to consolidate so much power so quickly. The VB was one of numerous federal "autonomous agencies" established near the start of the Harding administration as a means of engineering efficiency.[107] But by the late 1920s, the trend was receiving mixed reviews—even from initial proponents like Reed Smoot. Since 1913, Smoot noted in 1929, a new executive agency had been created roughly every year and a half. The result, he lamented, was bloated and "amorphous" governance. "History has demonstrated that agencies of government, once created, tend to perpetuate themselves indefinitely. . . If a government department or bureau should ever report to Congress that its jurisdiction should be curtailed or that it had fulfilled the purpose for which it was created and should be abolished, undoubtedly there would be a demand for an investigation to ascertain what was wrong."[108] From a policy standpoint, Charles Forbes helped ensure that the VB not only perpetuated but also expanded exponentially.

Forbes's eager aggressiveness in growing his agency's power and institutional girth—whatever his underlying motivations—had lasting effects quite apart from the creation of scandal: they served as primary forces in the early expansion of the Veterans Bureau hospital system. It is debatable whether, without his efforts, an autonomous veterans' hospital system would have emerged after World War I. Had he not pushed to gain control over PHS facilities and pursue a building program for the VB, veterans may have been housed in facilities owned by a variety of federal entities, which would have eventually reverted to the auspices of existing government branches. Instead, a vast system of hospitals was controlled by the VB, and accessible—specifically and indefinitely—to veterans.

"A pension roll . . . that will make the pension roll of the Civil War look like a tip to the waiter"

One person not "greatly worried over the possibility of being overhospitalized" was Frank T. Hines, who was appointed director of the Veterans Bureau after the resignation of Charles Forbes. Hines, the son of a Utah mining engineer, had enlisted in the army as a private in 1898 and participated in "20-odd engagements" in the Philippines during the Spanish-American War. After receiving a medal for bravery, he went on to earn degrees in mechanical and electrical engineering. By August 1917, four months after the United States entered the war, he had become head of the army's embarkation service, where he was credited with ensuring that US soldiers were shipped abroad for "$81.75 per man, which was about half what the British had demanded at the outset." In 1920, after he had moved up the ranks to brigadier general and been widely lauded for running army transport operations efficiently and economically, he resigned from his military post and took a job as the vice president of the Baltic Steamship Company, which moved freight and passengers from New York to Eastern Europe. When President Harding asked Hines to become director of the embattled Veterans Bureau in February 1923, he was forty-four years old and, as Silas Bent of the *New York Times* put it, "slender, brown-eyed . . . with the smile of a young boy . . . one of the gentlest and most urbane persons ever you saw."[109] His chief recommendations, according to another admiring reporter, "were ability to master details and a mind as orderly as a card index."[110] When Hines accepted Harding's request, friends wondered why he would leave his comfortable private sector post to "to take a 'killing' place in Washington." "You've taken a devil of a job," one told him. Hines, however, was doggedly determined. "I am not at all sure I can get away with this thing," he told Silas Bent shortly after being appointed. "But I am going to do my level best. I'm going to work 18 hours a day. I'll work twenty-four if need be."[111]

Like Charles Forbes, Frank Hines assumed his post at the Veterans Bureau declaring his determination to "meet the needs of veterans with the least cost to the government."[112] He promised to discourage "hard-boiled methods" and emphasize that beneficiaries were "entitled to the greatest courtesy and the kindest treatment."[113] The Veterans Bureau, he maintained, should "function as a large business organization."[114] Rather than retaining many poorly paid employees, he said, it should offer higher salaries and be "more compact." Still, he argued that beneficiaries "should not be cared for as babies" but given an opportunity to earn a living.[115] Hines said he viewed his job as "a problem in administrative geometry—to find the shortest distance between two given points: the service man and the money." After one month on the job, he had gathered that "there is overlapping, crossing of wires, red tape . . . and systematic delay," which resulted in great waste.[116] Within six months of being appointed, Hines had closed twenty bureau subdistrict offices located across the country, a move he argued would save the government $750,000 annually. Referring to the original legislation establishing the Veterans Bureau, the *New York Times* declared that Hines's move was "in keeping with the intent of Congress that these subdistrict offices shall not be retained after 1926."[117] Three months later, the *Times* reported that Hines had cut more than two thousand clerks and field agents from the VB payroll.[118] During his first year at the bureau, the new director earned a reputation as efficiency-minded and capable of "clearing away the obstructions in his path."[119]

Even as he worked to cut bureaucratic fat and spending, Hines collaborated with veterans' advocacy groups to lay the groundwork for a major expansion of the veterans' hospital system. In fact, his reputation as cost-conscious likely helped legitimize his requests for growing the bureau's health services. Soon after his arrival in Washington, he planned a nationwide survey to determine whether facilities at forty-eight veterans' hospitals were "adequate."[120] In December 1923, he announced that the VB needed $6 million for veterans' hospitals.[121] In addition to lobbying for money, Hines also joined veterans' advocates in arguing that all veterans should have access to the institutions. Congress heeded the call with the June 7, 1924, passage of the World War Veterans' Act (WWVA).

The sweeping, twenty-three-page act, which had the overarching goal of revising and clarifying aspects of legislation related to the functioning of the VB, had a dramatic effect on the nature of veterans' hospital care. Previous legislation allocating funding for hospitals and creating the VB provided the framework necessary for the creation of a medical system intended solely for veterans. The WWVA greatly expanded the pool beneficiaries who could access that system.

It not only loosened restrictions regarding "presumed" service connection of illnesses such as tuberculosis but also stipulated that those who had served since 1897 and suffered from a variety of health conditions—"regardless whether such ailments or diseases [were] due to military service or otherwise"—were eligible to receive care in veterans' hospitals. Still, the notion that a system of preference should exist was central to the shape of veterans' health care. According to the World War Veterans' Act, former service members could be treated at the expense of the VB "without regard to the nature or origin of their disabilities," but only if "existing Government facilities" permitted and if they were otherwise "financially unable to pay."[122] The act thus clearly delineated the principle that veterans whose ailments could be traced to duty would receive medical care with no means test—as an entitlement—while others would receive it based on financial need—primarily as welfare.

In the months leading up to the proposal of the WWVA, a flurry of new legislation made it clear that the post–World War I period would mirror the post–Civil War era, when veterans' access to benefits gradually became less dependent on whether or not they could prove that disabilities were connected to service. In July 1919, for example, the government granted access to publicly sponsored vocational rehabilitation not just for those who had incurred a disability in the line of duty but to any former service member whose disability was "incurred, increased, or aggravated while a member of such [military] forces, or later developing a disability traceable in the opinion of the board to service." Four years later, in 1923, Congress amended the War Risk Insurance Act to stipulate that if the VB issued a veteran a disability rating of at least 10 percent due to tuberculosis or neuropsychiatric disease within three years of discharge, the condition would be considered service-connected.[123] Those and other piecemeal legislative measures resulted from the administrative challenge of tracing chronic conditions to service, and to strong advocacy efforts on the part of veterans' groups. They helped pave the way for broader changes to come.

By the time the World War Veterans' Act came up for debate, the Veterans Bureau had become a vast bureaucracy. Since its inception in 1921, the agency had disbursed more than $40 million for hospital-related expenses. In January 1924, it had 157,000 claimants and was paying for the care of more than 18,000 hospital patients: approximately 7,800 of them were being treated for tuberculosis, 6,200 for neuropsychiatric conditions, and 4,400 for general medical and surgical issues.[124] Between 1919 and 1921, advocates worked to ensure that former service members could receive care while remaining in close proximity to loved ones. In so doing, they pushed for a Veterans Bureau hospital system that consisted of relatively small institutions scattered throughout the country. By 1924, there were more than forty Veterans Bureau hospitals that specialized in tuberculosis, neuropsychiatry, or general medicine and surgery.[125]

Ironically, by the mid-1920s, the problem of a lack of beds had been replaced by the problem of what some said were too many beds. There were plenty of examples of supply—and provisions of previously approved hospital plans—exceeding demand. In February 1923, George H. Wood, president of the Board of Managers of the National Home for Disabled Volunteer Soldiers, said the branches of his service did "not have the number of patients from the Veterans' Bureau" previously expected. For example, a $50,000, thousand-bed annex had been built at the Western Soldiers' Home in order to provide care for two hundred Veterans Bureau patients. Wood reported that he received a letter from Charles Forbes in July 1922 (once the building was complete) "cancelling all reservations." Now, "Annex R" stood "completely closed, with no patients in it." Wood surmised that "there is no demand in that district. In fact, I might say that the number of patients treated by the Veterans' Bureau has decreased in the last year, and has not increased, while the number of hospitals for their care has been so decidedly increased . . . that they have a superfluity of facilities."[126] By January 1924, when the World War Veterans' Act was under discussion, approximately 25 percent of the Veterans Bureau's sixteen thousand hospital beds were empty.[127]

But the problem could not be summed up simply as oversupply. Demand for hospital services varied by locale, specialty, and—in the case of a diagnosis like tuberculosis—the season. So while some facilities were sparsely populated, others were filled to capacity. Furthermore, although the number of neuropsychiatric patients in VB hospitals steadily increased between 1919 and 1924, the number of tuberculosis and general medical cases decreased overall during the same period.[128]

In debates regarding the World War Veterans' Act, advocates argued that huge numbers of empty beds had more to do with rules about disability ratings and diagnoses than they did with "overhospitalization," or real levels of demand. There were plenty of veterans who needed treatment, said VB director Frank Hines, but the bureau denied their claims because their disabilities were not considered connected to service.[129]

Hines relied on a pragmatic argument to justify why VB hospitals should be opened to such patients: empty beds led to decreased efficiency; expanding access to more veterans was the most viable option for improving services across the board. "It is better if the government uses the facilities to their full load which you have spent some $41,000,000 to build than to have vacant beds," he said.[130] In other words, now that the veterans' medical system existed, access to it had to be expanded in order for it to be most effective.

Providing care to more veterans made sense from an administrative standpoint as well, according to a representative of the Veterans of Foreign Wars, which was, in the early 1920s, dominated by elderly former service members, and eagerly "seeking to make inroads with Great War veterans."[131] The VFW's Edwin Bettelheim noted that the reviews of records necessary in order to prove service connection were time-consuming and costly. "Rather than go through all the administrative work of investigating and segregating, Bettelheim said, the VB should "take care of the man as he comes knocking at your door."[132] Treating all veterans who sought care, as opposed to only some, advocates counterintuitively argued, would help alleviate wastefulness.

Bettelheim and others also argued that the neediest and most worthy cases would receive care first and assured legislators that demand would remain manageable. Wasn't it worth spending $4 or $5 million per year, Bettelheim asked, "to take care of these men that will become a charge on some community"? It was illogical to assume that "veterans will be out and try to get all the hospital treatment they can."[133] In fact, said the VB's Frank Hines, a vast majority of the 4 million people who served during the war would "prefer to go to hospitals of their own selection and under their own doctors." Hines predicted that the number of people being discharged from veterans' hospitals would balance the numbers being newly admitted and that even once all veterans were granted the right to hospitalization, the patient load "will not, as we go along, be very much greater than the load we have carried in the past." The VB director went so far as to guarantee that it would be unnecessary to build any new facilities as a result of the proposed legislation.[134]

Legislators rejected such optimistic forecasts and voiced deep skepticism about the premise of the proposal. Above all, Republicans and Democrats alike were astonished by the sheer magnitude of the request. "Would it be true to say that we are adopting a new principle, if we establish the precedent of undertaking to furnish hospitalization for 4,000,000 of our people during the terms of their lives?," asked Robert Luce (R-MA). Alfred L. Bulwinkle (D-NC) was also baffled and expressed the incredulity many southern whites would doubtless harbor regarding such a request: "You do not recommend that every man who walks up to a hospital with a discharge in his hand with some ill, regardless of his financial standing, shall be admitted to that hospital?"[135] The measure would cost "billions of dollars," said James H. MacLafferty (R-CA). After all, "during a man's life there would be a vast amount of sickness that could not be connected with the service."[136] Homer P. Snyder (R-NY) conceded that there was a "crying need" for better policy in the short-term, "but whether it should be carried to the extent of all time is another story."[137] John E. Rankin (D-MS) was most definitive in his disapproval. "You are throwing the door wide open," he told Bettelheim. "You are going to have a pension roll here that will make the pension roll of the Civil War look like a tip to the waiter."[138] Luce questioned the contention that no new facilities would be necessary in order to fulfill the mandate in the proposed legislation: "Don't you see, if we establish the principle of free hospitalization for all veterans, it would then be incumbent upon us to furnish the facilities."[139]

Congressional representatives also disagreed on an ideological level with the proposal. Rankin, like those who had fought against granting blanket pensions in the nineteenth century, argued that offering special treatment to ex-soldiers amounted to creating a privileged class. "Why limit it to soldiers?," he asked:

> Why should we come up here 25 years after the war closes and say to this man . . . "you say you served a few weeks or months in the training camp. Of course you did not get across; you did not get hit. But you come up here 25 years after the war is over and you contract measles or you break your leg, and you can go into the hospital now and stay there the rest of your life." Because when you get them in there, believe me, there will be many a one who will stick. Here is another man who had a wife and children to support. He contributed whatever we required of him. He would have gone if the draft had demanded it. He is down and out, and has some incurable disease. Possibly he has reached the age of 70. You say to him, "oh no you are precluded from this." He is just as likely to become a public charge as I am. If you are going to put that on the ground that these men are likely to become a public charge, do not let us narrow it down to the men who have served a short time in the Army, Navy or Marine Corps.

The legislation in question was a "veterans' proposition," Bettelheim succinctly responded, "and it is not our province to advocate something for others."[140]

Robert Luce shared Rankin's sentiment but was most perturbed by the degree of government intervention called for by the legislation. "We are opening up . . . a very important problem," he said. "Because it involves an immeasurable expense over 50 to 75 years, but also involves a long step toward that centraliza-

tion of activities which some people call socialism." By granting millions of former service members access to government hospitals, he suggested, communities
would no longer be encouraged to collectively provide the institutions necessary to care for their neighbors. "You are throwing away . . . the idea of local
responsibility."[141]

In the face of such skepticism, a few distinct historical circumstances paved
the way for the passage of the World War Veterans' Act. A major factor contrib-
uting to its ultimate approval and leniency was the emergence in the early to
mid-1920s of a particular "subgovernment," wherein a congressional committee,
veterans' advocacy groups, and the Veterans Bureau formed a consolidated and
highly effective political force.[142] Congress established the Committee on World
War Veterans' Legislation on January 14, 1924, following a House debate during
which Bertrand Snell (R-NY) justified its necessity by arguing that "it is impossible to get all veterans to agree . . . we are not taking anything away from
[Spanish-American or Civil War veterans], their legislation will go to the same
committees it always has, we are simply now trying to help out the World War
veterans."[143] Headed by Royal C. Johnson, a South Dakota Republican, Legionnaire, and fiercely committed veterans' advocate, the World War Veterans' Committee provided a forum where the Legion, Veterans of Foreign Wars, Disabled
American Veterans, and other advocacy groups could present proposed legislation and receive a prompt and sympathetic hearing. Its existence meant that
advocates could "concentrate their . . . work on relatively few legislators and
staffers."[144] The World War Veterans' Act, for example, resulted from the "amal-
gamation of corrections, additions, and other changes" on which advocates and
legislative committee members could all agree.[145] Although representatives like
Luce and Rankin may have harbored reservations about legislative proposals,
they and other committee members showed a willingness to work through them
until they could gain the congressional backing necessary for passage.

The World War Veterans' Act also met with approval because the majority of
its measures were aimed at an impetus most elected officials could support: ensuring that the Veterans Bureau could function more smoothly—that it could
more efficiently allocate material benefits like medical care, insurance, and vocational training. When it came time to vote on the act, legislators trumpeted
the bill as a stunning accomplishment, and (as was the case regarding legislation
establishing the VB), even those who initially voiced skepticism about some
details of the bill eventually expressed strong support for it. "I am glad today that
the House of Representatives is going on record, and I doubt not practically

unanimously, before the disabled men of this country to the effect, 'Fellows, we have said in the past that nothing was too good for our disabled men, now here is what we proposed to do at the present time. It is yours and you are welcomed to it.'" said James MacLafferty. John Rankin boasted that each member of the Committee on World War Veterans' Legislation had worked out particulars in the act "actuated by a desire to do the best he could for the disabled ex-service men." Although the bill was not perfect, these legislators argued, it went a long way in enhancing the rights of worthy veterans. Robert Luce joined his fellow committee members in a chorus of self-congratulations, "indorsing what has been said about their absolute freedom from partisanship and also testifying as to their lack of self-assertion, their anxiety to reconcile conflicting views, their unanimous desire to dispense not only justice but also equity." Like the bill establishing a Veterans Bureau, the WWVA passed in the House with no opposing votes.[146]

At a time when hospitals were only just beginning to emerge as desired sites of care and their long-term costs were virtually unknown, providing access to government institutions seemed to many to be a fair price to pay to ensure the well-being of former service members.[147] In fact, rhetoric surrounding health benefits contained in the World War Veterans' Act (passed in June 1924) was starkly different from that pertaining to a more well-known piece of legislation, the Adjusted Compensation Act (passed in May 1924). The latter granted veterans of World War I the right to collect a payment in 1945 equivalent to approximately $1 per day for their time in service. Adjusted compensation, or the provision of a cash "bonus" for all former service members—even those who had served just a short time—drew the ire of many who saw it as "class legislation."[148] In his State of the Union address in December 1923, Calvin Coolidge unapologetically noted that he did not "favor the granting of a bonus" but recommended "that all hospitals be authorized at once to receive and care for, without hospital pay, the veterans of all wars needing such care, whenever there are vacant beds, and that immediate steps be taken to enlarge and build new hospitals to serve all such cases."[149] Coolidge and others could, in good conscience, support the seemingly humane ideal of providing access to hospital care for veterans, even as they rejected the rationale of cash payments.[150]

Furthermore, politicians who had supported the bonus legislation felt it their responsibility to offer an extra entitlement to ill and wounded veterans and expressed relief that the WWVA was virtually uncontroversial. "Those of us that took a stand for the service men recently in the matter of adjusted compensation have heard some criticism," said James MacLafferty. "That is an open question, but, thank God, on this question there is no debate necessary." John Rankin joined MacLafferty in his "gratification over the fact that there will not be much criticism of the members of the Veterans' Committee" regarding their support for the World War Veterans' Act.[151]

The ongoing congressional investigation of Charles Forbes and the Veterans Bureau helped the advocates' cause. Released the day before the WWVA became law, a congressional report regarding allegations painted a dark picture, noting that it would "probably never be known how much money was spent for makeshift expedients."[152] Evidently, at least some of the millions of dollars allocated for veterans' services and programs had never been used for their intended purposes. The World War Veterans' Act was a fresh start—a way to make things right. It did "a great deal to clear the situation," as one congressman put it, "and covers many deficiencies that have been discovered in the actual enforcement of the law."[153]

As it turned out, legislators who had worried about the expansiveness of some provisions of the World War Veterans' Act were more accurate than VB director Frank Hines, who maintained that the legislation would result in somewhat of an increase in the VB's number of patients but that there would be a general balancing out of discharges and admissions. By 1930, an "increasing number of hospital admissions each year" had brought about a "growing problem of hospitalization of veterans of the world and other wars, and the necessity for the expansion of government facilities."[154]

The establishment of the Veterans Bureau marked a turning point in the history of veterans' entitlements. After 1921, a multifaceted agency focused solely on providing services and payments to former service members existed separate and apart from other federal departments. It served as a seed for the growth of what became "the single most powerful social policy agency in U.S. history."[155] Advocates cited the pragmatically appealing twin goals of administrative efficiency and fiscal responsibility in order to convince lawmakers to establish the new bureau, and later to extend health services to all veterans, not just those who had incurred their disabilities or illnesses in the line of duty. They fought for their demands based on the notion that the federal government had thus far failed to offer acceptable services, presenting the situation as a catastrophe that could only be alleviated by providing veterans with an unparalleled level of government assistance via an independent agency.

When the VB was established, veterans' groups wished it to be powerful and permanent. Budget-conscious congressional representatives, however, held out hope that it would be a temporary fix to a crisis situation. The agency's first director, Charles R. Forbes, ensured that advocates' hopes were fulfilled and that the new bureau would replace the Department of the Treasury as overseer of hospital building and administration. Pronouncing a determination to sidestep government bureaucracy and prioritize corporate efficiency, he used his independent agency to aggressively grow the number of available veterans' hospitals.

In fact, there was no single moment when the US government definitively legislated a veterans' hospital system. But its roots were planted once Congress approved the Veterans Bureau and vested it with the authority to build institutions and administer medical services. The subsequent, aggressively proactive lobbying of veterans' groups and others, as well as the passage of the 1924 World War Veterans' Act, resulted in generous allotments for the construction of new facilities and a more far-reaching national system of veterans' hospitals than many originally thought necessary or advisable. Looking forward, it gradually became clear that the government would offer a distinct and increasingly valuable entitlement to former service members, and the Veterans Bureau would continue on a growth trajectory. In the short term, however, a host of questions remained about how a young federal agency would run an expansive medical care system and satisfactorily respond to the needs of its many thousands of beneficiaries.

CHAPTER SIX

I Never Did Feel Well Again

Entrenching a Federal Health System

There was rarely an indisputable case. Elam Shirk had served in the army for eight years, including twelve months in France, when he was assigned to be a meat handler at Walter Reed Hospital in 1919. There, he worked with sides of beef upward of 130 pounds and threw out his back. "From then on," he wrote in a letter to a congressional committee in December 1923, "I was never the same man." But Shirk "braved [the] pain, anxious to get out," and after an army medical exam of "fifteen minutes," which he called "a farce," he was released from service with no official disability. In January 1921, four months after being discharged, Shirk took another medical exam, this time to qualify for the civil service and work as a letter carrier. Although it revealed that he had "heart trouble," the Postal Service allowed him to assume his duties. Within a month, Shirk found himself "a complete wreck . . . unable to walk or arise from [his] bed." And he found it difficult to believe that his maladies had developed anywhere but in the military: "This I had when leaving the service," he alleged, "and the doctors that examined me deliberately passed me by." By November 1921, Shirk was back at Walter Reed Hospital, as a patient, his care funded by the Veterans Bureau. Doctors placed him in a brace from his hips to his shoulders and suggested that he wear it permanently. Shirk reported feeling "strapped together" and claimed that it was "agony to work." He was furious that the Veterans Bureau "says I am not handicapped, also no connection with the service."[1]

Edwin Jackson Algeo preferred "home treatment" for his advanced pulmonary tuberculosis, rather than seeking care in a Veterans Bureau hospital in his home state of New York. Institutions there, he maintained, were subpar. But he was disturbed that the VB's home treatment program assumed that veterans would use their disability compensation to pay for outside services, such as x-rays, which caused an undue financial hardship. In his case, there was little money left after he spent $60 of his $73.40 monthly payment on room and board and up to $12 on doctor's bills. The VB, Algeo said, was "economizing at the cost of lives."[2]

Shirk and Algeo joined more than a thousand fellow veterans who shared their stories in letters to a Senate committee investigating the US Veterans Bureau in 1923 and 1924. Newspaper accounts of the congressional investigation focused on the supposed corruption of the agency's recently ousted director, Charles R. Forbes; reports of drunken debauchery at the government's expense sold copy. But veterans' complaints indicated that dissatisfaction with bureau medical care did not begin or end with one man.[3] Indeed, frustration with the VB and its health services persisted throughout the long tenure of Forbes's replacement, Frank T. Hines, who was known for his careful managerial practices.

At the time Algeo and Shirk wrote their letters, the same question that had loomed over veterans' health services since the closing months of the war remained: how expansive and lasting would this burgeoning system be? At least three forces coalesced in the 1920s and early 1930s to bring about tremendous growth in services and spending, and to lay the groundwork for the veterans' health system that endured through the following century. First, administrators proved willing to respond to the demands of veterans and their advocates, who challenged bureau practices surrounding disability ratings and access to care, not least of all when it came to seeking relief for chronic conditions. Second, former service members and local officials relied on VB health institutions as part of a loose welfare network during a time of mounting economic and social challenges. And finally, bureaucrats and government officials made compelling cases for building hospitals. In 1920, there were approximately 43,000 total admissions of veterans to federal, state, and civil hospitals at the expense of the federal government. By 1932, that number had more than tripled, to about 148,000.[4] Around that time, the historian Charles A. Beard pointed out that the gradual expansion of veterans' benefits was hardly unique to the post–World War I era. "As time thins the ranks and wage earners become infirm on account of advancing years," he observed, "the scope of the scheme is widened to include those who are suffering from disabilities no matter how acquired."[5]

An examination of how and why veterans' health services expanded in the years following World War I demonstrates not only how a federally sponsored health system became a lasting reality in the United States but also the messiness of policy formation and implementation. Once the Veterans Bureau was established and federal legislation expanded its powers, former service members proved determined to push the federal government to make good on its promise to ensure their well-being. And bureaucrats in charge of organizing and administering a veterans' health system faced challenging questions about, among other things, how to judge and rate disabilities, who should access care and why, what services to offer, and how to govern relations with local social service organizations. The bevy of orders, rules, and memoranda they articulated—one compendium of regulations and procedures governing the Veterans Bureau from 1922 through 1928 was 2,300 pages long—demonstrates the power of a bureaucracy to define the boundaries of federal policy.[6] And they indicate that a bureaucracy is a tool not only of its managers and department heads but also of its beneficiaries. The Veterans Bureau was at the center of a circular process in the 1920s: in response to veterans' demand for services, advocates and legislators shaped legislation for an expandable agency; administrators then built bureaucratic structures; veterans' experiences within the bureaucracy subsequently shaped their demands for services and further legislation; administrators, advocates, and legislators responded by restructuring legislation and the bureaucracy.

The dynamics of the expansion of health and medical services for veterans in the interwar years highlight the potentially massive, though often subjectively defined, personal and societal long-term consequences of war. Veterans' experiences within the bureaucracy showcased how policy fluctuations and debates about medical treatment and cure played out in individuals' lives. They illustrated that the process of defining service connection, disability, and indigence could be contentious, especially at a moment when poverty and need dominated the lives of many Americans. For some, the Veterans Bureau and its health services became an important part of a porous, locally administered social safety net. Demands for benefits represented an attempt by poor and working-class Americans to obtain a modicum of security from their government.

Veterans' Demands and Tensions over Government Responsibility

In February 1922, John J. O'Brien found a one-page circular from the Veterans Bureau enclosed with his regular government insurance statement. It listed eleven items beneath a bolded heading, "THE UNITED STATES VETERANS' BUREAU IS: 1. Paying out *over* $1,000,000 in cash every day, including Sunday. . . . 2. Providing, without cost, hospital care and treatment to 30,000 veterans. . . . 5. Con-

ducting an insurance business for over six hundred thousand ex-service men. . . .
6. Conducting over fifty thousand medical examinations every month . . ."[7]

O'Brien was infuriated. "Will you kindly tell me where the ex-service man who has been gassed and who has become tuberculous [*sic*] comes in, if he has not made a claim within one year after he left the service?," he wrote in a letter to then VB director Charles R. Forbes, referring to a policy then in place stipulating that a claim for a service-connected disability had to be filed within a certain period. "Thousands of men," O'Brien alleged, were "ill, neglected, disabled, and without any aid from the government."[8]

O'Brien was far from alone in his frustrations. By April 1922, within a couple of months of mailing out the circulars, the VB had received hundreds of them back with similar sentiments scrawled furiously in the margins, along the bottom of the document, or attached in separate notes. Veterans and their advocates wanted to know why "men couldn't get government aid because of the tape being too long and red."[9] In spite of the allocation of hundreds of thousands of dollars, they alleged, "the best of care is not given the men at hospitals."[10] Along with an insurance payment of $6.50, Edgar A. Sentman, of Wingate, Indiana, sent the VB a letter that was more desperate than hostile: "Am sorrow to say son was and ex-service boy and was over sees and was shell shocked and was in a deranged mental condition, for which we failed to get treatment and is know in the U.S. army again somewhere I think in the philipen islands. We have been trying to get in touch with him for the past four months we fear for his safety owing to his condition and do not see how he could get in the army again but will hope for the best."[11]

Veterans' correspondence went beyond claims of neglect. Some alleged that the circular was aimed at undercutting efforts to win an ongoing legislative battle for a cash bonus. "Is this more anti-bonus propaganda?," wondered Orley A. Rhodes.[12] Others took an almost opposite perspective. "A great percentage of this enormous expenditure is wasted because of false claims filed by ex-service men," one veteran remarked.[13] "There seems to be a great incentive to be disabled," another noted sardonically.[14] The expenditures touted in the circular equated to a "waste of money and a disregard for the pocketbooks of the American people," according to one concerned former service member.[15] Amid statements of disappointment and anger, a minority of veterans expressed gratitude and satisfaction. Paul M. Prugh, of Eaton, Ohio, reported receiving "the promptest of service, with the best of attention, at all times."[16] A St. Louis, Missouri, church pastor, who had served during the war as a chaplain, wrote that he felt like "the beneficiary of so many and varied blessings. . . . I have no regrets and should my country ever need me, I am ready to answer at the first 'roll call.' "[17]

In letters of reply to individual veterans, the embattled Forbes pointed out that the mailed circular was not intended to imply that the situation was perfect but merely to offer a blanket response to the many requests he had received for "information . . . as to what the government had done and was doing for ex-service men."[18] Forbes's administrative notes jotted on letters regarding unanswered claims and other systemic shortfalls suggest that the director and his central office colleagues worked to refer cases to the proper divisions or district offices for further action.

Veterans' gripes with the system were diverse and varied—ranging from allegations of excess to deprivation—but they had one thing in common: they were focused largely on negative feelings about the Veterans Bureau. In fact, disabled veterans' "contempt and loathing" for that agency were "beyond their power of expression," according to the protagonist in a 1924 autobiographical novel by Laurence Stallings, whose battle wounds resulted in the amputation of one leg in 1922 and the other twenty years later.[19] Highlighting problems that would grow more challenging over time, those strong emotions were due in part to the fact that patients, doctors, and administrators had widely varying views, expectations, and definitions of government-sponsored medical care.

Federal laws set general rules regarding who could receive care in veterans' hospitals. The World War Veterans' Act attempted to clarify previous legislation by stipulating that the VB was liable to treat veterans suffering from a variety of conditions, including "neuropsychiatric or tubercular ailments," regardless of whether they were "due to military service or otherwise." In addition—and most drastically—the act stated that the director of the VB was authorized, "so far as he shall find that existing Government facilities permit," to treat veterans of any war, occupation, or expedition since 1897, not dishonorably discharged, "provided that preference to [*sic*] admission . . . shall be given to those veterans who are financially unable to pay for hospitalization."[20] Officially, throughout the early 1920s, the bureau prioritized care for veterans with service-connected "compensable" injuries or illnesses—those who had received a disability rating of greater than 10 percent. VB hospital administrators could admit patients in need of emergency care and sort out paperwork later, but they could also deny those who lacked proof of honorable discharge or had non-service-connected conditions, especially if space in a facility was limited. Veterans fought determinedly to prove that they were injured and ill, and that their ailments could be traced to service. Meanwhile, administrators and doctors struggled to keep up with demand.

A few cases are illustrative. Between 1921 and 1923, two pictures emerged of Donald C. McDaniel—one presented in medical reports and affidavits from friends and another in one-page Veterans Bureau ratings sheets. McDaniel enlisted in his home state of Georgia in July 1918 and was discharged a year later, after serving in France as a private with the 161st Engineers. McDaniel was working as a "railroad man" in July 1921 when he arrived at Sawtelle National Soldiers' Home in Los Angeles with various ills. Doctors performed a medical exam then offered treatment at the home while the Veterans Bureau reviewed his claim. According to bureau records, the veteran's conditions included a swollen eye, a sore throat, "heart neurosis," and dental problems.[21]

Had Sawtelle's examiner deemed McDaniels's case nonemergent, or otherwise unworthy of treatment, he could have been sent away from the home while he awaited the decision on his disability claim. Such was the case for Bartley O'Reilly, who was discharged from a veterans' hospital in New York while the VB considered whether to cover the costs of dental, optical, and other services. "I had my teeth pulled in France," he wrote to VB officials, "and never put in." After visiting the hospital twice to check on the status of his claim, he wrote to Washington: "I am stopping with my aunt here until I hear from you, which I hope will be soon."[22]

Veterans who, unlike O'Reilly and McDaniel, sought care outside of government institutions enjoyed no guarantee that the services they received would be reimbursed. Willard L. Ellsworth reported to Portland, Maine, orthopedist, Edville G. Abbott in September 1922, suffering from "pain and stiffness of spine, arthritis of spine; short and painful sciatic nerves. Unable to sleep and tired easily upon any physical exertion." Abbott assessed that the injuries "resulted from the concussion of a high explosive shell during his war service." Between September 1922 and March 1923, Ellsworth rendered payments amounting to more than $620 to Abbott for treatments to relieve his pain.[23] He then wrote to his senator Medill McCormick (R-IL) to ask that he support him in his effort to receive reimbursement from the VB for the medical bills. Ellsworth argued that he had only sought care from Abbott because he felt the VB had failed him; during six months under the care of the private doctor, he said, "I have made more progress than I did in four years under the Veterans' Bureau." Ellsworth was adamant: "*I have had several years of needless suffering*. Is it not my paramount right to regain the health which I lost because of my service? The Veterans Bureau was either unable, or uninterested enough to restore me to complete health. Am I to be penalized then because I am *seeking*, and *finding*, complete restoration to health?"[24] In response, L. B. Rogers, assistant director of the VB Medical Division, noted that the bureau was not authorized by law to reimburse private physicians. But there were "one or two conditions" under which it might: if treatment had been rendered "in the case of a medical emergency" or if a claimant was "at the time he contracted the expense ignorant of his right to treatment by the U.S. Veterans Bureau." Although it seemed that Ellsworth's case fit neither condition, Rogers assured Senator McCormick that the veteran's claim would receive "careful and thorough study."[25]

The cases of Ellsworth and others show that veterans had their own interpretations of the government's promises to provide for them, which could be disputed. Thomas L. McCarthy, for example, requested in 1922 that the Veterans Bureau reimburse him for care he received at a private tuberculosis sanatorium. But the claim was denied for at least two reasons. First, his condition was not judged to be due to service, which, prior to the 1924 passage of the World War Veterans Act, meant that he could not access free care. Second, like Ellsworth, McCarthy was evidently not "ignorant" that he could be cared for in a government institution or "a suitable hospital."[26]

But admission to a government facility was no guarantee that the VB would judge patients' conditions as service-connected or, by extension, that care would be rendered indefinitely. Donald McDaniel, the railroad man with eye, heart, and dental problems, was treated at Sawtelle National Soldiers' Home for a variety of conditions but was then informed that none of them were due to service. Doctors diagnosed him with dacryocystitis in his left eye—commonly exhibited as inflammation and swelling—and "neurasthenia cardiac neurosis and asthenia." Within weeks of the exams, McDaniel received the news from the VB central office that because his vision had been rated 20/30 when he first enlisted, his eye condition "existed prior to enlistment and was not aggravated by the service." Additionally, he was told that his "neuropsychiatric disability" was "not of service connection and does not come under Public 47"—a reference to a law stipulating that claims for service-related tuberculosis and neuropsychiatric disease had to be filed within two years of discharge.[27]

In response to the ratings decisions, McDaniel sent affidavits from fellow veterans substantiating his claim that his service had brought about a precipitous deterioration in his physical and mental well-being. Joseph Waters and Lyle T.

Smith, who served with McDaniel in France, reported to the VB that their comrade had been hospitalized in the winter of 1918 in France for a "bad eye and seemed over-fatigued." A woman named P. J. Brosnan noted that since she had met McDaniel around the time of his discharge, "he was extremely nervous, had eye trouble, and was unable to do much work." VB administrators were unconvinced; the evidence was "determined to be insufficient to warrant the reopening of the case." On March 19, 1922, McDaniel had another physical exam and was diagnosed with dacryocystitis (again) and neurasthenia, but the final prognosis helped explain why he would find little relief from the government in the near future: "No affective disturbance. Hypochondriacal trend." Not only could the veteran's conditions not be clearly traced to service, according to VB examiners, but they also did not drastically impede his ability to work. The battle continued in 1922 and 1923. George A. Kramm said that during the ten years he was acquainted with McDaniel prior to the war, "he was in good health, but that after his return he noticed that he was suffering from a nervous breakdown and stomach trouble." Other friends noted that McDaniel "appeared run down in health and has spells of vomiting and nervousness" and that he was subject to "cough and vomiting spells," was "unusually nervous, worked very little, and appeared to be in a general rundown state of health."[28]

The VB's subsequent ratings decisions—which were prompted by the new evidence submitted by McDaniel but all based on the physical exam completed in March 1922—exemplified why many veterans came to believe that their ratings were based not mainly on their level of suffering but instead on arbitrary government statutes. In response to the veteran's claims, the VB affirmed the original decision: none of his ailments were worthy of compensation or connected with his time in service. By May 1923, the assessment on his ratings sheet no longer referenced Public Law 47 regarding the timely filing of claims; instead, it justified lack of service connection by noting that McDaniel's "case does not fall under the terms of the first proviso, Section #2, of the Amendatory Act, Public 542, 67th Congress."[29]

Veterans voiced frustration that medical exams often contradicted ratings, and that their access to treatment and compensation payments could be abruptly reduced or halted. "I was wounded and gassed in the war, drew compensation for a time and then was informed by the wise guys up at Washington that my disability had decreased and that my compensation would be discontinued," Missourian Charles Strickel wrote to the bureau's central office in 1922. "You see they knew all about me," he added sarcastically. "They were in Washington and

I was here."[30] John J. Murphy wrote to Senator George H. Moses (R-NH) in July 1924 to express similar misgivings. His monthly compensation of $30, which was awarded because he injured his back at Camp Travis, Texas, in 1918, was eventually cut to $20, and then to $10. A dejected Murphy noted, "my condition is no better, but worse if anything, than at the time $30 a month was received."[31] When Peter Echo was asked to report to the VB's Philadelphia office for a general examination, he "was informed from the doctors . . . that I had serious disabilities." Nonetheless, Echo's disability rating was dropped from 50 percent in 1921 to 10 percent in 1923. In 1922, after the rating was lowered, he was denied a request for hospitalization.[32]

The cases of McDaniel, Strickel, Murphy, and Echo make it clear that former service members gained access to treatment and compensation not mainly based on their own understandings and representations of illness and injury but instead on doctors' and bureaucrats' sometimes inconsistent impressions and diagnoses and on legal interpretations of a bevy of fluctuating federal laws regarding disability and work. They were at a loss to understand how the VB could judge their conditions "without letting a man open his mouth to prove his disability," as veteran Bartley J. O'Reilly put it.[33]

VB administrators' responses to such complaints show how veterans' demands could foster bureaucratic reorganization and expansion. Between 1921 and 1924, patients like McDaniel might be in contact with or receive medical examinations at more than 120 VB "suboffices" around the country or at hospitals run by the Veterans Bureau, the Public Health Service, or Soldiers' Homes. The agency then sent paperwork regarding their cases to one of fourteen district offices throughout the country, which each contained "medical rating sections" made up of doctors who were specialists in "various branches of medical service." Finally, the VB forwarded "problem cases" and the claims of those with the most severe disabilities to the central office in Washington, DC, where a medical board of review or board of appeals studied the relevant records and came to a final decision. Between July 1921 and June 1922, the central office reviewed more than 45,000 claims—McDaniels's among them.[34] By 1923, VB director Frank Hines was publicly acknowledging the problem that veterans had been raising. He was eager, he said, to combat "deserved criticism that the bureau was making 'paper ratings.'" As such, the VB established ratings boards in late 1923 in all regional offices "so the bureau and claimant may meet." Local offices would be responsible for rating disabilities, though appeals would still be handled by the central office.[35] During 1924 debates about the World War Veterans' Act, Frank Hines trumpeted the value of "decentralization" so claimants could feel they were being heard and answered by the agency.[36]

Although it indicated responsiveness, the solution did little to quell the growing concerns of doctors, who loathed the idea of acting as go-betweens for patients and claims review boards and believed the process led to higher rates of hospitalization. Haven Emerson, medical adviser to the Veterans Bureau and later director of Columbia University's School of Public Health, told attendees of the American Hospital Association's 1921 annual meeting that hospitals should not be used to "maintain and continue the status of total temporary compensation but to diagnose and treat the sick, and in so doing to accomplish so much by treatment that a prompt and reasonable reduction in compensation due to diminished disability may be determined." Emerson argued that in the VB model, the patient viewed the doctor as a gatekeeper of government benefits, which "caused that alteration in the normal relation between the sick and the well, between patient and doctor, between patient and hospital."[37] In essence, Emerson implied, in the veterans' medical system, patients were not seeking cure eagerly enough because they could gain financially from claiming ill health. They were, he alleged while addressing the Mississippi Valley Tuberculosis Conference, "eager to be found sick."[38] That posed a challenge for doctors, who saw healing as their primary purpose. It also served as one potential explanation for the growth in the number of patients treated in bureau hospitals.

Doctors and patients alike found it difficult to fathom that men like Bartley O'Reilly and Donald McDaniel received disability ratings from a far-flung administrative office, sometimes long after physical examinations. A manual for medical examiners of the Veterans Bureau noted that doctors should not express their opinions regarding service connection or the amount of compensation a patient deserved, "nor will the examiner make any promises as to the treatment which the patient will receive." Those sorts of decisions, according to the manual, should be left to a medical rating board.[39] According to a memo from VB medical director L. B. Rogers to hospital staff, the policy stemmed from the concern that the bureau was "incurring much criticism as a result of officers in hospitals expressing their personal opinion to claimants and other persons interested, as to the percentage of rating that should be received on the disability."[40] Strictly speaking, Rogers said, bureau disability ratings were based on section 302 of the War Risk Insurance Act and the degree of "reduction in earning capacity."[41] "Very few, and in fact practically none of our medical examiners in the field," he contended, "are at all familiar with the subject of disability ratings." Such work was "highly technical and requires special education and training."[42]

While federal legislation provided a general framework for determining who could obtain care and compensation, disability ratings more directly determined individual access to benefits. In order to simplify the rating process and to respond to widespread complaints about the agency's amorphous classifications, the VB revised its disability schedules in the mid-1920s. When the agency was established in 1921, it used rating tables originally devised by the Bureau of War Risk Insurance. They specified levels of "medical impairment" as "temporary total," "permanent total," "permanent partial," and "temporary partial."[43] The definitions of those terms were shrouded in some secrecy; VB officials regularly denied requests from congressional representatives and leaders of advocacy organizations like the American Legion to view them.[44] By 1925, director Frank Hines acknowledged that the rating schedules were in need of updating. Securing the aid of actuarial experts and implementing the changes, Hines reported, was a monumental challenge: "In volume, comprehensiveness, and complexity the new schedule must necessarily go far beyond any work previously attempted along occupational lines, and . . . must be largely a pioneer effort on the part of the United States Veterans Bureau."[45]

The VB enlisted the help of insurance experts who had been involved in devising the Workmen's Compensation, Insurance, and Safety Act of California—one of the more intricate and generous state workers' compensation laws on the books—to rework its ratings tables.[46] By 1927, Hines could report that a new schedule provided a "relatively liberal allowance . . . for actual disablement which in turn has resulted in a material increase in the average value of awards and the monthly disbursements."[47]

Before the ratings overhaul was complete, Hines spearheaded a sweeping effort to "review all temporary awards with a view to putting them on a permanent basis wherever possible," to avoid the administrative expense and difficulty of repeatedly performing medical examinations.[48] Beneficiaries who were rated as permanently disabled with any condition aside from tuberculosis would only be reexamined at their own request. Those rated as permanently disabled with tuberculosis were reexamined every eighteen months.[49]

Both the "decentralization" of ratings, and the move toward "permanent" ratings were aimed at improving services, but the changes had another direct result: an immediate expansion in the VB's administrative capacity. Agency officials believed that fewer physical exams would mean fewer complaints about "paper ratings" and would foster "a notable economy in cost of administration."[50] If they accomplished those results, they also made veterans' hospitals indefinitely accessible to thousands more veterans. In 1922, 13 percent of disabilities were rated as permanent; by 1925, more than 48 percent of veteran beneficiaries were classified as permanently disabled.[51]

While many saw the rationale in allowing disability ratings to determine access to cash payments, patients, administrators, and representatives of social service organizations voiced concerns regarding using them in order to restrict access to care. In 1923, F. A. Fearney, chief of the regional rating division based in Boston, was especially worried about a rule then in place dictating that veterans who had disabilities of less than 10 percent could not obtain free treatment. "The present rating schedule . . . works many hardships upon the ex-soldier who has disabilities of service origin," Fearney told the central office Medical Division in 1923. He suggested that such claimants—even if they were rated at less than 10 percent—be permitted free hospitalization. The government, he noted, "would gain by this action in reducing its future liability on certain disabilities." Fearney cited a specific case of a priest who had served overseas and been diagnosed with six disabilities of service origin, all at less than 10 percent. "The government with one hand decorated him for his bravery, and with the other restrained him from receiving treatment under the law for service incurred disabilities."[52]

That a great many veterans sought care for chronic illnesses rather than visible wounds of battle meant that VB doctors, administrators, and patients faced the same difficult questions plaguing the army and PHS medical systems: Who should have access to care? When should a patient be considered cured? To what extent was the government responsible for ensuring that a patient could be productive following treatment? How should productivity be defined? Throughout the 1920s the VB hosted conferences and forums to seek advice from medical experts on tuberculosis, neuropsychiatric diseases, and an array of other chronic conditions. Laws and general orders were revised countless times to reflect changing beliefs and ideals, bringing about both confusion and a lack of consistency in treatment. The undeniable reality was, as the 1924 VB annual report noted in reference to neuropsychiatric illnesses, "as one gets farther away from the cessation of the war, there are more and more of these whose disabilities have been continuous since discharge that will not recover." And at least some of those patients would "require custodial care in an institution the remainder of their lives."[53]

"The service that I rendered . . . was just as true"

Veterans' health services expanded in the 1920s in part because of rising demands from marginalized groups. Their struggles for access to care forced VB administrators and staff to confront confounding questions regarding entitlement—as had army, BWRI, and PHS officials before them. In June 1925, 241 women and 1,791 black men were receiving hospital treatment sponsored by the bureau. At that point, the latter group constituted 8 percent of the total veteran hospital population of about 26,610.[54] By 1932, numbers of minority veterans in government hospitals had increased alongside numbers of their white, male counterparts, though they remained relatively low; by the end of the fiscal year, more than 3,300 African American men and 330 women were under treatment. Approximately 80 percent of the 11,300 black former service members admitted to hospitals were treated for general medical conditions, 11 percent for tuberculosis, and 10 percent for neuropsychiatric disease. Likewise, 77 percent of the 1,127 women admitted as veteran-patients in 1932 had general medical conditions, while 15 percent sought care for neuropsychiatric diseases.[55] All told, between June 1923 and June 1941, the number of women veterans remaining in hospitals at the expense of the government almost doubled, from 220 to 404, and the number of black men receiving hospital care quadrupled, from approximately 1,300 to 5,540 (figure 6.1). In the same period, the total number of veterans remaining in hospitals increased more than twofold, from 23,600 to 58,160.[56]

In some cases, advocates teamed with government officials and local boosters in the 1920s to extend access to care. Secretary of War John W. Weeks wrote to the president of the National Home for Disabled Volunteer Soldiers in June 1923 after receiving a visit from a woman veteran who notified him that a great many "former enlisted women" had "developed serious troubles." Why, he wondered, were "these young women . . . not entitled to the same consideration given to males who enlisted at the same time and under the same general conditions."[57] In March 1924, the Los Angeles Chamber of Commerce urged the director of the Veterans Bureau to build a medical facility for female veterans near the city, justifying the request by pointing out that "large numbers" of the women who "were subject to the hardships of service the same as the men" had "since the war broken down from the ravages of tuberculosis and other diseases."[58]

Mainstream veterans' advocacy groups joined the call for facilities for women veterans. In the American Legion, the Disabled American Veterans, and the Veterans of Foreign Wars, white women were treated as a class apart, but they fared

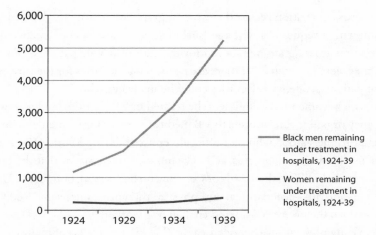

Figure 6.1. Number of minority veterans remaining in hospitals, 1924–39. *Annual Report of the Administrator of Veterans' Affairs for the Fiscal Year Ended June 30, 1941* (Washington, DC: GPO, 1941), 48

better than veterans of color. For example, from the Legion's inception, women who were regularly commissioned as nurses in the US Army, Navy, or Marine Corps were eligible for membership. Indeed, the organization's official policies consistently noted the necessity of obtaining rights for "service men and women," and all-female posts were established in various locations. In 1921, a report from the Legislative Committee to the annual convention noted, "your committee has not been unmindful that women as well as men who served in the Great War are eligible to [*sic*] the benefits of hospitalization, compensation and vocational training."[59] Behind the scenes, too, American Legion officials pushed VB administrators to make more facilities accessible to women beneficiaries. Percy J. Cantwell, secretary of the Legion's New England District Rehabilitation Committee told the agency's medical director in February 1925 that he was "deeply interested, as are many other legionaires" in the matter of hospital facilities for "female beneficiaries."[60] Around the same time, Edwin Bettelheim of the Veterans of Foreign Wars told Frank Hines that there were 2,700 women in the New England area with "no hospital facilities to take care of them" since "none of the Veterans Bureau Hospitals had thought of making provisions to receive and care for the female sex."[61]

The VB's central office was also concerned with ensuring that services were available for women veterans. In the spring of 1923, veterans' hospital administrators across the nation received a two-paragraph letter from the VB's Medical Division with a request: "advise the Bureau at your earliest convenience of the facilities now existing at your station for the care of female patients." Furthermore, they were instructed, "If there are no available facilities for the care of this class of patients, state what facilities could be made available."[62]

But which women were eligible to be treated in VB facilities, and how would the agency organize care? Access to VB medical services for women was initially restricted to the 34,000 who had officially enlisted during World War I: army nurses, marinettes, yeomanettes, and navy nurses.[63] That meant that the bureau barred from its facilities thousands of women who had served, both in the United States and abroad—occupational and physical therapists, dieticians, Red Cross nurses—since they were considered civilian war workers.

The Women's Overseas Service League (WOSL), made up of members who had served abroad during wartime in social service organizations as well as the military, brought public attention to their fight for access to hospitals and Soldiers' Homes. The group pointed out that when women returned home after serving outside the country with nongovernmental groups like the YWCA, the Red Cross, the Salvation Army, and the Jewish Welfare Board, they "signed releases absolving from further responsibility the organizations which had sent them." Such women were "more or less helpless because of hardships endured in the war," and many "are or were self-supporting women and persons of limited means." The problem was health-related, above all else, the group maintained. "Thousands of women are breaking down as a result of their service during the war and means must be devised for looking after them properly," proclaimed Anne Hoyt, chairman of the WOSL's 1925 New York City convention. "At present in the majority of cases there is no way of getting aid from the Government, and tuberculosis and other manifestations of impairment of physical faculties due in large measure to hardships undergone in the service of their country are beginning to take a heavy toll."[64]

Women who sought care from the government faced the same sorts of access restrictions as their male counterparts, and they had a similar range of health conditions. Service-connected disabilities of "compensable" degree received priority for treatment, though women with non-service-connected conditions could be treated if facilities were available.[65] In addition to receiving medical care, women beneficiaries were eligible for disability compensation, but individual cases proved complex. A 1923 report broke down into four categories disabilities for which 323 women beneficiaries were receiving compensation: 181 had problems with the "circulating system," 16 with "endocrinea," 82 with the "nervous system," and 44 had "psychiatric diseases."[66] Medical officer H. C. Watts of District 12, which covered the San Francisco area, wrote to the central office in January 1924 to share information about "the various females now hospitalized who will need continuous hospitalization." Louise Herbster had carcinoma of the breast, which had metastasized to her lung. Although her disability was not service-connected, Watts said, she was "in such a condition that we cannot discharge her." Dorothy Easterly was receiving care for double mastoiditis—an infection behind each of her ears. Additionally, she was, according to Watts, "suffering with neurasthenia and is in such a condition that it would not be advisable to have her transferred to any other institution." Thea Hauge had heart problems, including myocarditis and hypertrophy, which were determined to be service-connected, as well as a tumor in her left breast deemed to be not of service origin.[67]

Of course, before Hines mandated in 1924 that permanent ratings should be used whenever possible, diagnoses and ratings of Hauge and other women—like male beneficiaries—often changed over time. A 1925 report regarding seventy-seven women in the New York region receiving compensation for neuropsychiatric disabilities showed that a beneficiary might be examined and rerated as many as seven times within four years. For example, she might be classified as "temporary partial less than ten percent (neurasthenia)" in 1921 and "temporary total N.P. rating" in 1925.[68]

Achieving the goal of offering treatment to all bureau beneficiaries in VB hospitals, rather than contract or other government facilities, posed a special challenge when it came to women patients. All of the women Watts referred to in the San Francisco area were housed in private hospitals, demonstrating a larger trend: more than 30 percent of women admitted for hospital treatment in 1925 received care in state or civil institutions (versus approximately 14 percent of male patients).[69] According to a June 1924 report, government hospitals offered relatively limited facilities for women VB patients. According to a VB memo, in 1924, just nineteen beds were available in government hospitals across the nation for women patients with neuropsychiatric diseases: eight in a veterans' hospital in Palo Alto, California; one at Fitzsimmons Army Hospital in Denver, Colorado; and ten at St. Elizabeths Hospital in Washington, DC. Beds for women tuberculosis patients were slightly more numerous: there were 146 beds in veterans' hospitals, 58 in Soldiers' Homes in Wisconsin and California, and 27 in army hospitals in Washington, DC, and Colorado. Beds for women suffering from general medical conditions were also sparse: 33 were available in veterans' hospitals, 18 in Soldiers' Homes, and 9 in army hospitals. In all, 310 government beds were available for female veteran-patients in 1924.[70]

Women veterans and their families, at least in some cases, preferred private facilities to government ones. Four women veterans who were receiving treatment at a Soldiers' Home in California in 1923, for example, objected "strenuously to being retained there."[71] Families of female service members viewed other types of government institutions negatively, too. "There is a definite feeling on the part of the relatives of these patients against their admission to a state hospital," a Boston-based district medical officer reported to Frank Hines in 1924. The administrator was referring to "three psychotic cases among our women beneficiaries," one of whom was "extremely violent at times and at times suicidal. . . . It is believed that the Bureau should take special action in these cases in providing special care in institutions outside of state hospitals."[72] Likewise, Rep. Edith Nourse Rogers (R-MA) wrote to Frank Hines on behalf of the all-female Jane A. Delano American Legion Post in August 1930 to point out that too many women were being sent to government hospitals who "were merely tired out with their work," seemingly because there was nowhere else for them to go. Government hospitals—especially St. Elizabeths—Rogers maintained, could be depressing, and she urged the director to find a way to ensure that women could remain home or in "hospitals for nervous cases" that did not have the stigma of larger federal institutions.[73]

Serving female veteran-patients was a problem of infrastructure and not scale, according to Frank E. Leslie, medical officer in charge at a neuropsychiatric VB hospital in Palo Alto, California. Women "mental patients," he said, constituted "relatively few . . . cases" but "were a great problem." At Palo Alto, a ward of eight beds was "set aside" on the second floor of a hospital building for women patients. It contained its own kitchen, dining room, and sitting room. Although the facilities were more advanced than the ones available for women in many other institutions, Leslie noted that "the present arrangements are not entirely satisfactory" since it was "necessary to conduct all female patients through male services." He proposed offering women treatment at Palo Alto, but in a separate building that would contain physiotherapy and hydrotherapy departments and a room for occupational therapy. Creating such facilities, Leslie suggested, was an important part of the therapeutic regime. "The grounds surrounding this building," he said, "should be arranged with gardens and shrubbery or hedges so laid out as to protect female patients from interference or annoyance by male patients." Leslie recommended constructing a building that could house thirty or forty patients in order to "accommodate all female mental beneficiaries along the West Coast for some time to come."[74]

By the mid-1920s, Frank Hines was considering a variety of approaches to expand facilities for women; the question, from an administrative standpoint, was not *whether* to provide care but *how* to do so. VB officials considered building centrally located large institutions—one in the Midwest and another on the West Coast—strictly for female beneficiaries. But women physicians resisted the model for some of the same reasons that similar ideas were rejected for male veterans. Grace Patrick, a Kansas City doctor and chair of the Americanization committee of the Knights of Columbus Chapter of American War Mothers, wrote to the VB central office in May 1924 to suggest that "the best accommodations for women who served in the World War should be scattered over U.S.A. as annexes to or separate buildings adjacent to other buildings at the various hospitals . . . which would locate the women nearer to their respective homes and relatives."[75]

M. R. Stewart, a physician and senior surgeon with the VB, looked at the issue from an organizational perspective. She visited a veterans' hospital under construction at Excelsior Springs, Missouri, in the spring of 1924 to assess whether it should be devoted solely to women patients. In a memorandum to Frank Hines, she noted that women patients scattered in hospitals across the country—in North Carolina, New Mexico, Colorado, Oklahoma, Wisconsin, and Washington, DC—could be transferred to the new institution. But Stewart was concerned that "there will be some difficulty in filling this hospital to capacity."[76] She suggested surveying patients across the country to ascertain whether they "would accept transfers." Finally, she pointed out, "The opening of a woman's hospital by the U.S. Government will be establishing a precedent . . . its success will mean much to the Bureau and much to the women of the country," but "its failure would bring discredit to the Bureau which would be far reaching."[77] Hospitals for military veterans, Stewart argued, were not just venues for health care but powerfully symbolic political and social institutions.

Throughout the 1920s, the VB pushed ahead with the plan of locating women in institutions along with—though often "segregated" from—male patients. Women and men were often treated together in civilian hospitals and tuberculosis sanatoriums, but VB facility administrators had reservations, and varying degrees of enthusiasm, about the prospect of overseeing "mixed" institutions. R. L. Cook, the medical officer in charge at the veterans' hospital in Houston, reported to Frank Hines in May 1923 that there was "no opportunity for segregation or privacy" for women and that it was therefore "believed impracticable to make arrangements for the reception of female patients at this station."[78] O. C. Willhite, who oversaw the veterans' hospital at Knoxville, Iowa, reported in May 1924 that providing care for women would "necessitate, no doubt, a great deal of remodeling and in addition, it would rob the station of a tuberculosis building for male patients."[79]

Others were more adaptable. In June 1923, the Board of Managers of the National Home for Disabled Volunteer Soldiers released a statement to the organization's district medical offices: "While fully appreciating the fact that the present facilities of the Home had not been designed nor intended for the care and treatment of women . . . every effort must be made to meet this new demand."[80] Around the same time, the Soldiers' Home Board of Managers president, George Wood, noted that some facilities were better suited to the job than others. "There would be hell to pay if we sent the girls up to Battle Mountain," he said, referring to a sanatorium established in South Dakota in 1902.[81] Wood evidently concurred with the relatively common belief that, as one VB medical officer put it, "female patients require more care and better accommodations than do male patients."[82]

As authorities in the central offices of the Veterans' Bureau, National Soldiers' Homes, and the army attempted to decipher the level and extent of need among minority veterans, accessibility for women mirrored that of men; it varied depending on one's personal condition, and in some cases on the mind-set of local officials who acted as gatekeepers to care. In June 1925, L. H. Sinclair, acting manager of the Helena, Montana, regional office, wrote to bureau headquarters that "there has been no provision made for the hospitalization of female and negro beneficiaries." As such, Sinclair "respectfully requested that this office be authorized to make use of the nearest hospital which has facilities for the care of female and negro patients, without obtaining prior authority from the director."[83] Stopping short of suggesting that veterans' hospitals in the region be open to minority veterans, Sinclair suggested that he intended to at least find other facilities that were accessible.

Women, the Montana official's letter shows, were not the only minority group who faced barriers in accessing services through the Veterans Bureau. Accounts of struggles of black veterans to obtain hospital care in the 1920s—not to mention the very existence of the Tuskegee Veterans Hospital—demonstrate that there was no single standard of VB sponsored treatment, and that it was more available to some than others. They also show that individuals from marginalized groups joined a growing chorus of demands for more and better health services for veterans.

While many black veterans received services at Tuskegee Hospital in the 1920s, the majority sought bureau-sponsored treatment at other government institutions that generally embraced local practices when it came to the practice of segregation. Of the 1,791 veterans of color under the care of the Veterans Bureau in 1925, 508 were being treated at Tuskegee and another 101 were housed at St. Elizabeths in Washington, DC, which also served as a home hospital for the local population.[84] The remaining 1,000-plus individuals were scattered in veterans', army, and civil hospitals throughout the country.[85] According to a 1933 report, the agency had "no definite policy relative to the segregation of races" but "insofar as is feasible followed the custom in effect in the various localities in which hospitals are located." The VB offered black patients care in separate wards and, in some cases, separate buildings.[86]

That is, if they could get in to facilities at all. African American veterans faced extra challenges when they attempted to gain access to veterans' hospitals, even if they had valiant military records and service-connected disabilities. In February 1925, the VB faced questions from the NAACP when African American veteran Thomas Albert White, who had been gassed in France, was sent by the Veterans Bureau office in Pittsburgh to the tuberculosis hospital at Dawson Springs, Kentucky. Not only was White relegated to the Jim Crow car in the train on the way to the hospital, but once he arrived he was "told that no negro soldiers were allowed there and was sent back to Pittsburgh." After being rejected, too, from a government hospital in New York, White was sent home, where he was "failing rapidly." E. O. Crossman, medical director of the VB was quick to reply to the NAACP: hospitalization was being arranged at a sanatorium in Dayton, Ohio, he said, and the entire matter was being examined.[87] White's case demonstrates a larger truth, relevant not only to the story of the VB but to any federal program implemented locally: the determination of individuals to abide by customs and practices of segregation posed ideological and physical challenges for an already taxed national bureaucracy.

Solomon P. Suddeth faced similar barriers. When he was inducted by the draft board of Bradley County, Tennessee, in April 1918, he was 23 years old and working as a farmer. Assigned to the 366th Infantry, which participated in some of the bloodiest battles of the war, Suddeth was shot in the hand, which led to the loss of his middle and ring fingers. When he was discharged in March 1919, he returned to Tennessee, married a 27-year-old laundress named Mary Ann Boyles, and began working in a foundry. But like so many war veterans, he found his health slowly deteriorating as the months wore on. In 1923, he arrived at the National Soldiers' Home in Johnson City, Tennessee, with a variety of ailments. There was the hand injury, but he was also suffering from chronic pulmonary tuberculosis and what administrators at the home referred to as "chronic tonsillitis." Suddeth was a resident of the home for about six months, from July through December 1923.[88]

By late December, the veteran was at the Salvation Army on 7th Street in Washington, DC, composing a letter to Campbell B. Slemp, secretary to President Calvin Coolidge.[89] "I am a disabled veteran having been wounded overseas and in addition to my wound, I have lost my health otherwise," he wrote. Suddeth told Slemp he had been awarded compensation, which had been discontinued. "But I am not asking assistance to get my compensation it is a secondary matter to me just now what I want and need is hospital treatment and the same has been denied me." Suddeth's desperation was palpable:

> I am really suffering and need attention yet I am denied hospital treatment because the tuberculosis with which I am suffering is held not of service origins, due to some regulation yet I am suffering with my wounds. I lost two fingers from my right hand due to gun shot wounds received over seas and at times I can hardly use my hand or arm, in spite of this I am denied hospital treatment. I hate to worry you Mr. Slemp But my condition compels me to ask that you do what you can for me that I may go in the hospital at once.

Slemp found the case compelling enough to send Suddeth's letter on to VB director Frank Hines and request that he "look into the matter." Five days later, Hines replied that he would request that the district medical officer overseeing the Washington area contact Suddeth at the Salvation Army address and "arrange for his immediate hospitalization if same is deemed necessary pending the arrival of the records of his case from Atlanta." About a month after Hines replied to Slemp, the veteran had been admitted to Walter Reed Hospital.[90]

But earlier, urgent pleas foreshadowed tragedy. Suddeth died at Walter Reed on January 23, 1924. A few weeks later, his remains arrived back in Cleveland, Tennessee, where his young widow and two sisters attended his funeral at the town's First Baptist Church.[91] Suddeth may have contracted tuberculosis and died whether or not he had served and whether or not he had sought care in veterans' health facilities. But he looked to his military experience as the root cause of his deteriorating health. By virtue of the existence of the VB, he had a place to turn for care, and an entity to fault in the face of disappointing health outcomes.

Around the time of Solomon Suddeth's death, Henry H. Davis contacted legislators with similar complaints, but he used political language, linking his plight directly to bigotry. Davis noted that when he began his service in September 1918 at Camp Meade in Maryland, his "living quarters was a tent" and that he soon became ill. After his "hands and arms begune to swell . . . [to] twice the normal size," he was sent to the base hospital, where he was "operated on for some infections" and confined to bed for five weeks. From then on, Davis said, doctors continued to test his blood and offer him pills, but he "never did feel well again." Still, when he was released from the army on May 8, 1919, his "discharge shoad a reckord of physical conditions good and no one explain to me how that I might secure medical treatment if necessary." Simply put, Davis said, "I went into suvilion life sick."[92]

Within days of his discharge, Davis was "forsed to go to bed" in a Baltimore clinic, where he was diagnosed with incipient pulmonary tuberculosis, tuberculosis of the spine, and a form of arthritis called spondylitis. In Baltimore, Davis received a visit from a Red Cross nurse who explained, as he put it, "what the government had provided for me." The nurse's advice prompted him to visit a Public Health Service hospital, where doctors diagnosed hookworm. During a bedside visit, PHS doctors assured Davis that his disabilities had originated in service or were, at least, agitated while he was in the military. Despite that he was told that he "would never be able to do eny form of labor" again, Davis recalled that a ward surgeon exhibited little sympathy, and told his colleagues: "He is a negrow and he don't nead nothen" other than "a job with a pick and shovel." Three years later, Davis reported, "I am now helpless and pining away with the disobility of T.B. and for the like of medical attention and no way to support myself or my family."[93]

Davis reported that the doctor he saw implied that "my coller kep me from being a born citizen of U.S. States of America, and the act of congress did not prepair nothen for the black man." That, he argued, was a "durty deal . . . I do not denie being a black man but I do want to say that the service that I rendered to the flag of the U.S. was just as true and onest as the whitest man the sun ever shined on." Some day, Davis said, "the negrow haters . . . will want the good will and onest service of the black man again . . . but . . . I don't think that I will ever bee able to render eny more of my service to the U.S."[94] Davis was far from alone in his sentiments. Dissatisfaction with inadequate health treatment and benefits fostered widespread discontent among many African Americans—patients, professionals, and activists alike.[95]

The stories of Solomon Suddeth and Henry Davis show that the problems faced by white former service members were amplified for African American veterans and that black veterans demanded that their government fulfill its stated obligations. For them, there were sometimes insurmountable barriers to government assistance that could foster deep feelings of betrayal and lead to negative health outcomes. They felt that their disability ratings did not adequately represent the extent of their injuries and illnesses; that they were denied proper medical care; that they needed to justify the service they rendered as valiant; and that they could not trust their doctors or VB administrators. When minority veterans struggled against those challenges and fought for more and better services in the 1920s, they helped lay the groundwork for an enduring veterans' health system.

Veterans' Medical Care as Part of a Social Service Network

As Henry Davis's account indicates, the health-related services veterans accessed in the 1920s and 1930s were part of a larger, disparate American welfare state comprising local charities, private businesses, individual citizens, and municipal, state, and federal governments. Veterans who sought care at Soldiers' Homes, hospitals, and prisons, and from local service providers, coped not only with dire medical conditions but also with challenging social circumstances. As economic conditions worsened in the late 1920s and early 1930s, veterans' health struggles became enmeshed in the experience of American poverty.

The notion that veterans' medical care might qualify as anything resembling charity was not only distasteful but simply incorrect, according to some former service members. Many resented being made to feel as though they were simply needy and had not earned—either through service or by virtue of paying monthly insurance premiums—the government benefits they were receiving. "I don't feel like I have got anything for nothing," one ex-soldier told VB administrators. "Please don't forget what the veterans has paid the U.S. what he is still paying and what he has offered for the world," another wrote.[96]

The VB medical system was, first and foremost, a massive public health program that touched families, homes, and communities. "In dealing with the United States Veterans' Bureau beneficiary," VB nurse Harriet Baird noted in December 1925, "you not only have the man himself, you also have the problems of his home and family." On a "lonely country road," Baird met "a claimant living in a tent" who had recently experienced a hemorrhage and had a 104-degree temperature. The nurse rushed to the nearest town to call the bureau's Los Angeles office, which authorized transport to and care in a local hospital.[97]

The VB home nursing service was the agency's version of the visiting nursing services founded across the country in the late nineteenth and early twentieth centuries to alleviate the health consequences of urbanization and treat underserved people in rural areas. Public health nursing allowed educated women to take what would come to be known as an environmental approach to illness, assessing health on an individual basis but also as a product of conditions at work and home. Such a model was predicated on the idea that visiting nurses could bring "'care, cleanliness, and character' to the homes of the sick poor."[98]

But VB nurses in the field faced major challenges in achieving that lofty goal. When nurse Baird visited Mr. G., a victim of tuberculosis who opted for home treatment but hoped to keep his illness a secret from his family, she found that he was sharing a bed with his wife and two-month-old baby, and that his four other children stayed in the same room. When Baird asked Mrs. G. whether her husband was sick, the wife replied, "He takes some kind of spells; he will be standing talking to us when the blood will run out of his nose and mouth; then he will have to go to bed for several weeks." When Baird advised Mrs. G. that "sick people should have their own bed and room, if possible, and exercise precautionary measures with children," the veteran's wife responded that she was glad to provide her husband a bed on the porch.[99]

In some locations, VB personnel and offices were part of a network of interdependent service providers focused on the needs of the working (and nonworking) poor. That was overwhelmingly apparent in Massachusetts, by one account one of the "most decentralized" state models of poor-relief, in which "public welfare remained an overwhelmingly local responsibility," resulting in a "confused, bewildering, administrative pattern."[100] In February 1928, W. T. Eddy of the Office of the Agent for Soldiers' Relief in Fitchburg, Massachusetts, wrote to Frank Ryan, governor of the National Soldiers' Home in Togus, Maine, to inquire whether William Yokela had recently resided at the home. Although the city agency had bought Yokela a ticket to Togus, Eddy said, "it has been reported to us that he has been seen on the street here since that time." Eddy also inquired about the condition of another Fitchburg resident, George A. Leazott, who was "supposed to be suffering from epilepsy" and wondered about "the probability of his treatment affecting recovery." Since the city agency was assisting Leazott's family while he was a resident in the home, Eddy said, "we would very much like to know if we may expect that Mr. Leazott is likely to be restored to an ability to provide for him family [*sic*]."[101]

In the 1920s, government officials' skepticism about whether young veterans could benefit from being placed in Soldiers' Homes gave way to a mutually beneficial partnership. Throughout the decade, the VB funded improvements to various homes and paid a per diem rate for every patient offered care in the facilities. In 1919, there were approximately 2,500 patients considered sick in the hospitals of all ten branches of Soldiers' Homes. By 1930, home hospitals served more than 5,500 patients. The rising population indicated a larger trend. The average number of residents in National Soldiers' Homes decreased from 17,600 to 12,500 between 1913 and 1921, as Civil War veterans died. But after 1921, as World War veterans were discharged and Spanish-American War veterans aged, numbers on the rolls increased, reaching 19,500 by 1930.[102]

Administrators like Togus's governor Ryan viewed their responsibility to veterans expansively and worked with local officials and service providers in an attempt to ensure that they understood and responded to the social needs of veterans and their families. In January 1928, Margaret W. Bridgman, of the Associated Charities of Albany, New York, wrote to Ryan about a resident named Louis Willett who had "required hospitalization for a considerable length of time" but who recently told his wife he planned to return home. Bridgman noted that while Willett was a patient at the home, the War Chest, a locally administered charity, was providing assistance for his family, and they were "getting along very well." Bridgman hoped that the patient would remain in the home until he was "built up": "We wish to impress [Mr. Willett]," she said, "that upon his return the help of the War Chest will be withdrawn and he will be forced to take care of his own family and return to work." Since Bridgman was sure Willett was "unable to do this," she asked Ryan if he could "try to persuade [him] to stay as long as you advise him."[103] Responding, Ryan acknowledged that Willett's "heart trouble" was ongoing and that it was his "endeavor to cooperate in as personal a way as possible with all agencies of your character and with the members themselves [so] the best possible results be obtained."[104] Ryan, too, offered intimate details about patients in an attempt to solicit help from local charities. In his letter to Bridgman, he referred to another patient, James Cady, who had a "nervous condition." Ryan had urged the patient to remain in the home for at least a few months but told Bridgman that there was a hurdle to overcome: Cady was "much upset that his letters to his wife return to him 'not found.'" Ryan wondered whether Bridgman might "be able to induce Mrs. Cady to write [her husband] immediately and regularly." If that were possible, "he would probably remain here."[105]

Local officials turned to the VB as an institutional bulwark, not only against lingering health maladies and broken families but also against the scourges of indigence and vice. Farmington, Maine's municipal court judge, Reginald D. Seavey, wrote to the Soldiers' Home in Togus in January 1934 about a case "which I believe needs a little more consideration than the usual court procedure." Local resident Arthur Roderick was "intoxicated all the time," and "jail sentences are useless . . . for the instant he gets out his first thought is to find something to drink." Seavey, who was holding Roderick in custody for the time being, wondered whether he might be "treated at the hospital for both mental and physical troubles." Roderick, who had served in the army during World War I, had been admitted to the home in 1930 and diagnosed with inflammation of the stomach lining and arthritis. He had since drawn the attention of others in the veterans' welfare network, aside from Seavey. In April 1931, the home commander received a letter from Red Cross headquarters in Washington, DC, noting that Roderick had recently appeared there "as a transient and asked for $10.00 for maintenance." Following the letter, Roderick was admitted to Togus once again; this time his listed conditions included bronchitis, cicatrix (indicating complications related to the healing of a wound), and oral health issues. His intake form also noted: "Very little work during the past few years." Togus implemented its own regiments and disciplinary system in an attempt to rein in potentially unruly residents. By October 1935, Roderick was found guilty during disciplinary hearings at the home for "obstructing medical treatment by being under the influence of liquor on the grounds." Soon after, he was dropped from the rolls.[106]

For Roderick and others, the health-focused institutions and personnel of the Veterans Bureau became in the 1920s and 1930s important elements in an amorphous welfare network. Community organizations and officials turned to them as additional safety nets and valuable resources. Meanwhile, when aiming to assist veterans like William Yokela, George Leazott, Louis Willett, and James Cady, nurses, administrators, doctors, and hospitals viewed the provision of medical treatment and social services as related and connected undertakings.

A Political Push for Expansion

The growth of the veterans' health system was a product not only of demands of social service organizations and veterans, but also the pursuit among politicians

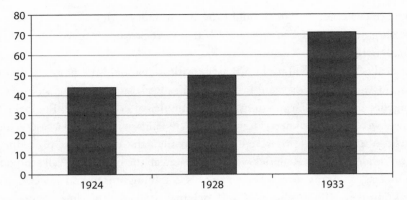

Figure 6.2. Total number of veterans' hospitals, 1924–33. *Annual Report of the Director, United States Veterans' Bureau, for the Fiscal Year Ended June 30, 1924* (Washington, DC: GPO, 1924), 45; *Annual Report of the Director, United States Veterans' Bureau, for the Fiscal Year Ended June 30, 1929* (Washington, DC: GPO, 1929), 13; *Annual Report of the Administrator of Veterans' Affairs for the Year 1933* (Washington, DC: GPO, 1933), 13–14

of the benefits of federalism. Throughout the 1920s and 1930s, local officials and citizens pushed for federal spending on veterans' facilities in their communities in order to create local jobs and boost economies. Their efforts were successful, in part, because the boundaries of veterans' health entitlements remained ill-defined.

From the 1920s on, a steady increase in the number of VB beds and buildings accompanied a rise in the agency's number of beneficiaries. Between 1924 and 1928, the VB went from overseeing 44 hospitals with about 15,600 beds, to overseeing 50 hospitals with a total bed capacity of more than 22,000.[107] By June 1933, the expanded agency was operating hospitals at 71 locations in 43 states and Washington, DC, with a total of 40,213 beds (figure 6.2).[108]

The VB's earliest facilities were simply inherited from the Public Health Service or branches of the military. Some of those institutions had existed long before the war; others had been created at the behest of enterprising politicians and local boosters in the months surrounding the Armistice. In September 1918, a few days after US and French soldiers fought a decisive victory in the Battle of St. Mihiel, David Kincheloe (D-KY) lobbied for federal funding for a veterans' tuberculosis hospital in his wooded, eastern Kentucky district. Kincheloe had approached officials of the Bureau of War Risk Insurance and the Public Health Service about hospital plans in the preceding months, "knowing that there was some talk of this kind of an institution." He pointed out that the proposed site, Dawson Springs, was on the main line of the Illinois Central Railroad route between Louisville and Memphis; it was centrally located; and, perhaps most importantly, a group of the town's businesspeople had come together and obtained 10,000 acres of land, the title of which they were willing to pass on to the US government at no cost. In March 1919, Kincheloe could report to his constituents a big win: Public Law 326 provided $1.5 million in federal funding to construct a tuberculosis sanatorium in Dawson Springs.[109]

Veterans' advocates and congressional representatives realized the potential benefits—economic and social—of federal largesse and sent letters and petitions advocating for the construction of medical facilities for former service members in their communities. A 1921 plea from an American Legion post in North Dakota to congressional representative George M. Young (R-ND) was typical. In a petition, chapter members announced their intent "to enlist [Young's] sympathy with those of our disabled buddies who still lie in pain and suffering in our country's hospitals." In order to get "back of our disabled buddies and . . . better their lot," the advocates suggested, the representative could vote for a variety of bills, including one providing millions of dollars for hospital construction.[110]

The calls continued from advocacy organizations nationwide throughout the 1920s. The Soldiers' Home at Sawtelle, California, was "inadequate to care for many who are seeking entrance," a Los Angeles chapter of the Daughters of Union Veterans of the Civil War reported to the Committee on Military Affairs. Therefore, it petitioned "the Government to immediately erect another hospital at the National Home . . . sufficiently large to accommodate those who need care and medical attention . . . no time [should] be lost in making this very urgent, necessary and important improvement."[111] Such petitions and letters came in groups when specific legislation was being considered and took the form of concerted campaigns. A Stanton, California, Legion post backed up the claims of the Daughters of Union Veterans requesting that a new hospital be built at the Sawtelle home: "It would seem that our government, so vast in its resources, might extend its hand . . . to further generous acknowledgement to those who sacrificed their lives, in time of war, that the nation might continue to live."[112]

In addition to pleas from advocacy groups, members of Congress received urgent calls for facilities from state legislatures. In April 1922, the secretary of the commonwealth of Massachusetts sent an order to the House Committee on Public Buildings and Grounds pointing out that "as a result of the World War, a large number of citizens in the Commonwealth who saw active service are today suffering from various disabilities ... some are physically incapacitated; others are mentally incapacitated." In order to answer the needs of the "many worthy veterans [who] find themselves without proper care," the Massachusetts official urged Congress to create a "government hospital to be devoted to the care, restoration, and relief of disabled veterans."[113] Other states echoed Massachusetts's request. In February 1927, Fern Ale, secretary of the Senate of Indiana sent a resolution to the House Committee on Ways and Means noting that as a result of the passage of the World War Veterans' Act, "there has been a substantial increase of admissions to hospitals," a pattern that was "expected to continue for years to come." Any of the 1 million veteran residents of Indiana who needed care had to travel to neighboring states, since Indiana had "not been allowed a veterans' hospital." The state's legislature justified an institution there because federal legislation made it necessary, other states already boasted similar resources, and, in a more immediate sense, "savings alone in transportation would be ... a stupendous amount."[114]

Amid the many calls for an expansion of the veterans' hospital system, there were some pleas for restraint. A Palo Alto, California, resident named J. R. Collins told the House Committee on Public Buildings and Grounds in February 1922 that he represented the "Committee on Protest" against the construction of a veterans' hospital in his town. "Halt the machinery for the building of a pile which means nothing to our invalid boys in the way of giving them back their health and vigor and making them enthusiastic patriots instead of resigned-to-their-fate charges, waiting their turn for early taps," Collins dramatically argued. But he demonstrated more concern with having a large population of ill and disabled veterans assume residence near his home than he did with the notion that building hospitals created dependency among veterans. The state of California, he suggested, should donate land in the Santa Cruz Mountains, which boasted a better climate and conditions for tubercular ex-soldiers—"where the oxygen oozes from the very leaves of the trees."[115]

Beginning in the early 1920s, a second phase of veterans' hospital building began as proposals and plans for locating facilities were debated, evaluated, and implemented not mainly in the halls of Congress but by medical experts on the White Committee and VB director Charles Forbes.[116] Although the White Committee honored requests for hearings from more than a hundred groups, including senators, congressional representatives, state and municipal committees, and chambers of commerce, its members argued, "these scarcely provided the data on which to build a rational Federal program." By 1923, the committee claimed that its recommendations for building or improving nineteen hospitals across the country were based not on local booster efforts, or the "hundreds of projects offered for sale and gift to the Government," but on data regarding the number of draftees in a given area; results of army surgeon general physical examinations; the number of government hospital beds already available in given locations; climate; and available railroad facilities.[117] As the White Committee painstakingly considered the nationwide hospital situation, Forbes ensured that Public Health Service facilities would be transferred to the VB and successfully advocated that an additional $12 million be spent on developing other facilities. He fought for passage of the second Langley Bill, which allowed him to make decisions about developing specific hospital projects; in correspondence with President Harding, he claimed that his recommendations for sites were based on studies undertaken by groups of neuropsychiatric and tuberculosis experts.[118] By June 1922, work was beginning at Forbes's behest on ten hospital projects throughout the country—some of them "new construction" and others improvements on previously existing facilities purchased by the government.[119]

The activities of both the White Committee and Forbes brought about an expansion in institutional capacity and reflected a transfer of power away from Congress, which authorized the appropriation of millions of dollars but then left decisions about how to spend the money in the hands of a specialized committee and a newly appointed bureaucrat in an independent agency. The main power check in place was that project proposals were subject to the approval of the president. Operating exclusively of each other, rather than in concert, both the White Committee and Forbes successfully justified their facilities in memoranda to President Harding with statistics and charts—showing, for example, which districts had the most need—and by arguing that there was no "consistent program for the complete hospitalization of the veterans of the World War."[120] Although the White Committee and the tenure of Charles Forbes were both relatively short-lived, the idea they each bolstered—that plans for the location of veterans' hospitals should be data-driven and overseen within the federal bureaucracy—endured.

By the mid-1920s, a third stage of a hospital building program had begun, this one marked by the power of the Federal Board of Hospitalization to approve and reject projects. The board, which was established in 1921 so federal officials from military branches, the Public Health Service, the Department of Indian Affairs, and the Veterans Bureau could coordinate efforts pertaining to hospitals, initially had questionable legal status and influence.[121] It was, according to board member and commissioner of Indian affairs Charles H. Burke, "in a position approaching the ridiculous."[122] But the passing of the White Committee and the exposure of Forbes's alleged embezzlement enhanced the power of the FBH. In 1923, its meetings saw a "stream of members of Congress and representatives of private groups making their pitch for a hospital."[123]

The existence of the FBH allowed Frank Hines to publicly minimize his degree of procedural power, which was, in fact, considerable. In 1927, for example, Hines met with the Committee on World War Veterans Legislation to urge the allocation of $10 million to improve existing hospital facilities, justifying his request by noting that it was based on a program endorsed by the FBH.[124] Likewise, when a fellow member of a Washington, DC, chapter of the Freemasons requested in 1930 that Hines "use your good offices to so great an extent as to establish a hospital" at Selma, Alabama, the VB director diplomatically replied that "the matter of the definite location of this hospital rests with the Federal Board of Hospitalization."[125] But in both cases Hines was underrepresenting his own authority: from 1923 through 1945, he served both as the head of the Veterans Bureau and chairman of the FBH.

The process for determining funding and a definitive building program was anything but straightforward. In the mid- to late 1920s, members of Congress carefully suggested that hospital building was above politics. "It has been the uniform practice to designate a lump sum, putting its distribution in the control of the director of the bureau," said a 1928 report from the World War Veterans' Committee chair, Edith Nourse Rogers.[126] Public Law 600, for example, allocated $35.2 million in 1928 to be used "for medical, surgical, dental, dispensary, and hospital services and facilities ... [to be] disbursed by the United States Veteran's Bureau." It contained no particulars regarding which institutions or regions would receive the funding.[127] Such "lump sum" appropriations, which generally emerged from Rogers's World War Veterans' Committee, were based at least in part on FBH recommendations. And the board's recommendations were shaped by requests from the VB director, veterans' advocates, and members of Congress. By the late 1920s, some members of the World War Veterans' Committee worried anew about allowing "the needs of victims of war [to] be met according to the power of personal pressure" and that "the exigencies of candidacies and campaigns" threatened to cause an unjustified expansion of veterans' hospitals.[128]

All told, Congress authorized more than $92 million for new hospital construction for the use of veterans in the 1920s; by 1930, only nine states were without Veterans Bureau hospitals.[129] Throughout the decade, Hines advocated for liberal appropriations from Congress with few conditions in part by arguing that well-informed members of the Federal Board of Hospitalization would ensure that the money was spent appropriately. During public hearings in 1929, for example, he fielded a congressman's query regarding where in Kentucky a new veterans' hospital would be located by noting that the federal board would decide the matter "on Saturday."[130]

As was the case in the immediate aftermath of war, veterans' hospital projects were consistently approved in the mid- to late 1920s not just because of money grabs and patronage but also because the administrators overseeing the system placed few definitive limits on who could have access to care. When fielding requests for services from veterans' advocates, Frank Hines often alluded to the existence of a priority system and noted that the World War Veterans' Act stipulated only that the VB provide hospitalization for all veterans via *existing facilities* rather than guaranteeing that the agency would build new ones. Still, since the act did state that all veterans were conditionally eligible for care, there was room for interpretation, and the bureau served an ever-increasing number of veterans with non-service-connected disabilities and illnesses throughout the 1920s. In 1925, 17 percent of patients were admitted to hospitals for non-service-connected disabilities. That number jumped to about 63 percent in 1928.[131] By 1931, 76 percent of hospital admissions were of veterans with non-service-connected injuries or illnesses (figure 6.3).[132]

The conditional nature of the health care entitlement for veterans with non-service-connected disabilities led to constant confusion. By 1928, Hines reported, Congress had still not clarified "the extent to which [it will] provide hospital accommodations for veterans whose disabilities have not been adjudicated to be of service origins."[133] In his 1930 annual report, Hines referred to the tensions that continued to arise from the somewhat vague provisions of the World War Veterans' Act: "With a potential load of more than 4,000,000 veterans, it is apparent to what proportions this may extend if it is to be the policy of our government to give the non-service connected class a mandatory, rather than a qualified right to hospitalization and establish facilities for them proportionate to the probable need."[134] The bureaucrat who had advocated for the World War Veterans' Act to include all veterans as potential beneficiaries evidently came to understand throughout the 1920s the full implications of that provision.

In the late 1920s, the disparate state of veterans' medical care helped justify

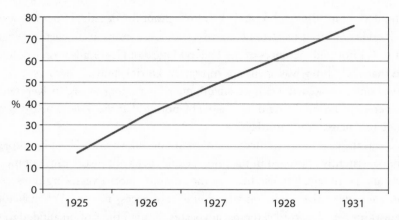

Figure 6.3. Percentage of veteran-patients admitted for non-service-connected disabilities, 1925–31. *Annual Report of the Director, United States Veterans' Bureau for the Fiscal Year Ended June 30, 1928* (Washington, DC: GPO, 1928), 8–9; *Annual Report of the Administrator of Veterans' Affairs for the Year 1931* (Washington, DC: GPO, 1931), 14

calls for growing the VB bureaucracy. Motivated by some of the same factors as his counterparts who lobbied for the creation of a Veterans Bureau in the early 1920s, Hines argued that consolidating the VB with the National Home for Disabled Volunteer Soldiers and the Bureau of Pensions could bring about "harmonization."[135] Echoing almost verbatim government reports of a decade prior regarding the Public Health Service, Bureau of War Risk Insurance, and Federal Board for Vocational Education, he pointed out that the tasks of the Pension Bureau, Soldiers' Homes, and VB were "so closely related" that they should all be overseen by the Veterans Bureau.[136]

Justifying his argument economically, Hines noted that placing Soldiers' Homes under the control of the bureau, rather than making them serve as institutions where veteran-patients could be treated for a fee, would "materially affect the future veterans' construction program of the Government." In many states, Hines argued, veterans were eligible for care in either a VB hospital or Soldiers' Home, and there was a "duplication of facilities." After consolidation, there would be greater institutional coordination, and fewer new buildings would have to be constructed, representing a "definite economy."[137]

But legislators were wary, not least of all because the hospitals the VB oversaw were relatively expensive compared to Soldiers' Homes. By placing more institutions under the agency's control, legislators feared, costs would increase across the board. In response to claims that Soldiers' Homes spent only $2.39 per day on each patient, while Veterans Bureau hospitals spent more than $4, Hines argued that bureau hospitals were more costly because they had been responsive to patient complaints and offered superior care and services. In comparison with Soldiers' Homes, VB hospitals had lower staff-to-patient ratios and better food. Also the VB resisted using patients as laborers. "One fails to find what is being accomplished in the homes in the treatment of disabled ex-service men," Hines said, "so that it is impossible to compare the results with the results obtained in the United States Veterans' Bureau." Hines suggested that homes offered custodial care while hospitals were curative: "I doubt if you can logically make a comparison between a home and a hospital." Besides, he maintained, the difference in costs between bureau hospitals and Soldiers' Homes actually equated to yet another argument for bringing the two under one bureaucratic head: "if [Soldiers' Homes] have a method whereby they can operate at a less cost than the Veterans' Bureau can operate and still give proper service, then we should have the advantage of that personnel and the plans of their doing so."[138]

Beyond practical considerations, Hines pointed out that by unifying the Bureau of Pensions, Soldiers' Homes, and the VB, the government would be "bringing about a uniform policy in dealing with all veterans of all the wars." As things stood, World War veterans viewed the Veterans Bureau as "their organization" while Civil War and Spanish-American War veterans viewed the Pension Bureau as "their agency." That meant that older veterans were more likely to receive care in Soldiers' Home hospitals, which had a long affiliation with the Pension Bureau, rather than VB hospitals. "This divided responsibility for the rendering of medical treatment is not conducive to the standardization of methods of treatment . . . nor to the best control of the medical problem of the veteran," Hines said. "There should be no difference in the method of treatment of veterans of different wars; it should be uniform." He noted that hospital and domiciliary care could be complimentary—especially for patients with chronic conditions, if they were coordinated. If both were overseen by one agency, "ex-service men transferred from hospital to domiciliary care in the national soldiers' homes could then receive rehabilitation training so that both the individual and the Government could obtain from him any potential economic worth which he possesses." While "undergoing rehabilitative employment," individuals would be medically supervised so that "in the event of a nervous breakdown they could very readily be transferred to a hospital status."[139] By fighting for coordination between hospitals and domicile care facilities, Hines embraced the ideal of modern, medicalized institutional care but also maintained that it should be used as a last resort.

In spite of opposition from heads of the other two agencies concerned, as well as the Department of the Interior, which oversaw them, legislators were drawn to Hines's focus on streamlined economy: in 1930, the Veterans Bureau was combined with the Bureau of Pensions and National Home for Disabled Volunteer Soldiers under one behemoth agency called the Veterans Administration. One immediate administrative upshot of the consolidation was the appearance of a larger population of veteran-patients. Between 1931 and 1932, the hospital load went from about 35,000 to approximately 43,800. About four thousand of the veterans counted in that total were Soldiers' Home patients who had previously been tallied as domicile patients.[140] As the American economy soured in the late 1920s and early 1930s, the VA's expenditures, and its growing hospital patient load, drew increasing attention and ire.

The first decade of the existence of a veterans' health system serves as a case study of challenges associated with the rise and implementation of a broad federal program. In the 1920s, Veterans Bureau administrators, staff, and beneficiaries faced questions about medical diagnoses, disability ratings, and treatment plans; how and when to limit or expand access; how to manage social norms regarding segregation and gender in a supposedly egalitarian publicly sponsored system; and how to ensure that VB hospitals could operate as part of a locally administered welfare network. Legislation establishing the agency in 1921 and the World War Veterans' Act of 1924 set rough administrative parameters, but federal employees and veterans defined how the system would operate.

In many ways the VB health system took shape only after it existed. During the Veterans Bureau's first decade, as the official boundaries of the agency's new medical system remained vague, the program proved highly malleable. By 1930, the foundation had been set for a lasting veteran's health system because of at least three factors: veterans' heavy demands for health and medical care, a perceived widespread economic and social need, and a political drive to bring federal funding to local communities.

The growth of the veterans' health system in the 1920s paved the way for a backlash in the early 1930s. As the economy worsened, doctors and politicians argued that veterans' entitlements had become excessive. Access to the privilege of government-sponsored medical care, they said, should be more strictly limited.

CHAPTER SEVEN

State Medicine

Enduring under Fire

The United Spanish War Veterans of Topeka, Kansas, felt swindled. In 1933, a 58-year-old former service member who traced his malaria and diabetes to the time he spent in Cuba suddenly stopped receiving his $60 per month compensation. After an appeal, the VA agreed to pay him $9 per month. Another veteran, who sustained "a severe head wound" at the Battle of Marilao River in the Philippines, had his payments cut from $60 to $20, though he continued to suffer from chronic bronchitis, chronic arthritis, an "ulcerated stomach from eating embalmed beef," chronic kidney and bladder trouble, and dysentery "from drinking water from the town well in Calacoon into which (an investigation disclosed) had been thrown bodies of dead insurgents."[1]

In December 1933, more than one hundred Kansas veterans shared similar accounts of struggles with a litany of ills—rheumatism, scurvy, dysentery, deafness—and the related challenges they faced seeking what they felt was their due from the government. "Did anyone serve three years in the Philippines and not incur any disabilities?," the veterans asked, getting at the crux of some complicated questions surrounding veterans' entitlements. Was it service that made one worthy of privileges, or the impact of that service? How could the government determine the origins of a chronic illness? What qualified as proper compensation?

The Topeka letters were prompted by drastic cuts in benefits at the height of the Great Depression—supported by government bureaucrats and medical elites and spearheaded by a popular democratic president named Franklin D. Roosevelt, who had his own ideas about how the government might go about guaranteeing the security of citizens. As economic conditions worsened in the early 1930s and veterans increasingly demanded VB services and treatment, doctors and prominent politicians called for cost control and efficiency. They expressed doubt that veterans who claimed to be injured and ill were willing and able to be rehabilitated or were worthy of entitlements. But veterans' advocates effectively fought against arguments that they were no different from fellow Americans who were financially devastated by the Great Depression. In spite of impassioned efforts to impose strict limits on veterans' access to health care, the system weathered the economic and political storm, emerging in the mid-1930s intact, and in many ways primed for further expansion.

Despite growing hostility to veterans' entitlements, the 1935 Social Security Act—a landmark in American social policy—built around and upon them. During debates about social security, policy makers represented veterans' benefits dichotomously, as a means of enhancing their arguments for or against expansions in government, federally sponsored racial segregation, and workers' rights. Ultimately, the Social Security Act entrenched a principle encapsulated in the new veterans' health system and central to American health and social policy: citizens who belonged to certain groups would gain access to state-sponsored privileges in large part because of their history or potential as workers, and as a means of enhancing independence. Like Progressives and advocates of the 1920s and 1930s who helped shape the veterans' health system, architects of the 1935 legislation argued that access to health care was integral to "economic security." But the act was shaped by a different set of actors, covered a different population, and came about at a different historical moment; although it funded care for poor mothers and children, as well as community-level public health measures, policy advisers' efforts to include a national "public medical program" or system of health insurance were ultimately unsuccessful. Indeed, the original Social Security Act helped ensure that—for most Americans who were not military veterans—the federal government would aim to guarantee economic security without providing access to health care.

Opposition to "State Medicine"

By the early 1930s, there were conflicting interpretations of the nature and extent of veterans' disability benefits. On the one hand, there were heart-wrenching accounts of suffering and need, like those conveyed by the Topeka, Kansas, veterans in 1933. But on the other hand, there was skepticism.

The latter sentiment was encapsulated in a cartoon from a 1933 book by Walter Reed Army Medical Center patients Edward C. Wells and John Moss, which depicted smiling, smoking men waiting in line for movie tickets. "This treatment is considered very beneficial," the cartoon's caption read. "The aches and pains get a recess, congress-men relax, and the boys 'get away from it all' for

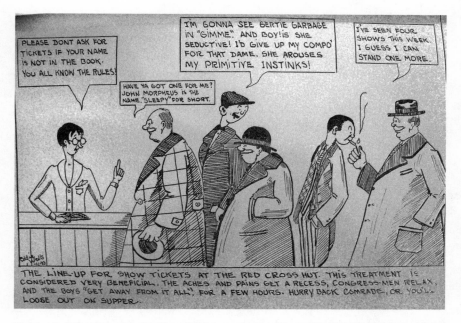

Figure 7.1. "The Line-Up for Show Tickets at the Red Cross Hut." Eddie Wells and John Moss, *We're Not Heroes: Cartoons of Life in a Veterans' Hospital* (1933), Book Collection, US Army Heritage and Education Center, Carlisle, PA

a few hours. Hurry back comrades, or you'll loose out on supper!" Another cartoon showed an overweight veteran, referred to as an "undernourished comrade," requesting an eggnog from a nurse and being denied. "Is [the nurse] going to get away with that? No Sir! Just wait until he hits the congressional office building" (figure 7.1).[2] Patients in veterans' hospitals, Wells and Moss implied, were offered an exorbitant array of amenities, and they only needed to appeal to politicians to receive more.

In the social milieu of the early 1930s, when millions of Americans were jobless, government officials, politicians, and professional doctors shared Wells and Moss's cynical sentiments. It bordered on ludicrous, they believed, that thousands of veterans—many of them without service-connected disabilities—were being housed and cared for at the government's expense. To some, veterans' hospitals were beginning to look more like an unearned gratuity than a legitimate entitlement.

Feelings of resentment escalated in part because veterans were demanding a relatively rare and valuable service. The turn-of-the-century trend toward accessing medical care in institutions and clinics rather than at home continued and accelerated in the first decades of the twentieth century. By the late 1920s, middle-class Americans viewed professionalized health care as a desired, and expensive, commodity. That much was clear in the more than twenty reports released between 1927 and 1932 by the Committee on the Costs of Medical Care (CCMC), a group of approximately fifty physicians and social scientists who— funded mainly by foundations that had a "certain vision of medical care for the public good"—studied the dual problems of access to and costs of health services.[3] The CCMC reported that "the proportion of families which consult a physician shows a consistent rise with income and the proportion of families receiving surgery and hospital care in the highest income groups is twice that in the lower." Furthermore, people in families with incomes of at least $10,000 were more than seven times more likely to use private nursing care than people in families with incomes of $1,200 or less. Members of "well-to-do families" participated in more than twice as many office consultations and treatments with physicians as low-income individuals. "The receipt of medical care goes hand in hand with the recognition of its need," the CCMC maintained. "But recognition of need is correlated with economic level and is lower for the poor than for the rich."[4]

As general "recognition of need" and costs increased, so too did visible animosity toward government involvement in medical care. In 1932, eight of the nineteen physician representatives on the CCMC refused to sign the group's final report, which argued for "the extension of all basic public health services— whether provided by governmental or nongovernmental agencies—so they will be available to the entire population according to its needs." They maintained that "government competition in the practice of medicine [should] be discontinued." The state should be restricted to providing for the "indigent," promoting public health, supporting the army and navy and other governmental departments, and, finally, caring for "veterans suffering from *bona fide* service-connected disabilities and diseases, except in the case of tuberculosis and nervous and mental diseases." By expanding care for the indigent, the report noted, unfair competition would be minimized and the government would be "relieving the medical profession of this burden."[5] In theory, these physicians supported the idea of government intervention to bolster citizens' health but only so far as it served to alleviate a "burden" on professional doctors.

That idea was encapsulated in the statements and actions of Ray Lyman Wilbur, a physician who served in the late 1920s not only as secretary of the interior but also as chairman of both the CCMC and the Veterans Bureau's Medical Council, a group of notable physicians who met occasionally with bureau administrators to provide advice regarding major questions and problems facing the agency. In 1928, Wilbur explained the goals of the CCMC to the VB Medical Council: "We are trying to see what can be done from the standpoint of study and organization to make it possible for all members of the population to get a reasonable share of what medical science can do for them and also to see that they get it no matter what their economic condition may be."[6] Wilbur's leadership of the VB Medical Council implied that he felt the CCMC's aims correlated with those of the bureau. But his support for the CCMC's majority report, and making health services more widely accessible, was in spite of his deep misgivings about the "state medicine" available to former service members.[7] He worried in 1933 that there had been an "exuberant mushroom growth of veterans' hospitals and as exuberant mushroom growth of legislation opening the doors of these hospitals to more and more classes of patients." Wilbur further maintained, "Congress is not selected on a basis that makes it an ideal board of directors for a national hospital system."[8] Years later, he lamented that the VB hospital-building program forged in the 1920s was "a new encroachment in a field we had thought of as belonging to medicine itself." Even as he and other physician advisers to the VB "saved the country many millions of dollars by our recommendations," he argued, some bureaucrats and veterans' advocacy groups resisted calls to limit services and access. "The very presence of the hospitals was a temptation to expenditure," Wilbur maintained.[9]

Although partnerships had been established between the VB and the medical profession throughout the 1920s and 1930s, the American Medical Association (AMA) and its affiliates consistently argued that federal management of medical care was destined for failure and that the purview of a government-controlled veterans' health system should be highly limited. At a January 1922 AMA meeting, Frank Billings noted that his experiences assisting the White Committee with plans for a national network of hospitals for veterans afforded him a clear view of "social medicine." "Inefficiency of the work," he said, was partially due to a lack of facilities and personnel, but "the chief cause of the failure was the centralization of the work and its direction in Washington."[10]

Some physicians running private practices saw themselves as a class apart, and somewhat threatened by, doctors working for the Veterans Bureau, who earned their salaries as government workers via the civil service system.[11] The VB attempted to ensure that self-employed physicians felt vested in the system not only by creating the Medical Council chaired by Ray Lyman Wilbur but also by requesting that local medical societies attend research presentations at VB facilities, share their "modern viewpoints in medicine," and "inspect the actual conditions under which the bureau is affording relief to its beneficiaries."[12] But some medical groups remained wary. Within a year of the establishment of the VB, the California State Medical Association "recommended a new system of medical treatment for disabled soldiers." Veterans would first call on physicians in their communities before, if necessary, moving on to larger diagnostic centers. Only those classified as "hopeless chronic invalids" would receive care in government institutions. The main point was to provide the "highest class of medical aid and hospital treatment and . . . guarantee individual attention and care."[13] Government assistance, the group suggested, should serve as a last resort.

Soon after the passage of the World War Veterans' Act of 1924, doctors expressed heightened fears about the potential largesse of the veterans' health system, arguing that it threatened local institutions, practitioners, and quality of care. A 1924 editorial in the *Journal of the American Medical Association* noted that the recent act "might work an unjust imposition on the medical profession" since it covered "thousands of veterans of the various wars . . . who are abundantly able to pay for medical service." Many would doubtless be "willing to take full advantage of the provisions in the act, so far as it relates to the receiving of free medical and hospital care." The effect was "hard to predict . . . but it is quite possible under the act to expand facilities to an almost unlimited extent." The issue deserved "constant and watchful attention."[14] Memphis, Tennessee, physician E. C. Ellett was more definitive. The World War Veterans' Act was "iniquitous legislation" that would "impose an expense on the taxpayers before which all other items of governmental expense will seem insignificant." Ellett, a former service member and American Legion member, argued that the legislation, which "tends to pauperize about five million Americans, most of whom are at their most productive age," should be repealed.[15] A 1926 editorial likewise referred to the veterans' medical system as "state medicine" and noted that the World War Veterans' Act required a beneficiary to "abandon his home physician and the hospitals of his own place of residence, and to enter a government institution, for treatment by physicians paid by the government." Worse still, demand on government services would only increase as veterans aged. The legislation "must be based on some hitherto undiscovered principle of federal liability or create a new concept of it." By drawing patients away from small towns and toward cities where government facilities were located, the editorial predicted, the program would drain communities of doctors.[16] "The government cannot be niggardly in the reward it gives for military service, but treatment and hospitalization for disabilities not incurred in the line of duty cannot be regarded as a recompense for such service," a later editorial maintained. The government system represented "unfair competition" with "the private practitioner and hospital."[17]

In the early 1930s, as the VA served an increasing number of patients in the midst of the Great Depression, the AMA continued its sustained attack by arguing that free medical care for veterans constituted an ideological and economic threat. In the veterans' health system, a patient became "a ward of the state." Not only did that represent an "insidious approach to state medicine," but it also struck at "fundamental principles of the democracy under which we live and for which our veterans fought." Furthermore, it meant that former service members might not receive high-quality medical care since the VA system did not allow for "free choice of physician and responsibility to the patient rather than to any other employer." On a more general level, there was the prospect that "socialistically and communistically minded demagogues will demand that the state administer care to all individuals as it has attempted to care for veterans."[18]

Some maintained not only that the government was overstepping its bounds but also that the VA's disability compensation model was inherently flawed from a clinical perspective. Lamenting the VA's increasing expenditures on patients with conditions related to "psychoneurosis," physicians Charles D. Aring and J. Fremont Bateman argued that by offering veterans disability compensation according to the severity of their conditions, the VA was discouraging them from seeking a "cure." "If the monetary reward is the greater the more severe the neurosis, what has the psychiatrist to offer in comparison?" It was hardly an ideal model, according to the doctors. "Possibly, we have here a 'prevue' of state medicine, medicine as it is administered by politicians."[19] The AMA's Committee on Legislative Activities voiced similar concerns about "abuse of the hospitalization privilege by the financially independent veteran, who was frequently . . . paid approximately $85 monthly while in the hospital, rendering it very difficult for the doctor to cure him."[20] Ray Lyman Wilbur also emphasized the impact of a government-run system on treatment methods, as well as physicians. "The minute we allow a bureaucracy to step in between the physician and the patient," he said, "we take the one step that will degrade our profession so that we cannot render ideal professional services to patients."[21] In 1931, the AMA passed a resolution urging Congress and the American Legion to "abandon the policy of rendering hospital and medical benefits to veterans of the World War with nonservice connected disabilities." Instead, AMA members argued, the government should provide "disability insurance," which would allow former service members to cover hospital expenses—presumably outside the purview of the VA.[22]

A different perspective could be found in the pages of the *Journal of the National Medical Association* (NMA), the premier national organization of black doctors. The NMA viewed the veterans' health system as both a potential source of professional development and an important vehicle for bettering the health of African Americans, who had relatively limited access to modern medical institutions and treatment methods. "With the large list of men seeking admission to veterans' hospitals, getting a Negro veteran into any hospital is now about as difficult as getting a job," Peter Marshall Murray, president of the NMA, wrote in 1932. Murray objected to the fact that most black veterans were receiving care in majority-white hospitals rather than institutions where they could be treated solely by black doctors and nurses. He thus pushed the NAACP to put aside its ardent demand for equality through integration and rally behind an initiative to construct more facilities solely for black veterans.[23] "Since there is a need for more bed space for our ex-service men in the South, and we are advised that they are being crowded into segregated quarters in connection with other institutions, we say unreservedly, let the Government build them another unit in some southern state, patterned after No. 91 [Tuskegee], and staffed and manned by men and women of our own race," a 1932 *Journal of the National Medical Association* editorial suggested.[24] By the late 1930s and 1940s, black health professionals and activist groups (including the NAACP and the NMA) were working tirelessly for unconditional systemic integration.[25] They focused not only on whether people with particular injuries and ailments were worthy of care but also on the veterans' health system's potential to improve the health of poor and middle-class people, and its role in a larger civil rights struggle.

But as the national economy shrank and VA expenses grew, there was widespread support for strictly limiting veterans' medical services. "Medical men, even those with large practices, are feeling the pinch of poverty," the *Saturday Evening Post* reported in January 1933. Congress "threatens to make [the situation] worse by building all over the land elaborate and costly hospitals for the care of sick and disabled veterans." The *Post* argued that the agency was "setting up destructive competition" with local hospitals.[26] In January 1932, Paul Fesler, president of the American Hospital Association, shared with Veterans Administration officials his hope that beneficiaries "may be cared for in local hospitals."[27]

Likewise, Senator George W. Norris told VA authorities that he was "receiving letters from ... constituents in which it is urged that, in view of the need for economy at the time, civilian hospitals should be utilized to care for our veterans instead of appropriating large sums of money for additional hospital and domiciliary facilities."[28]

But as many administrators, veterans, and doctors who encountered questions about disability ratings knew, it was difficult to enshrine into law the seemingly simple idea that the VA should treat only those with service-connected conditions. That fact was even more pronounced in the early 1930s, when Veterans Administration hospitals became one prospective line of defense against chronic illnesses like cancer and heart disease, which were quickly overtaking epidemic diseases as the primary health threats facing Americans. According to the Bureau of the Census Mortality Statistics, by 1932 there was a "very marked decline" in the overall death rate in the United States, but a few conditions were becoming increasingly threatening. Between 1900 and 1932, death rates due to cancer increased from 63 to 102 per 100,000, and death rates due to heart diseases climbed from 132 to a staggering 209 per 100,000.[29]

Debates about veterans' care reflected those broad trends. Martin Cooley of the Veterans Bureau's Medical Service noted during congressional hearings in 1930 that chronic conditions were "possibly the result of our complex civilization, of the high-geared life we live today, which breaks down the human machine very rapidly and scraps it." But Cooley argued that the Veterans Bureau should pay for the treatment of patients with heart disease, cancer, and a variety of other diseases, for "they are particularly diseases of stress and are as much entitled if not more entitled to presumption of service origin as other diseases." Ultimately, Cooley maintained, there was "no disease or injury that is particular to warfare," but it was "possible" that someone who served in the military may be more likely to experience heart trouble later in life.[30]

Cooley's testimony highlights a larger point: in the aftermath of battle, governments and citizens were left to decipher the unknowable health impacts of war. In the post–World War I years, for example, health experts, bureaucrats, and policy makers debated the long-term results of exposure to gas, but it took decades before a consensus existed.[31] Gathering longitudinal data took time, and scientific findings were contentiously called into question. Throughout the 1920s, physicians working with veteran-patients argued that a variety of chronic, debilitating respiratory conditions were directly linked to exposure to mustard gas. In 1921, J. B. Hawes, a regional consultant in diseases of the chest for the

US Public Health Service, made the point that exposure to gas caused "serious and progressive mechanical difficulties."[32] A 1925 report by Army Medical Corps doctor Edward Vedder noted that "if complete recovery does not take place at an early stage, the later effects of gas poisoning, if not permanent are at any rate of very long duration, and lower the standard of health of the individual for an indefinite period." Vedder cited eight common complaints among people who had been exposed to mustard, including cough ("usually worse in the morning and frequently worse in winter"); shortness of breath; chest pain or tightness; morning nausea or vomiting and a lack of appetite; headaches; and symptoms of neurasthenia, including insomnia and nervousness.[33] In 1922, physicians working for the Veterans Administration argued that the health impact of exposure to mustard "promises to be permanent and to produce distinct functional impairment."[34] About a decade later, a report by Harry L. Gilchrist, medical director of the American Expeditionary Forces Gas Service, confirmed those assertions, noting that examinations of eighty-nine former service members exposed to mustard revealed that twenty-seven had "definite anatomic or symptomatic residua" traceable to exposure to gas."[35]

But some military medical officials who argued that gas was a humane alternative to other weapons, and that the military had effectively protected personnel during the war, expressed suspicions about veterans' rights to government benefits. Chemical weapons, according to army doctor Leon A. Fox, "relieved the misery of war." To prove his point, Fox asserted that almost 90 percent of soldiers who were gassed during the war made a "complete recovery."[36] Former Army Medical Department physician A. P. Francine, who was a consultant in gas to the Fourth Army Corps during the war, argued that during his service, "gas discipline was generally good and our type of gas mask effective." People had "a much distorted mental picture" of the effects of gas. In fact, "anyone who saw closely the use and effect of gas would far rather be exposed to a gas attack than take a chance with a half inch of red hot flying steel . . . it would appear incapable of leaving any pathological after-effects."[37] Frank T. Hines, administrator of the Veterans Administration, concurred with that flawed logic as he offered his support for rearmament in 1938 during a speech at the Chemical Warfare School in Maryland. "Post-war studies," he said, had "upset another popular impression, by demonstrating that gas cases rarely develop unforeseen complications after a period of years has elapsed."[38] Army doctor Amos Fries, who stood in "staunch defense of chemical warfare" throughout the 1920s and 1930s, offered further justification for denying long-term health impacts of chemical weapons: "The idea that warfare gases cause tuberculosis and a host of other respiratory diseases has opened up to the malingerer or the fraud who served overseas a chance to claim complete disability and thereby get the great benefits the United States has wisely and considerately given to its seriously crippled veterans."[39]

The loosening of restrictions surrounding veterans' access to treatment and compensation was a product of hazy conceptions of chronic diseases—both epidemiologically and socially—but also of a desire to use medical outcomes as a means of undermining or bolstering the sanctity of military strategies. Officials like Fox, Fries, Hines, and Amos attempted to justify the use of chemical weapons, and the tactics employed for defending against them, by arguing that the long-term health impacts of exposure were minimal. In order to decipher whether veterans deserved state-sponsored privileges, legislators of the interwar years tried to grasp the prevalence and causes of health conditions that were both enigmatic and politically charged. The impossibility of that task fostered a gradual move away from ideals of prewar planners aimed at tying government benefits strictly to service-related disabilities.

Decades after the war, studies revealed a correlation between exposure to mustard gas and a variety of illnesses.[40] In 1993, long after most Great War veterans had died, a report from the VA and Institutes of Medicine concluded that at least seven diseases—asthma, chronic bronchitis, emphysema, chronic laryngitis, corneal opacities, chronic conjunctivitis, and keratitis—were due to "mustard agents."[41] Although it came too late for many, the report served as exoneration for American Expeditionary Forces service members who battled respiratory and other conditions for the greater part of their adult lives.

"We probably had gone too far"

In the face of rising hostility toward entitlements, and in response to a massive economic depression, many veterans remained steadfast in their demands, often justifying them by highlighting postwar health struggles. The most visible effort came in the late spring of 1932, when approximately twenty thousand former service members made their way from all corners of the nation to Washington, DC, for a mass rally that came to be known as the Bonus March. The protesters hoped to compel legislators to alter the 1924 bonus law so they could be granted cash payments for their time in service immediately, rather than in 1945 as the initial legislation stipulated. Setting up camp for weeks, they made a point of highlighting the health problems veterans faced. According to a contemporary observer of one of the veterans' marches, some participants wore bandages on their heads and enacted "stage properties of wartime disabilities." As they "began to hobble painfully . . . no one seemed to question the authenticity of these sudden physical disabilities. It made a good show."[42] But the "show"—if that is what it was—did not achieve the desired ends. On July 28, Herbert Hoover ordered federal troops to use bayonets and tear gas to forcibly evacuate the marchers from their encampment. The episode was a demonstration, according to some historical renderings, of gross and incomprehensible callousness on the part of the Hoover administration and General Douglas MacArthur, who carried out—indeed, went beyond—the president's orders.[43]

But considered in a larger context, the violent and tragic end to the Bonus March was not so simple. It was due not only to the actions of individuals like Hoover and MacArthur but also to long-simmering skepticism regarding veterans' demands on the state. By 1932, sympathy for veterans was evaporating among many, including health experts, bureaucrats, and elected officials.

That was evident not only in medical journals but also in the catacombs of the federal government. In October 1932, a few months after the Bonus March, VA administrator Frank Hines sent a letter to members of the Federal Board of Hospitalization, asking whether they could support cost-cutting measures surrounding veterans' health benefits. Would it be advisable, he asked, to decrease pay offered to veterans while they received hospital care? Also, should access to Soldiers' Homes and veterans' hospitals be limited by age and origin of disability?[44]

The frank replies Hines received foreshadowed—and offered justifications for—the deep cuts to come. Too many veterans "prefer to stay in hospitals than be outside," argued Robert U. Patterson, who had worked with Charles Forbes to lay the foundations of the veterans' health system and was serving in the Army Surgeon General's Office. The pay beneficiaries received while under treatment was too generous, Patterson wrote, and veterans with non-service-connected disabilities, who were otherwise able to work, were inexcusably seeking institutional care. Patterson also argued that if veterans with non-service-connected disabilities and illnesses needed hospital care, they should seek it from "*local* civil charitable organizations" who handled "other indigents or those in the vagrant class." Echoing arguments put forth by civilian doctors, Patterson further maintained that "by giving them care to which they are not entitled (in the opinion of a great many people), congress is depriving the medical profession of the country of a legitimate source of income to which they are entitled." George H.

Wood, formerly the president of the Board of Managers of the National Soldiers' Homes, also supported Hines's ideas for cutting costs. He suggested limiting Soldiers' Home access to veterans who were at least 62 years old and added that the magnitude of the responsibility of offering care to all veterans, regardless of whether their ailments were service connected, was "almost appalling. . . . I can see no limit to your program of hospital construction." PHS Surgeon General Hugh S. Cumming concurred: "In the case of individuals who were discharged in good mental or physical condition into the general body of our citizenry, I consider that the government owes them no more than any other of her citizens."[45]

Letters from Wood, Patterson, and others reflected a larger movement for fiscal restraint and the belief that in spite of a decade of federal beneficence—the passage of bonus legislation in 1924, for example, and the loosening of the definition of service connection for tuberculosis and mental illness—veterans remained selfishly relentless in their demands. To these bureaucrats, the Bonus March was not a justified call for rights but an indication that one group of Americans was unfairly taxing an already overstretched economy. The National Association of Manufacturers, the Chamber of Commerce, and conservative veterans argued in 1931 and 1932 that veterans' benefits must be strictly limited to individuals with service-connected illnesses and injuries—a precedent many felt had been wrongly and unnaturally eroded throughout the 1920s. The political power of veterans' organizations and the dynamics of a lame-duck Congress ensured that their calls initially went unheeded. But the American Legion warned that in the dark days of the depression "the cause of the veteran is by no means out of danger . . . [from] those who would pounce upon the issue of economy as a means of wiping out existing veteran legislation."[46] Veterans' groups expected funding cuts in the early 1930s, but the policies to come exceeded their most dire predictions.

Two weeks after taking office in 1933, having won more than 57 percent of the popular vote, Franklin D. Roosevelt made it clear that before fulfilling his promise to offer relief through employment programs and industrial regulations, he would focus on slashing spending. He and his budget director, World War I veteran Lewis Douglas, devised legislation intended to cut the unprecedented $22.5 billion federal deficit. Aimed at two populations that were particularly costly for the federal government—veterans and government employees— their Economy Act had a massive impact on the VA health and pension programs that doctors, bureaucrats, and many others viewed as overly costly and wasteful.

It repealed "all public laws granting medical or hospital treatment, domiciliary care, compensation and other allowances, pension, disability allowance, or retirement pay" for veterans of any war covered by provisions of the World War Veterans' Act.[47] FDR's congressional allies abided by his request to pursue immediate action on the legislation, "steamrolling the Bill through Congress with rules stipulating minimal debate and sharply limiting amendments."[48] Executive orders issued eleven days after the act's passage clarified sections pertaining specifically to medical care. One stipulated that the administrator of the VA was thereafter authorized to offer honorably discharged veterans of various wars "medical, surgical, and dental services," provided they were "suffering with diseases or injuries incurred or aggravated in the line of duty in the active military or naval service."[49] FDR's efforts represented a sweeping reconception of a decade's worth of complex political battles for expanded entitlements.

The new law and successive executive orders had a swift and pronounced effect. Three months after their implementation, the total number of hospitalized veterans decreased from about 43,000 to 33,000, a drop of roughly 23 percent; the vast majority of those released from treatment—86 percent—had been receiving care for ailments not of service origin.[50] In his introductory message to the 1933 VA annual report, Frank Hines backed the president's efforts. "We probably had gone too far," the administrator lamented, pointing out that "there was not that marked distinction regarding benefits paid to veterans with combat and service disabilities as against benefits flowing to those who undoubtedly were in need of help but, nevertheless, who did not claim their disabilities were due to service." Roosevelt's legislation offered a corrective, he said, by ensuring that veterans' benefits would be "placed upon a fair basis and upon sound principles."[51]

Frank Hines was not the only supporter of the president's drastic legislation. Individuals and advocacy organizations wrote to members of Congress in support of greater parsimony, indicating a rising skepticism of what many considered "self-serving patriotism of the veterans' lobby."[52] "In spite of our lack of organization and lobbyists, we, the people, are in the majority," L. E. Dowling, of Marietta, Ohio, wrote to a state senator days after the introduction of the bill that paved the way for the passage of the Economy Act. "Resist and defeat the selfish interests of minority groups who seek the continuance of political extravagance and veteran graft." E. Frank Williams, of Orrville, Ohio, focused directly on the allocation of compensation to veterans "on account of injuries received after discharge from active military service." Those individuals, he said, had no "more right to a pension or compensation than has a civilian that has never been in the service of the army or navy."[53] The American Veterans Association, formed in 1932 by American Legion members "disgruntled" by the organization's support for more liberal benefits, was one of the most organized and vocal lobbies supporting cuts in entitlements for veterans.[54] A letter to members of Congress that was signed by members of the association—more than eighty educated elites from universities, newspapers, hospitals, medical societies, and railroads and other businesses—argued: "The time has come when present abuses and inequities of veterans' compensation should give way to a constructive program which would be unassailably fair to the truly war-disabled and their dependents. The matter should no longer be dominated by sentiment."[55]

Those who took an opposing stand against Roosevelt's budget cuts were aware of the efforts and backgrounds of their opponents, and they did not hesitate to make class-based arguments for reinstating benefits. A January 1934 resolution from a group of veterans denounced the American Medical Association for "its cruel, heartless, and unprofessional act in bringing about the depriving of our ex-service men of all wars of free hospitalization and domiciliary care by the U.S. government."[56] In letters to Congress regarding the Economy Act and later legislation, veterans referred to themselves as "poor working class people" and "the working man," employing the rhetoric of public figures like Smedley Butler and Wright Patman, who publicly argued at the height of the Great Depression that corporations had reaped the financial rewards of the Great War on the backs of disadvantaged service members and workers.[57] A March 1934 telegram from Max Adler, of Bridgeport, Connecticut, summed up the sentiments of many of his counterparts: "I being a disabled veteran spent five years in a veteran hospital lost compensation self supporter give us a square deal help us who helped this country."[58] Veterans should receive benefits, Adler argued, in return for their service and sacrifice.

While decrying the Economy Act, veterans' groups emphasized the plight of disabled veterans above others. "The main purpose of all veteran organizations is the welfare of the sick, needy and disabled," said a letter from a New York City chapter of the Veterans of Foreign Wars. Noting that, because of the Economy Act, "many unfortunate veterans are caused untold suffering and many deserving cases are neglected," the VFW post urged the reinstatement of rights to hospital and domiciliary care for "all deserving veterans."[59] Likewise, a New York American Legion post urged legislators that "hospitalization under Federal Government auspices be afforded all veterans not dishonorably discharged who require hospital treatment and who are not reasonably able to pay for their own treatment."[60] The president's Economy Act, a Legion official argued in April 1934, "appears only another effort to again make [veterans and their dependents] . . . suffer the horrors of war." He pointedly asked an Arizona senator, "Can we depend on you to protect the disabled sick and helpless?"[61]

By depriving those in need of hospital and domicile care, veterans argued, the Economy Act had usurped an earned right. Since the law's passage, members of the United Spanish War Veterans post of the National Soldiers' Home in Washington, DC, told legislators they had been forced to deduct money from their pensions to remain in the home. "The privileges of this Home was one of the inducements of our inlistment, thus creating an implied contract," the veterans argued in January 1934. "We feel that we are entitled to the privilege of the United States Soldiers' Homes."[62] Their argument mirrored that of World War veterans, who pointed out that the War Risk Insurance Act guaranteed access to medical care.

If claims of unlawful injustice were not enough, veterans also aimed to convince legislators that without the VA health and pension system as a safety net, they might become charges on local and state systems. Spanish-American War Veterans made particularly cogent arguments in this respect. At around 60 years old, they said, "our bodies are physically unfit to engage in activities which require full human efforts on account of varied sickness incurred during the time we were in active service." At the same time, those who enlisted during the Spanish-American War argued that it was especially difficult to prove that their health problems were due to service because of the nature of their diseases and the availability of military records. By linking benefits strictly to service connection, these veterans argued, the Economy Act, "humiliates [us] by making [us] objects of charity."[63] Elderly veterans loathed the idea of seeking financial and medical assistance outside of the purview of the VA. Members of an Iowa chapter of the United Spanish War veterans focused on a similar issue but made an economic argument. Cuts in federal benefits, they said, equated to shifting "the burden from the government to the City and County tax payers."[64] Likewise, members of a Brooklyn United Spanish War Veterans post wondered, "Are the states of which [veterans] are residents . . . in a position to care for the many thousands who would have to turn to [them] for relief?"[65]

In limiting access to VA hospitals to those with service-connected disabilities, the Economy Act created a mountain of paperwork and cases to be reviewed but failed to pay heed to the root of the problem: former service members continued to believe and argue that conditions like rheumatism and deafness could be directly linked to their time in the military. It was their word against the skepticism of politicians and administrators. John D. Kirchenstein, for example, made numerous appeals to the Veterans Administration in the 1930s for cash benefits and medical care to alleviate the effects of a mustard gas burn to the lungs that he claimed led to chronic coughing and caused him to miss work often. Even with the notarized affidavits of fellow veterans, who verified that he had been the victim of a gas attack near Château-Thierry in the summer of 1918, and of doctors, who confirmed that he had been treated since his discharge from the military in 1919 for chronic lung conditions likely caused by gas, his application for benefits—including repayment for a $150 hospital bill—was repeatedly denied.[66] Looking back on his experience in the war, Harold Lafferty similarly noted that although his military record contained no evidence that he sustained any injury during the war, his service led to "nervous facial twitches" that likely contributed to a later onset of "mental problems."[67] Edmond Sorenson recounted a story similar to Kirchenstein's. "I was gassed in France—had lung troubles later, which persisted for a long time—applied for educational benefits after discharge, but was turned down, not of service origin. I needed it badly but went to work and made it in spite of this—wasn't easy."[68]

The arguments of the Economy Act naysayers—and well-publicized tales of neglect that advocates argued resulted from the policy—led the new rules to be overturned almost as swiftly as they were implemented.[69] A series of laws passed between the summers of 1933 and 1934 reinstated many veterans' benefits, including access to medical facilities, to pre–Economy Act levels. Public Act 141, supported by House Democrats concerned with pleasing veteran constituents and passed over President Roosevelt's veto, stipulated that "any veteran of any war not dishonorably discharged who is suffering from disability, disease, or defect, and who is in need of hospitalization or domiciliary care and is unable to defray the necessary expense therefor" would be granted access to VA facilities as long as space was available.[70] The impact, again, was immediate: in 1934, VA hospital rates rose by 19 percent. Virtually the entire increase took place in the population with non-service-connected disabilities, which went from 18,931 in June 1933 to 27,055 in June 1934. Ever the pragmatist, Frank Hines noted in the 1934 VA annual report that it was "unquestionably true" that changes in recent laws had brought veterans and their dependents "material benefits." But it was also true that they had brought about "inconsistencies, inequalities, and complications which will require correction."[71] In other words, from an administrative standpoint, things were hardly better than they had been before 1933. In spite of Roosevelt's efforts, the "mushroom growth" of hospitalization that Ray Lyman Wilbur lamented in 1932 continued virtually unabated throughout the 1930s. By 1937, four years after the passage of the Economy Act, the number of patients under treatment in hospitals—approximately 46,000—exceeded pre–Economy Act levels. In June 1941, more than 58,000 veterans were hospitalized at the expense of the Veterans Administration. While the number of diagnoses for "general" and neuropsychiatric conditions consistently increased in the 1930s, the number of tuberculosis cases decreased. On the most general level, those patterns revealed that health trends among veterans mirrored those of the general population; even before the 1940s (when tuberculosis could be countered with antibiotics), deaths due to the disease decreased as overall living standards improved. In addition, aside from being susceptible to conditions that were specifically due to service, veterans, like the general population, were increasingly prone to illness as they aged (figures 7.2 and 7.3).[72]

Aside from presenting practical and logistical challenges, veterans' health benefits faced an ideological identity crisis. Did the measures qualify as social insurance or social assistance? Had recipients *earned* the right to health care by virtue of their exposure to military life and its related health threats? Or was access to hospitals granted as a means of offering *unearned* assistance to one group

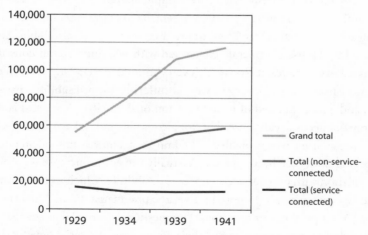

Figure 7.2. Number of veterans remaining in hospitals, 1929–41. *Annual Report of the Administrator of Veterans' Affairs for the Fiscal Year Ended June 30, 1941* (Washington, DC: GPO, 1941), 49

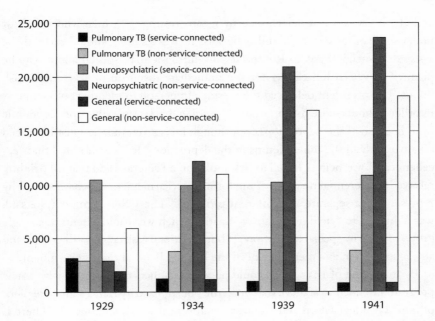

Figure 7.3. Number of veterans remaining in hospitals, by condition, 1929–41. *Annual Report of the Administrator of Veterans' Affairs for the Fiscal Year Ended June 30, 1941* (Washington, DC: GPO, 1941), 49

at the expense of the greater population? By including means testing as a device for determining eligibility for those who had non-service-connected ailments, policy makers marked veterans' benefits—in some cases—as a form of welfare or social assistance, defined by one policy expert of the time as being based on "selecting people for payment because they are in need," and resting on a belief in "the right to a minimum standard of living based on membership in a civilized community."[73] Veterans like the ones from Topeka who argued that their economic and physical conditions were directly related to their previous service rejected such a classification.

But FDR and others highlighted the parallels between veterans' benefits and welfare, juxtaposing them with the much-favored social insurance model, wherein the government ran a universally accessible program designed to "protect citizens from predetermined outcomes that negatively impact their ability to participate in society." Crucially, they pointed out, social insurance systems were based on the needs of the entire population rather than portions of it or individuals; they were funded "by everyone and [offered] benefits to everyone";

and eligibility was not determined by means testing.[74] "A man who is sick or under some other special disability because he was a soldier should certainly be assisted as such," Franklin Roosevelt said during a 1935 speech about why he planned to veto a bill calling for the immediate disbursal of a veterans' cash bonus. The president delivered the message in person to members of Congress in order to underscore its importance. "But if a man is suffering from economic need because of the depression, even though he is a veteran, he must be placed on a par with all the other victims of the depression." Roosevelt noted that "excellent care" was being offered to sick and disabled veterans and that they rightly received "preferential treatment." But former service members discharged healthy represented "a separate and different problem." The US government, he said, was obligated to "yield not to the sympathy which we would extend to a single group or class by special legislation . . . but . . . extend assistance to all groups and all classes who in an emergency need the helping hand of their government."[75]

By the spring of 1935, FDR could present members of Congress with a new program intended to achieve that goal: the Social Security Act, a signature piece of New Deal legislation and a milestone in American social policy.[76] "There is before this Congress legislation providing old age benefits and a greater measure of security for all workers against the hazards of unemployment," Roosevelt noted during his anti-bonus speech. Aimed at developing "safeguards which are so manifestly needed for individual security," the act's most costly and lasting provisions offered federal funding to assist portions of vulnerable groups.[77] Titles I, III, IV, and V provided grants to states to offer assistance to the elderly, the unemployed, mothers, and children; Title II established a federal reserve account for old-age pensions; Title VI established means by which states and localities could receive federal aid to undertake public health work.[78]

During congressional debates prior to the passage of the act, the veterans' health and benefits system became a policy chameleon—represented by politicians and advocates as a bastion of shame or pride, depending on their larger ideals and goals. "We have had the most disgusting experiences in the matter of public health," said NAACP attorney Charles Houston, during 1935 hearings about measures to be included in the Social Security Act. That was true not only for "ordinary" African American citizens, he said, but also for black veterans, who were segregated from white patients in VA hospitals and mixed among each other within wards, regardless of their health condition. "If this Federal Government which calls upon Negroes to defend it in time of war is going to contribute money for public health, and we hope it does contribute money for public health

... then I say to you that so far as institutions are concerned, so far as the administration of personnel is concerned, then we ask that guaranties of no discrimination be written into the act."[79] For activists like Houston, VA hospitals and the structure of the Social Security Act were two battlefronts in a larger war against Jim Crow.

Harold Knutson (R-MN), too, framed some of his concerns about social security within a discussion of shortfalls of the veterans' health and benefits system. In 1917, he pointed out, Congress created the Bureau of War Risk Insurance, "over my protest . . . and this bureau has already cost the American people endless hundreds of millions of dollars for its administration." Knutson was careful to note that his skepticism about the VA—the outgrowth, he pointed out, of the Bureau of War Risk Insurance—did not indicate that he had ill feelings about veterans' entitlements in general. The "administration" of the benefits, he argued, necessitated "money that should have gone to the veterans." Knutson worried that "in this social security legislation, it is proposed to repeat that expensive mistake, as you would set up another costly and cumbersome bureau to administer a new experimental pension system by and through which we will again spend hundreds of millions of dollars . . . to operate a new and unnecessary Government machine."[80] For Knutson, the VA was an embodiment of government waste—a foreshadowing of what could come with social security.

Others who held convictions that the government could act effectively on behalf of citizens' health and welfare represented veterans' benefits in a different light. Like President Roosevelt, Ernest Lundeen (R-MN) argued that the government should provide security for individuals but could not reconcile why all war veterans were considered a class apart. Why, he wondered, was the US government willing to spend hundreds of million of dollars on veterans' welfare, "but when anyone comes in here to speak for the workers of America . . . then we begin to talk about whether we can afford it or not, and where we are going to get the money"?[81] Similarly, Stephen M. Young (D-OH) expressed a desire to expand entitlements beyond the veteran population. "We can do better than the poorhouse, better than public or private charity . . . we can treat our old folks who have done their part . . . as the veterans of our wars are treated when they are broken in the fray or have bended under the burden of their years." Employing rhetoric similar to that of veterans' advocates, Young argued that elderly Americans "have also done their bit. . . . [A]re they not entitled to receive the means of comfort and decent living upon a ground and in a manner that will neither brand them paupers nor wound their self-respect?"[82] Lundeen and Young's representations of veterans' benefits were rooted in their larger political missions and ideologies. After serving in the Spanish-American War, Lundeen voted against declaring war with Germany in 1917 and became a member of the Minnesota Farmer-Labor Party—a prominent voice for workers' rights during the interwar years. He was, as a House colleague put it, "known to be a man of the common people."[83] Young, also an army veteran, had served on the Ohio Commission on Unemployment Insurance in the 1930s, and constituents viewed him as "a great friend of organized labor."[84] To both men, government programs for veterans encapsulated the right principles, but they were unjustifiably limited.

Both social security and veterans' health entitlements were products of their time, motivated in part by new realities and ideas regarding health and well-being, and based on some of the same fundamental policy principles. Generally, the Social Security Act supported the idea that entitlements may be necessary as a means of enhancing financial independence and strengthening traditional family structures built around a male breadwinner. It bolstered one of the primary unifying principles of numerous diverse New Deal programs and policies: an unabashed rejection of "the dole"—the notion that a citizen should get something for nothing.[85] Like veterans' legislation before it, social security provided entitlements based on citizens' social and professional backgrounds, and to those who posed a potentially heavy burden on local and private systems. As was the case for veterans' benefits, some citizens—including entire occupational groups comprised largely of women and people of color—initially faced barriers in access.

But the testimony of Lundeen, Young, and others highlighted crucial differences between the principles that shaped veterans' entitlements and those underlying social security. In spite of its limits, supporters of social security represented it as universal and argued that a great majority of citizens would face the challenges of old age and unemployment. Veterans, however, constituted a distinct minority of the population. Unlike veterans' benefits, which many prewar planners had hoped would be highly limited and temporary, Social security's architect envisioned it as a "slow-growing tree" that "could not provide much shelter in the near term," but "once grown, it would be strong enough to weather bad times as well as good."[86]

The federally sponsored old-age benefits at the center of the original Social Security Act in particular departed from veterans' health and welfare of the interwar years in another crucial respect: they were predicated on the sanctity of pensions. The veterans' health system came about, in part, because Progressive reformers in 1917 railed against the idea that former service members should receive monthly payments for the remainder of their lives, which they feared could compromise their drive to become productive members of society. But in the larger context of the Great Depression, and in the shadow of the expanding welfare states of other developed countries, policy makers of the 1930s viewed pensions differently than their counterparts prior to the war had. Unlike recently discharged service members, the elderly were past their prime working years. As advocates for the aged consistently pointed out, it was simply not feasible for them to look to an employer for economic security. The old-age pensions of the Social Security Act were also predominantly defined positively, as social insurance, rather than negatively, as symbols of dependency, because they were funded largely by employer and employee payments, rather than general revenues, and predicated on the idea that wage-earning workers had monetarily supported—and therefore deserved to benefit from—the system. Monthly social security disbursements were carefully calculated based on financial contributions during one's working years, which were significantly less challenging to quantify than disability or valor of wartime service.

Like those who advocated for an expansion of the veterans' health system in the 1920s and 1930s, some of the sociologists, economists, and public health advocates on the Committee on Economic Security, which designed the Social Security Act, viewed access to health care as a crucial pillar of financial well-being. They carefully considered research regarding the financial and social challenges of illness. They deliberated whether the Social Security Act should include a system of "public medical care," national health insurance, both, or neither. They also considered a variety of creative payment and insurance schemes that had been instituted by hospitals, physicians' groups, and workers in the prior decade, and they discussed what shape a national health insurance program might take. Should it cover physicians' costs, hospitals costs, catastrophic illnesses, or all three? Should coverage vary by income?[87]

But they faced insurmountable barriers in their efforts to ensure that the Social Security Act would include national systems of public medical care or compulsory health insurance. In January 1935, during meetings devoted to the topic of "Health in Relation to Economic Security," the Committee on Economic Security met with physician advisers, including representatives of the American Medical Association, who voiced their hostility toward even limited governmental intervention in health care. "We will all agree to the principle that something must be done to provide medical service for a certain class of society, but if it is entirely under governmental control I can't see how you can avoid the political phases that have been so inherent in the European situation," said Walter Bierring, president of the AMA, referring to other countries' efforts in the realm of government-sponsored health care and insurance. His colleague Stewart Roberts pushed the point forward. It was necessary to "help the people," he said, but "at the same time preserve the profession."[88] Bierring and other AMA officials spoke in favor of the Social Security Act, including funding for state health departments and other public health measures, but strongly opposed measures that could lead to "any interference with the traditional ethical practice of the medical profession."[89]

In contrast with the case of veterans' health care in the 1920s, there was no "grassroots" or "large-scale, activist, popular movement" lobbying for more accessible care as policy makers debated the Social Security Act in the 1930s.[90] In the end, President Roosevelt and others set aside proposals for national health care or insurance in large part because they were unwilling or unable to fight doctors' claims regarding prospective threats to the art of the practice of medicine, the economic well-being and autonomy of physicians, and, more broadly, the American way of life.[91] The federal government would, at least for the time being, provide limited aid to certain groups and grants-in-aid to states rather than administer national insurance or service-oriented programs geared specifically at access to health services.

Despite its uniqueness, the Social Security Act helped solidify a core principle of the veterans' health system. It further entrenched the idea that federal health and welfare programs in the United States would be "categorical."[92] Although Franklin Roosevelt denounced veterans' entitlements because they offered privileges to one group above others, the original Social Security Act was based on a similar premise, albeit applied on a much larger scale. It offered benefits to distinct groups based on their societal contributions and ability—or lack of ability—to work. With the long-term goal of universality, the architects of the legislation attempted to expand on, rather than replace, the variety of disparate government programs that already existed for the benefit of "special wards and special areas and special problems," as Isidore Falk, who was part of the Committee on Economic Security, recalled. "We may have deliberately decided that we would not touch the areas of, say, the veterans or the Indians or other special areas of concern."[93] Beyond building around existing selective services, the Social Security Act provided funds that would allow particular agencies—the Children's Bureau, the Public Health Service, the Veterans Administration, for example—

to pursue their missions and establish "administrative beachheads."[94] By the end of the 1930s, veterans' health care represented one important element in a "costly, extraordinarily complicated system, which . . . protected enough of the public to make the system resistant to change."[95]

Before social scientists from burgeoning fields like medical economics began quantifying and publicly pronouncing the costs of sickness and health care, and before national leaders of the American Medical Association had formed a united front against all forms of "state medicine," the government established the veterans' health system—haphazardly, piecemeal, bit by bit. Physicians like Ray Lyman Wilbur, who maintained in the interwar years that they were wary of widespread government intervention in the health realm because of their concern for the well-being of the practice and profession of medicine, contributed their time to help shape the VA. But during its formative years they did not have a seat of power when it came to policy formulation; their calls for limiting access largely failed. It did not help their cause that there was no one bill—no single "Veterans' Security Act"—to lobby against. Rather, during the interwar years a dizzying flurry of legislation, bureaucracy, and activism, which built on a long legacy of veterans' entitlements, served as an unshakable foundation for what would soon become the largest integrated health care system in the United States.

A decade and a half after mobilization, FDR, professional doctors, and others who aimed to reduce veterans' benefits argued that the American welfare state should be based on a social insurance, rather than a social assistance, model. Their efforts were predicated on the ideal that government-sponsored benefits should be directly tied to one's work life and limited to worthy citizens who had earned them. According to their interpretation, only those whose disabilities could be traced to military service had rightfully won access to publicly sponsored health care offered through the Veterans Administration. So-called able-bodied veterans, FDR and others argued in the 1930s, should be enveloped in the larger American citizenry.

But their efforts were for naught. The Economy Act experience showed how difficult it was to overturn laws granting benefits to a powerful and apparently worthy interest group, especially when there were complicated medical and ideological questions, as well as a vast physical infrastructure, to consider. It was difficult, after all, to trace the causes and roots of chronic diseases and challenging to disprove veterans' claims that their maladies were connected to service.

Even if service connection was denied, former service members and their advocates came to expect and demand that the government honor the somewhat vague guarantees of the World War Veterans' Act—that those with conditions deemed non-service-connected could be treated if facilities were available. There was widespread agreement with Roosevelt's belief that the system was wasteful and irrational, but virtually all of the benefits that his administration sought to limit were eventually reinstated. In a medicalized veterans' benefits system, laws like the Economy Act, which were intended to restrict access to care based simply on proof of service connection, would consistently generate questions similar to the one posed by the Topeka Spanish-American War veterans: "Did anyone serve . . . and not incur any disabilities?"

The Legacy of Great War Health Policy

In June 1942, six months after the United States entered World War II, Frank Hines, administrator of the Veterans Administration, declared that aging World War I veterans being admitted to VA hospitals for neuropsychiatric diseases required "considerably more continuous medical and nursing attention than a decade ago." Meanwhile, because of "the transition of our nation from a national-defense basis to a war basis . . . prospective hospital facilities would have to be expanded to meet the expected load of men disabled in line of duty."[1] In 1942, as in 1917, veterans of earlier wars demanded that the government make good on its promises to them, even as a new generation of men and women mobilized. On the eve of the Good War, they could request not just financial support and shelter in domicile care facilities but access to a vast—albeit troubled—national health system. The change was evident as service members returned from the front lines to communities across the United States. In 1945, in New York's Westchester County, the local health commissioner, William A. Holla, worried that veterans were "wandering on our streets, confused, sometimes unable to tell who they are or where they live." Such men, he argued, should be "in a veterans' hospital and kept there until cured."[2]

Holla's declaration reflected how policies, practices, and activism of the World War I era shaped postwar experiences for the following century. In the interwar years the federal government assumed the responsibility of quelling the effects of military service by providing access to health care. The establishment of the veterans' health system, intended to alleviate a potentially overwhelming economic and public health burden, represented the extension of a rare and increasingly valuable entitlement to millions of working- and middle-class Americans. But as some of the individual stories featured in this book demonstrate, this is not a tale of unyielding progress. In the wake of wars—which are "generally anathema to public health"—the nation and its veterans reckon with changing realities: new battle tactics and weapons that lead to previously unseen injuries and illnesses; confounding questions about how to determine service connection; expanding expectations of the possibilities of modern medical care; economic downturns that bring about budgetary constraints and increased demand for services.[3] Efforts to delimit and rein in health benefits have resulted in arcane rules and regulations, and sometimes shortfalls in care, but have never undercut the system entirely. In the 1930s and beyond, veterans retained their unique entitlements because they fought for them—physically and politically—and because they embodied the amorphous, unpredictable, pervasive, and in many ways indeterminable long-term health consequences of military service and war.

How did such a system come to be in the wake of World War I? After all, in 1917, when legislators, doctors and government officials attempted to plan for the rehabilitation of the war-wounded, they hoped to defend against long-term obligations—monetary or otherwise—to former service members. According to their rationale, by the time most soldiers were discharged as civilians, they would be fully self-reliant. The 1917 War Risk Insurance Act guaranteed that ex-soldiers could receive necessary medical services after being released from the military, but it failed to define who would manage and fund those services.

The immediate effects of prewar policies aimed at guaranteeing that soldiers would be discharged as fully healed civilians were most evident at institutions such as Walter Reed Hospital, where the army implemented sweeping rehabilitation measures, which were presented and perceived in a variety of ways. Army representatives portrayed military hospitals as camp-like sanctuaries of learning, healing, and growth. Some patients and their relatives, however, complained that care and conditions at the institutions were unsatisfactory. Hardships were compounded for service members of color.

Regardless of perspective, it soon became evident that for many, military hospitals would serve as mere starting points on a long path of institutional care. By the winter of 1918–19, government officials increasingly paid heed to claims from both soldiers and bureaucrats that the prewar hope of rehabilitating service members under the auspices of the military was unrealistic. Injured and ill soldiers, as well as temporarily enlisted medical personnel, opted for hasty discharges rather than prolonged hospital stays. At the same time, some former service members argued that they were being discharged from the military before they were fully capable of taking care of themselves—physically or economically. All the while, soldiers and veterans came forward with tuberculosis, mental illness, and other ailments they argued were service-connected. Throughout 1919, members of Congress acknowledged that medical care would have to extend beyond the purview of the military, and they dictated that multiple government agencies work together to provide services for an ever-expanding number of veterans. Even as Congress enacted legislation allocating more funding, however, those agencies struggled to define areas of jurisdiction and standards of treatment.

Advocacy groups like the American Legion and Disabled American Veterans helped ensure that the failure did not go unrecognized. In collaboration with government officials and medical professionals, they ceaselessly demanded three things: funding for a vast veterans' hospital system; a powerful new government agency that would oversee the institutions and ensure the proper administration of veterans' benefits; and, finally, access for all honorably discharged service members to veterans' hospitals. The Legion and DAV were successful because they built coalitions with bureaucrats and politicians and because they had a legal basis—in the form of the War Risk Insurance Act—for the claim that former service members had been guaranteed medical care, and that hospitals were justified and necessary. In a sense, they obliged the legislators of the 1920s to enact policies formulated in a very different, prewar era, when Progressives dictated that government should serve as a broker for citizens' rights in an industrial, capitalist economy. The groups' leaders capitalized on the social turbulence of the interwar years by arguing that increased government services could foster a certain brand of patriotism and stave off political radicalism among seemingly vulnerable former service members.

Under the auspices of an expandable bureaucracy, the veterans' health system grew quickly but haphazardly. Powerful forces coalesced in the 1920s and 1930s to lay the groundwork for expansion. Veterans with economic and physical needs demanded health care at unprecedented levels, reflecting a broader increasing tendency to seek treatment in institutions for chronic conditions that had origins that were difficult to trace. Simultaneously, bureaucrats and advocates worked to convince legislators that providing care at the federal level would alleviate economic and social destitution that was a drain on local communities. All the while, there was a tremendous political drive to bring federal resources—in the form of veterans' hospitals—to local communities and to satisfy the demands of veteran voters.

At the height of the Great Depression, physicians, the general public, and members of both political parties voiced frustration with, and opposition to, massive spending on veterans' entitlements. But when Franklin D. Roosevelt attempted to limit them, in part by restricting access to health services, veterans vehemently protested, and Congress hastily reinstated benefits. The episode made it clear not only that veterans constituted a powerful political constituency but also that rules regarding access to health services would be sharply contested—complicated by the impossible task of defining a term like "service connection" and the parameters of the physical consequences of war.

Roosevelt and others viewed the provision of hospital care for people with non-service-connected disabilities and limited income as social assistance—an unearned handout—rather than social insurance—an earned right. As he railed against the notion of universal veterans' benefits, he touted the merits of the Social Security Act, a signature piece of New Deal legislation that, among other things, provided old age and unemployment benefits to certain American workers, as well as support for people with disabilities. Like veterans' benefits, social security was a product of its time and initially covered only some Americans, though it grew to include people working in nearly all occupations. During discussions about the new entitlement program, policy makers represented veterans' health care in widely variable ways—as a case study of the bright potential, or grave dangers, of expanded government entitlements. In the end, the fundamental ideals guiding both social security and veterans' benefits reflected guiding principles of twentieth-century US social and health policy: citizens should gain access to state-sponsored privileges because of their professional history and potential.

During and after World War II, the VA experienced a phenomenon that would repeat throughout the following century: it was overloaded by demands from Congress and a new generation of veterans. Between 1944 and 1946, VA hospital admissions increased from approximately 194,000 to more than 346,000. In about the same period, the veteran population went from just over 5 million to more than 17 million.[4] As its number of beneficiaries expanded massively and quickly, the agency took on responsibility for overseeing a bevy of new entitlements, including the 1944 Servicemen's Readjustment Act, or GI Bill.

In early 1945, public sympathy for veterans that had ebbed in the 1930s was reinvigorated by a new generation of returning service members, and widely read articles critical of the VA helped bring about a fundamental restructuring of the agency's health program. Albert Deutsch's ten-part series, which ran in *PM* magazine in January 1945, indicted the agency as "a colossal bureaucracy" that oversaw the "tangling of human destinies in an excessive mass of red tape."[5]

A "man coming within the VA's scope is more likely to be regarded as a disability or disease, or a complex of both, rather than as a patient—a person—in need of curative treatment or rehabilitation," Deutsch charged. Furthermore, he said, VA doctors spent their days filling out paperwork rather than devoting time and effort to treatment and rehabilitation. They examined patients "as a garage mechanic examines an automobile—to appraise the extent of damage." Many had risen in the ranks by "seniority rather than ability."[6] Given the initial justifications for the necessity of the veterans' health system as a defense against pensions and long-term dependency, Deutsch's suggestion that the VA ran a "merry-go-round of medicine and pensions" in which a beneficiary's "ultimate recovery and rehabilitation [was] often overlooked or understressed" was tragically ironic.[7] Deutsch argued that Frank Hines, who had directed the VA since Charles Forbes left in a cloud of scandal in 1921, was "dollar-honest but incompetent."[8]

Albert Q. Maisel, who had written positively about military medical care during World War II, seconded Deutsch's negative reports about the VA.[9] In articles published in *Cosmopolitan* and *Reader's Digest* in 1945, he charged that VA doctors and nurses were undertrained and neglectful, and that an individual was treated as "a 'case' or a 'number' or a 'compensable.' . . . Our disabled veterans are being betrayed by the incompetence, bureaucracy and callousness of the Veterans' Administration, the agency set up over 20 years ago to insure the finest medical care for them."[10]

VA officials were disturbed by the accounts. Assistant medical director of the agency's Tuberculosis Division, Roy A. Wolford, dismissed Maisel's articles as flagrant misrepresentations. "There is a distinct ring of sensationalism and a show of gross ignorance, but no sincerity of purpose in what [Maisel] has written," Wolford told the Committee on World War Veterans' Legislation in June 1945. Maisel's article, he charged, would have a "far-reaching effect on the peace of mind of millions of veterans and their families . . . shake the morale of the patients in every veterans' hospital in the country . . . [and] malign and be a source of discouragement to every nurse and every physician in the Veterans' Administration—the very individuals who have with true sincerity unselfishly dedicated their lives to serve those veterans."[11] Frank Hines was more proactive than combative. While maintaining that VA hospital care was "on a par with any in this country," he announced in March 1945 that he would meet with leaders of veterans' organizations about the "question of veterans' hospitalization."[12]

Widespread perceptions and representations of crisis soon brought about changes in leadership and bureaucratic structure—as it had in 1921. Under a cloud of bad press, Hines hesitantly resigned his long-held post in June 1945. Harry S. Truman called on General Omar N. Bradley, a West Point graduate who had earned a reputation while commanding troops in Europe as the "G.I.'s General," to serve as the new administrator of the struggling agency.[13] Bradley was "devastated" to be tapped for the thankless job but took it out of a sense of obligation and professional opportunism; Truman assured him that he would direct the agency for no longer than two years then be virtually guaranteed a different federal post he coveted. Also, Bradley told the press after taking office, assuming leadership at the VA "gives me the chance to do something for the men who did so much for us." Still, at the time, he later recalled, "I knew absolutely nothing about the Veterans' Administration."[14] His first impressions were discouraging. One particularly "vivid memory" from his first days in office at the VA central office in Washington included "the sight of unopened canvas mail bags stacked to the ceiling in the hallways: hundreds of thousands of letters from veterans or dependents unanswered." The VA, he maintained, was wholly "unprepared to cope with [an] onrushing horde" of World War II veterans.[15]

Among the major systemic changes Bradley oversaw was a drastic restructuring of the veterans' health program. "Upgrading the quality of VA medicine," he believed, was "the most urgent challenge" of any the agency faced. He enlisted the assistance of longtime Army Medical Corps doctor Paul R. Hawley, who duly reported to his superior that the doctors approved by civil service to work at VA represented the "dregs of the medical profession." Hawley and Paul B. Magnuson, a renowned surgeon who had assisted with World War I mobilization and was well connected in the cloistered world of academic medicine, took it upon themselves to usurp control of VA health care from the Civil Service Commission. If the agency could establish partnerships with medical schools throughout the country, they and many others firmly believed, veterans would receive "medical care second to none," as Hawley put it, from educated professionals rather than lackadaisical service from elderly, poorly paid physicians unfamiliar with modern techniques and treatments.[16]

Convinced that "if the medical men of this country were given a chance to render service to the sick and wounded veterans and to the younger doctors, they would do it wholeheartedly," Magnuson made phone calls, wrote letters, and personally visited the deans of medical schools throughout the country. The eighteen distinguished doctors he met with in San Francisco were most skeptical of establishing partnerships with the VA. Reflecting sentiments surrounding the VA's growing purview in the 1920s and 1930s, they told him with hostility that they wanted nothing to do with what they deemed "a beginning of socialized medicine." "To my complete surprise and horror," Magnuson recounted, I found I was being looked on in this place as a sort of undercover advance man for a thing which was absolutely anathema to me!" After all, Magnuson had hesitantly taken the job at the VA because he viewed it as a chance to "do something about ... the complete bureaucracy in Washington that [was] building up to seize control of almost every phase of American life." The cornerstone of Magnuson's Deans Committee Plan was that private practitioners and medical schools would control staffing at VA hospitals, not work as hired government employees. He eventually convinced the San Francisco doctors, and many others. By 1948, more than sixty top medical schools across the country were affiliated with the VA and its hospitals.[17] From that point on, private physicians had some control over, and a stake in, the massive federally sponsored veterans' health program.

Since its inception, public views of the veterans' health system, and the way it has been consistently reimagined by policy makers, veterans, bureaucrats, and caregivers, have reflected ideals and apprehensions about war, government, and health care. In the second half of the twentieth century, the VA health system experienced anew two challenges it had faced in the 1920s and 1940s: phenomenal and unpredictable demand for services and skepticism and hostility from politicians, medical professionals, veterans, and the general public. The agency responded to claims of neglect and reflected changes in the larger health care field by expanding its research, education, and training efforts and diversifying care in hospitals, nursing homes, and ambulatory care facilities. Increased benefits and organizational restructuring were typically spurred not strictly by public generosity but by veteran advocacy, larger changes in the health and welfare landscape, and perceived crises. Activism and publicity surrounding the neglect and struggles of Vietnam veterans in the 1970s, for example, helped create an awareness of the unique challenges of readaptation to civilian life, giving the VA reason to expand access to community-based mental health counseling and programs aimed at combating substance abuse, homelessness, and the long-term consequences of exposure to chemical weapons, such as Agent Orange. In the same period, VA doctors worked to improve a cumbersome bureaucracy by pioneering an electronic health record system that served as a model for private sector institutions. Building on the institutional diversification of the 1970s and 1980s and responding to the needs of a new cadre of veterans of the Persian Gulf War, VA leadership in the 1990s replaced the agency's hospital-centered model with "integrated service networks," which relied on a variety of in- and outpatient facilities in particular regions.[18]

Throughout the VA's existence, government officials have trumpeted its cause even while pursuing fiscal responsibility. In 1988, for example, after mandating that some veterans pay for a portion of their medical care, President Ronald Reagan supported the elevation of the VA from being an independent agency to a cabinet-level office known as the Department of Veterans Affairs. A reorganized branch of the new VA—the Veterans Health Administration (VHA)—would administer health services. According to an Associated Press report, Reagan's White House spokesman maintained that the change in status "would not necessarily increase [the VA's] size or budget but would give it a greater say in the councils of government."[19] Veterans could not fully escape the sting of Reagan's vast cuts to entitlement programs, but they at least gained access to representation at the highest level of the federal bureaucracy. The change highlighted the centrality of war in the nation's twentieth-century history and, more directly, veterans' unique hold on political power relative to other interest groups largely comprising working- and middle-class Americans.

Amid organizational changes, battles about the righteousness and conditions of federal intervention have raged on. As the United States engaged in two lengthy wars in Iraq and Afghanistan at the beginning of the twenty-first century, the number of veterans eligible for treatment rose sharply, much to the chagrin of conservative legislators who argued—as some had in the 1920s—that access to publicly sponsored medical care should be strictly limited. The Cato Institute's Michael F. Cannon maintained in March 2006 that the Veterans Health Administration was hardly a model system since it was forced to "play politics with people's health" and cope with decreases in federal funding by "freezing enrollment, increasing waiting times, and rationing access to the latest prescription drugs."[20] In November 2011, when presidential candidate Mitt Romney told a gathering of veterans in a South Carolina barbeque shop that he wondered "if there would be some way to introduce private sector competition" to the VHA, *New York Times* columnist and economist Paul Krugman joined a chorus of skeptical veterans' advocacy groups. "What Mr. Romney and everyone else should know is that the VHA is a huge policy success story," Krugman argued, pointing out that it has achieved "rising quality and successful cost control." That is true, he added, because it is an "integrated" system, meaning it both provides and pays for health care. "Yes, this is 'socialized medicine' . . . but it works."[21] Indeed, according to a 2014 report, 84 percent of veterans were satisfied with VA inpatient care and 82 percent were satisfied with outpatient care. Those rates were about on par with perceptions of non-VA care nationwide.[22]

But Krugman's assertion has been called into question in the wake of wars, in part because lawmakers sometimes do what their World War I counterparts did: they enact policies as a means of demonstrating support for neglected veterans but overlook, or fail to accurately predict, answers to important questions about implementation. In the spring of 2014, for example, news reports of veterans enduring dire health consequences as a result of long wait times for VA health services wove a national scandal. Congress hastily passed the Veterans Access, Choice, and Accountability Act, intended in part to expand a program allowing certain veterans to receive care from private providers. Legislators gave the VA ninety days to implement the far-reaching law. In an attempt to meet that challenge, the agency contracted out the work to a private company. Veterans soon reported spending hours waiting on hold with a telemarketing center. Private providers, too, reported problems: they had to submit requests multiple times before receiving approvals. By the spring of 2016, National Public Radio reported, wait times had in fact "gotten worse" following the implementation of the Choice program. In general, the program had not "worked out as planned."[23] As was the case during and after World War I, there was plenty of public sympathy and a pronounced commitment to the nation's wounded warriors but massive faltering when it came to putting ideals into action. Since the early 1920s, when it took root, the veterans' health system has been the public receptacle for complaints and animosity regarding perceived injustices to veterans, but, in some instances at least, it is only a reflection of broader policies, practices, and values—its shortfalls a symptom of larger ills.

For all of the unique challenges it faces, the veterans' health system has come to represent one of the most expansive and resilient of the government's disparate efforts to guarantee access to professional medical care. Over the course of the twentieth century, an increasing number of Americans joined the "protected public." The poor and the elderly became eligible in the 1960s for Medicaid and Medicare, which granted them state assistance in accessing health services.[24] Legislation establishing mini systems of government-sponsored health care and insurance has, like the veterans' entitlements of the World War I era, been approved on both practical and ideological grounds: practically, veterans, the elderly, and the poor were potentially heavy medical burdens, less likely than others to be able to afford the costs of care. Ideologically, advocates maintained that members of each of those groups were underserved and relatively helpless;

they were rightful recipients of aid from their fellow citizens. Proponents of government intervention focused on constituents' practical needs, their worthiness of privileges, and the potential public health and economic burden that would emerge with inaction. Opponents who argued that government health programs constituted an overreaching of the state helped ensure that access and services would be conditional and limited, but they did not succeed in wholly undermining the programs. If the United States remained the only developed nation without a system of national health insurance throughout the twentieth century, its government nevertheless provided limited assistance in making health care accessible—albeit hesitantly, conditionally, and only for select groups of citizens.

Most recently, advocates have fought for the passage of the Patient Protection and Affordable Care Act (ACA) by employing a rationale similar to those who advocated for expansive veterans' health services in the 1920s: government intervention was not only laudable in a humanitarian sense, but it would cut costs, increase efficiency, and protect the public's health. In a July 2012 congressional floor speech in opposition to Republican efforts to repeal the ACA, House Democratic Leader Nancy Pelosi noted, "This bill creates four million jobs, it reduces the deficit, it enables our society to have the vitality of everyone rising to their aspirations without being job locked . . . let us move forward together to strengthen the economy and to strengthen the great middle class, which is the backbone of our democracy."[25] President Barack Obama, too, reiterated arguments focused on economic efficiency and security. "Each time an uninsured American steps foot into an emergency room with no way to reimburse the hospital for care," he told attendees of the American Medical Association convention in Chicago in 2009, "the cost is handed over to every American family as a bill of about $1,000."[26] Health and health care, Pelosi and Obama argued—as their Progressive Era counterparts had when making pre–World War I mobilization plans—was directly tied to economic security.

Likewise, opponents of the ACA cited concerns similar to those who questioned the expansion of the VA system: cost, government largesse, and the squashing of individual rights and initiative. In August 2012, when vice presidential candidate Paul Ryan addressed the Republican National Convention, he invoked ideals of fiscal conservatives of the 1920s regarding "local responsibility" and gave voice to a timeless argument against federal involvement in health care: "We do not each face the world alone. And the greatest of all responsibilities, is that of the strong to protect the weak." But, Ryan argued, "our rights come from nature and God, and not from government."[27] An October 2009 report by Matt Peterson of the National Center for Public Policy Research made a related point, referring specifically to the ACA's requirement that every citizen purchase insurance. The individual mandate, Peterson said, "would constitute a gross abuse of governmental power and a violation of every American's right to decide what is best for themselves and his or her family."[28]

Perhaps the most striking similarity between the policy debates surrounding a veterans' health program and the ACA is that in both cases conceptions about dependency—the creation of a "dependent class" as Mark Steyn put it in *National Review* in 2009—shaped opinions.[29] Some, including Public Health Service Surgeon General Rupert Blue, Robert Marx of the Disabled American Veterans, and Democratic Leader Nancy Pelosi, viewed federal intervention as a means of promoting self-reliance. Others—Utah Republican Reed Smoot, his Massachusetts counterpart Robert Luce, and Paul Ryan—tended to see it in the opposite light: government aid was something to be earned, a potential threat to community, and frighteningly paternalistic.

In a variety of ways, early proponents of veterans' health care faced less of a challenge than supporters of the ACA. Former service members represented a limited and, many agreed, worthy constituency. The ACA, by contrast, was designed with the ambition of making health insurance available to virtually every citizen—not least of all to those left behind by state- and employer-sponsored programs established in the twentieth century: the working poor, the young, and people with previously existing conditions who did not form a cohesive and powerful constituency. Time will tell how the legislation intended to cover those populations, like its twentieth-century predecessor aimed at veterans, will be shaped and reshaped by larger political and social realities.

In the meantime, it is worth remembering how the veterans' health system differs from other health policy initiatives that have come in its wake. Its establishment was based, in part, on federal liability, and on the premise that former service members had a unique and direct claim on the nation. "It was by the laws and action of the United States government that upon the . . . soldiers, sailors and marines were placed the great burdens, hazards and losses of . . . war," as the 1919 constitution of the Soldiers' and Sailors' Legion put it. "Only by the laws and action of the United States government can these burdens be removed," in part through the creation of "a more just and liberal policy toward the wounded and disabled."[30] In the interwar years, the nation and its veterans struggled to define the terms of that mandate. One hundred years later the struggle continues.

Notes

Abbreviations

AHEC	US Army Heritage and Education Center, Carlisle, PA
ALL	American Legion Library, Indianapolis, IN
BCH	Board of Consultants on Hospitalization, General Correspondence and Related Records, entry PI110 31 in Records of the Public Buildings Service (RG 121), NACP
CWCD	Correspondence of War College Division and Related Gen. Staff Offices, in Records of the War Department (RG 165), NACP
CWRIB	Correspondence with the War Risk Insurance Bureau and Veterans' Bureau, Entry NC-34 23, in Records of the Public Health Service (RG 90), NACP
DAVNH	Disabled American Veterans National Headquarters, Cold Spring, KY
DF	Director's Files, 1917–1935, Entry NM-60 2A, in RG 15 (NAB)
GPO	US Government Printing Office
JAMA	*Journal of the American Medical Association*
MSS 903	Robert S. Marx Papers, 1904–1974, Cincinnati Museum Center, Cincinnati, OH
NAB	National Archives Building, Washington, DC
NACP	National Archives at College Park, College Park, MD
NARA	National Archives and Records Administration
NMHM	National Museum of Health and Medicine, Silver Spring, MD
ODF	"Old Division Files," Records of the Medical Division, Entry A1-58, in RG 15 (NAB)
OHA 97	Angier and Hitchcock Collection, Otis Historical Archives, NMHM
OHA 245	Montgomery Collection, Otis Historical Archives, NMHM
OHA 355	Walter Reed Army Medical Center Historical Collection, Otis Historical Archives, NMHM
PGAF	Administrator of Veterans Affairs; Policy and General Administration Files, Entry A1-55, in RG 15 (NAB)
RFBH	Records of the Federal Board of Hospitalization, Entry 3, in RG 51
RG	Record Group
RG 15	Records of the Department of Veterans Affairs, accessed in NAB, NACP, and NARA at Boston
RG 46	Records of the United States Senate, Center for Legislative Archives, Washington, DC

RG 51	Records of the Office of Management and Budget (OMB), 1905–1980, NACP
RG 62	Records of the Council of National Defense, NACP
RG 112	Records of the Office of the Surgeon General, NAB
RG 159	Records of the Office of the Inspector General (Army), NACP
RG 200	Records of the American National Red Cross, NACP
RG 233	Records of the United States House of Representatives, Center for Legislative Archives, Washington, DC
RG 407	Records of the Adjutant General's Office, NACP

INTRODUCTION: War and Federally Sponsored Health Care

1. Leonard Poirier, interview with author, Somerville, MA, Feb. 24, 2014. On Vietnam era veterans' benefits, see Mark Boulton, *Failing Our Veterans: The GI Bill and the Vietnam Generation* (New York: New York University Press, 2014); Paul Starr, *The Discarded Army: Veterans after Vietnam: The Nader Report on Vietnam Veterans and the Veterans Administration* (New York: Charterhouse, 1974); Richard Milford Lewis Severo, *The Wages of War: When America's Soldiers Came Home—from Valley Forge to Vietnam* (New York: Simon & Schuster, 1989); and Karen Cleary Adlerman and Sar A. Levitan, *Old Wars Remain Unfinished: The Veteran Benefits System* (Baltimore: Johns Hopkins University Press, 1973). For a bibliographic overview of diverse works focused on the Vietnam War and memory, see Jerry Lembcke, "The War in Vietnam: Studies in Remembrance and Legacy, 2000–2014," *Choice* 53, no. 11 (June 2016). Lembcke warns: "Remembered as a war that was lost because of betrayal at home, Vietnam becomes a modern-day Alamo that must be avenged, a pretext for more war and generations of more veterans." Lembcke, "From Oral History to Movie Script: The Vietnam Veteran Interviews for *Coming Home*," *Oral History Review* 26, no. 2 (1999): 85. Lembcke argues that, in oral history interviews, "veterans indeed appear to graft onto their own biographies storylines from folklore and popular films, and then recount those stories as 'memories.'" Lembcke, "Why Students Should Stop Interviewing Vietnam Veterans," *History News Network*, May 27, 2013. Lembcke's insights serve as an indirect reminder that veterans do not hold a monopoly on the suffering caused by war, and their diverse stories do not wholly explain historical conundrums. Still, in a book about how and why a veterans' health system was established and grew over time, it is crucial to consider personal accounts and memories, not least of all because they helped shape and propel the development of veterans' health care in the interwar years and beyond. As Donald Ritchie argues in *Doing Oral History*, 3rd ed. (Oxford: Oxford University Press, 2014), it is "better to listen to the veterans' complaints than to write them off as mass delusion" (22–23).

2. On Rogers, see chapter 5.

3. The first quote is from Abraham Lincoln's second inaugural address, Mar. 4, 1865, available at www.loc.gov/rr/program/bib/ourdocs/Lincoln2nd.html. The second quote is from "President Wilson's Message on Healing the Hurts of Our Wounded," *Come-Back*, Dec. 24, 1918. As James D. Ridgway, "The Splendid Isolation Revisited: Lessons from the History of Veterans' Benefits before Judicial Review," *Veterans Law Review* 3 (2011), presciently notes, "it should not be assumed that historical artifacts of veterans' law—no matter how entrenched—exist to benefit veterans. Rather, every piece must be examined in a historical context" (145).

4. This volume builds on a growing body of work on the history of the veterans' health system, providing social and political context and connecting it with questions about how US health policies are made and developed. See, e.g., Bernard Rostker, *Providing for the Casualties of War: The American Experience through World War II* (Santa Monica: RAND Corporation, 2013); Rosemary A. Stevens, *A Time of Scandal: Charles Forbes, Warren G. Harding, and the Mak-*

ing of the Veterans Bureau (Baltimore: Johns Hopkins University Press, 2016); James D. Ridgway, "Recovering an Institutional Memory: The Origins of the Modern Veterans' Benefits System from 1914 to 1958," *Veterans Law Review* 5 (2013); Jesse T. Tarbert, "Scandal and Reform in Federal Veterans' Welfare Agencies: Building the Veterans' Administration, 1920–1932" (MA thesis, Case Western Reserve University, 2011); Marguerite T. Hays, *A Historical Look at the Department of Veterans Affairs Research and Development Program* (Palo Alto, CA: VA Office of Research and Development, 2010); Kenneth W. Kizer and R. Adams Dudley, "Extreme Makeover: Transformation of the Veterans Health Care System," *Annual Review of Public Health* 30, no. 18 (2009); Phillip Longman, *Best Care Anywhere: Why V.A. Health Care Is Better than Yours* (Sausalito, CA: PoliPointPress, 2007); Adam Oliver, "The Veterans Health Administration: An American Success Story?," *Milbank Quarterly* 85, no. 1 (2007); Scott Gelber, "A 'Hard-Boiled Order': The Reeducation of Disabled World War I Veterans in New York City," *Journal of Social History* 39, no. 1 (2005); Paul C. Light, *Forging Legislation* (New York: Norton, 1991); Rosemary A. Stevens, "Can the Government Govern? Lessons from the Formation of the Veterans Administration," *Journal of Health Politics, Policy and Law* 16, no. 2 (1991); and Mitchel B. Wallerstein, "Terminating Entitlements: Veterans' Disability Benefits in the Depression," *Policy Sciences* 7, no. 2 (June 1976). For a thorough institutional overview of the early years of veterans' care, see R. E. Adkins, *Medical Care of Veterans* (Washington, DC: GPO, 1967). A helpful earlier account is Gustavus Adolphus Weber and Laurence Frederick Schmeckebier, *The Veterans' Administration, Its History, Activities and Organization* (Washington, DC: Brookings Institution, 1934).

5. On the military and American society in the Progressive era, see Roger Possner, *The Rise of Militarism in the Progressive Era, 1900–1914* (Jefferson, NC: McFarland, 2009); Ben Baack and Edward Ray, "The Political Economy of the Rise of Origins of the Military-Industrial Complex in the United States," *Journal of Economic History* 45, no. 2 (1985); James L. Abrahamson, *America Arms for a New Century: The Making of a Great Military Power* (New York: Free Press, 1981); Ronald Barr, *The Progressive Army: U.S. Army Command and Administration, 1870–1914* (New York: St. Martin's, 1998); Edward M. Coffman, *The Regulars: The American Army, 1898–1941* (Cambridge, MA: Harvard University Press, 2004); and Peter Karsten, "Armed Progressives: The Military Reorganizes for the American Century," in *The Military in America: From the Colonial Era to the Present*, rev. ed., ed. Peter Karsten (New York: Free Press, 1986). On military mobilization, wars, and the state, see Robert P. Saldin, *War, the American State, and Politics since 1898* (New York: Cambridge University Press, 2014), esp. chap. 3 (on World War I); Paul A. C. Koistinen, "The 'Industrial-Military Complex' in Historical Perspective: World War I," *Business History Review* 41, no. 4 (1967); Paul Koistinen, *Mobilizing for Modern War: The Political Economy of American Warfare, 1865–1919*, Modern War Studies (Lawrence: University Press of Kansas, 1997); and David R. Mayhew, "Wars and American Politics," *Perspectives on Politics* 3 (Sept. 2005). For analyses of the overlapping of Progressive ideas with mobilization efforts and the state, see Douglas B. Craig, *Progressives at War: William G. McAdoo and Newton D. Baker, 1863–1941* (Baltimore: Johns Hopkins University Press, 2013); Jennifer D. Keene, *Doughboys, the Great War, and the Remaking of America* (Baltimore: Johns Hopkins University Press, 2001); and Christopher Capozzola, *Uncle Sam Wants You: World War I and the Making of the Modern American Citizen* (New York: Oxford University Press, 2008).

6. Particularly useful sources on the history of army health care include Shauna Devine, *Learning from the Wounded: The Civil War and the Rise of American Medical Science* (Chapel Hill: University of North Carolina Press, 2014); Margaret Humphreys, *Marrow of Tragedy: The Health Crisis of the American Civil War* (Baltimore: Johns Hopkins University Press, 2013); Carol R. Byerly, *Good Tuberculosis Men: The Army Medical Department's Struggle with Tuberculosis* (Fort Sam Houston, TX: Office of the Surgeon General, Borden Institute, US Army Medical De-

partment Center and School, 2013); Bobby A. Wintermute, *Public Health and the U.S. Military: A History of the Army Medical Department, 1818–1917*, Advances in American History (New York: Routledge, 2011); Sanders Marble, "Rehabilitating the Wounded: Historical Perspectives on Army Policy" (Falls Church, VA, July 2008); and Carol Byerly, *Fever of War: The Influenza Epidemic in the U.S. Army during World War I* (New York: New York University Press, 2005). See also these volumes in the United States Army Historical Series (Washington, DC: Center of Military History, US Army): Mary C. Gillett, *The Army Medical Department, 1775–1818* (1981); *The Army Medical Department, 1818–1865* (1987); *The Army Medical Department, 1865–1917* (1995); and *The Army Medical Department, 1917–1941* (2009). The fourteen volumes of *The Medical Department of the United States Army in the World War*, published shortly after the war by the Surgeon General's Office and cited throughout this book, contain valuable information for anyone interested in the health-related efforts of the US Army immediately before, during, and shortly after the war. They are accessible via the website of the US Army Medical Department: http://history.amedd.army.mil/books.html. On the early years of Walter Reed General Hospital, and references to other sources about the institution and military medicine, see Jessica L. Adler, "The Founding of Walter Reed General Hospital and the Beginning of Modern Institutional Army Medical Care in the United States," *Journal of the History of Medicine and Allied Sciences* 69, no. 4 (2014).

7. Important works on pre-twentieth-century policies surrounding health-related veterans' entitlements in the United States include Theda Skocpol, *Protecting Soldiers and Mothers: The Political Origins of Social Policy in the United States* (Cambridge, MA: Belknap Press of Harvard University Press, 1992); Patrick J. Kelly, *Creating a National Home: Building the Veterans' Welfare State, 1860–1900* (Cambridge, MA: Harvard University Press, 1997); Trevor K. Plante, "The National Home for Disabled Volunteer Soldiers," *Prologue Magazine*, Spring 2004; James Marten, "Nomads in Blue: Disabled Veterans and Alcohol at the National Home," in *Disabled Veterans in History*, ed. David A. Gerber (Ann Arbor: University of Michigan, 2012); Peter Blanck and Larry M. Logue, *Race, Ethnicity, and Disability: Veterans and Benefits in Post–Civil War America* (New York: Cambridge University Press, 2010); and Judith Gladys Cetina, "A History of Veterans' Homes in the United States, 1811–1930" (PhD diss., Case Western Reserve University, 1977).

8. An 1869 announcement of the opening of one home noted, "Soldiers are respectfully informed that the Asylums are neither hospitals nor almshouses, but *homes*" (emphasis in original). "Our Soldiers' Homes," *New York Times*, Sept. 19, 1869.

9. Linda Gordon and Nancy Fraser, "A Genealogy of Dependency: Tracing a Keyword of the U.S. Welfare State," *Signs* 19, no. 2 (1994), identify four "registers of meaning" associated with the term "dependency": social, economic, psychological, and political. They define economic dependency as "reliance on some other person(s) or institution for subsistence" (312).

10. On medicalization, which Peter H. Conrad defines as "the process by which nonmedical problems become defined and treated as medical problems, usually in terms of illnesses and disorders," see Conrad, *The Medicalization of Society* (Baltimore: Johns Hopkins University Press, 2007), 4. Throughout the book, I explore the historical forces that fostered an emphasis on all things medical—professionals, institutions, diagnoses—even when veterans faced nonmedical challenges. But I also highlight stories of debility, "the place where impairment, disability, chronic illness, and senescence meet," as Beth Linker puts it. In at least some cases, veterans were part of an "unhealthy disabled" population that actively sought medical interventions. Linker, "On the Borderland of Medical and Disability History: A Survey of the Fields," *Bulletin of the History of Medicine* 87, no. 4 (2013): 526.

11. *Annual Report of the Administrator of Veterans' Affairs for the Fiscal Year Ended June 30 1941* (Washington, DC: GPO, 1941), 49.

12. For a brief synopsis of the number of service members during various wars, see Department of Veterans' Affairs, Office of Public Affairs, "America's Wars," www.va.gov/opa/publica tions/factsheets/fs_americas_wars.pdf.

13. As Glenn C. Altschuler and Stuart M. Blumin put it in *The G.I. Bill: A New Deal for Veterans* (New York: Oxford University Press, 2009), "the innovations of the interwar period form an immediate and influential background to the proposals that would find their way into the G.I. Bill in 1944" (32). Likewise, Kathleen J. Frydl, in *The G.I. Bill* (New York: Cambridge University Press, 2009), notes that "the political stewards who orchestrated (the GI Bill) were veterans of World War I." (37). Stephen R. Ortiz echoes that sentiment in *Beyond the Bonus March and G.I. Bill* (New York: New York University Press, 2010), noting that in the wake of the Great War, "the federal government succeeded in setting up a seemingly judicious and incorruptible new veterans' system," which would later be expanded (16).

14. The Veterans Bureau, established in 1921, was reconfigured and renamed the Veterans Administration in 1930. In 1988, the agency gained cabinet-level status and became the Department of Veterans Affairs. These bureaucratic changes are explored throughout this book. In 2014, 9.1 million beneficiaries were enrolled in the VA health care system. They had access to a variety of types of institutions, including 150 hospitals, more than 800 outpatient clinics, and 300 Vet Centers. Selected Veterans Health Administration Characteristics, FY2002 to FY2014, VA National Center for Veterans Analysis and Statistics, www.va.gov/vetdata/Utiliza tion.asp (accessed June 22, 2016).

15. James D. Ridgway, "A Benefits System for the Information Age," *Veterans Law Review* 7 (2015): 36.

16. Marina Larsson, "Restoring the Spirit: The Rehabilitation of Disabled Soldiers in Australia after the Great War," *Health & History* 6, no. 2 (2004): 49.

17. Beth Linker, *War's Waste: Rehabilitation in World War I America* (Chicago: University of Chicago Press, 2011), 3. Literature on disability, soldiers, and veterans has expanded over the last two decades. David Gerber's seminal volume, *Disabled Veterans in History* (Ann Arbor: University of Michigan, 2012), which is transnational in scope, offers crucial perspective on disability history, specifically as it relates to veterans. John Kinder, *Paying with Their Bodies: American War and the Problem of the Disabled Veteran* (Chicago: University of Chicago Press, 2015), and John Casey, *New Men: Reconstructing the Image of the Veteran in Late Nineteenth-Century American Literature and Culture* (New York: Fordham University Press, 2015), each examine veterans' experiences in the United States with an eye toward gender, culture, and conceptions of disability. Other recent work focuses on the connection between military rehabilitation efforts in various countries with attitudes toward disability, as well as disability policy. See Joanna Bourke, *Dismembering the Male: Men's Bodies, Britain, and the Great War* (Chicago: University of Chicago Press, 1996); Ana Carden-Coyne, "Ungrateful Bodies: Rehabilitation, Resistance and Disabled American Veterans of the First World War," *European Review of History* 14, no. 4 (2007); Deborah Cohen, *The War Come Home: Disabled Veterans in Britain and Germany, 1914–1939* (Berkeley: University of California Press, 2001); and David A. Gerber, "Disabled Veterans, the State, and the Experience of Disability in Western Societies, 1914–1950," *Journal of Social History* 36, no. 4 (2003). Important works on the understudied topic of disability policy history in the United States include Edward D. Berkowitz, "Domestic Politics and International Expertise in the History of American Disability Policy," *Milbank Quarterly* 67, suppl. 2 part 1 (1989); Berkowitz, ed., *Disability Policies and Government Programs* (New York: Praeger, 1979); Berkowitz, *Rehabilitation: The Federal Government's Response to Disability* (Chicago: Northwestern University Press, 1976); Richard K. Scotch, *From Good Will to Civil Rights: Transforming Federal Disability Policy* (Philadelphia: Temple University Press, 2001); Berkowitz, *Disabled Policy: America's Programs for the Handicapped: A Twentieth Century Fund Report* (New York:

Cambridge University Press, 1987); and Deborah A. Stone, *The Disabled State* (Philadelphia: Temple University Press, 1984). On Civil War pension policies and disability, see Peter David Blanck and Michael Millender, "Before Disability Civil Rights: Civil War Pensions and the Politics of Disability in America," *Alabama Law Review* 52, no. 1 (2000).

18. On the history of chronic disease, see, e.g., George Weisz, *Chronic Disease in the Twentieth Century: A History* (Baltimore: Johns Hopkins University Press, 2014). The trend was mirrored in the world of veterans' health, where former service members with long-term health challenges placed more demands on hospitals than those with acute injuries did.

19. There is a general consensus that hospitals went from serving as moralistic, charitable institutions in the nineteenth century to focusing heavily on medical problems and which technologies could alleviate them in the early twentieth century. But scholars differ as to why such a change came about. See, e.g. David Rosner, *A Once Charitable Enterprise* (Cambridge: Cambridge University Press, 1982); Morris J. Vogel, *The Invention of the Modern Hospital: Boston, 1870–1930* (Chicago: University of Chicago Press, 1980); Charles Rosenberg, *The Care of Strangers: The Rise of America's Hospital System* (New York: Basic Books, 1987); and Rosemary Stevens, *In Sickness and in Wealth: American Hospitals in the Twentieth Century* (New York: Basic Books, 1989). For a global and long view of the history of hospitals, see Guenter B. Risse, *Mending Bodies, Saving Souls: A History of Hospitals* (Oxford: Oxford University Press, 1999).

20. See the essay on sources for references regarding long-term impacts of tuberculosis, exposure to poison gas, and mental illness.

21. This volume concentrates particularly on the army and soldiers. The US Marines, Coast Guard, and Navy also built massive forces relative to their pre–World War I numbers. But 4.1 million of the approximately 4.3 million service members inducted between April 1917 and December 1919 joined the army, which the federal government relied on to provide rehabilitation services for its own personnel and members of other military branches. The 4.1 million calculation is from Albert G. Love, *Medical and Casualty Statistics*, vol. 15, part 2, of *The Medical Department of the United States Army in the World War*, ed. M. W. Ireland (Washington, DC: GPO, 1925), 15. Between April 1917 and December 1918, the US Marine Corps grew from 13,725 to its peak wartime strength of 75,101 officers and enlisted personnel. Although marines were "essentially part of the Naval establishment," and as such had access to naval hospitals, there were only six such hospitals in the United States, overseen by a relatively small Navy Medical Corps. Both near the front and at home, some marines and sailors were treated in army hospitals. Edwin N. McClellan, *The United States Marine Corps in the World War* (Washington, DC: Historical Branch, US Marine Corps, 1920), 10. The official army order allowing navy personnel to be treated in army reconstruction hospitals was handed down on May 27, 1918. A. G. Crane, *Physical Reconstruction and Vocational Education*, vol. 13, part 1, of *The Medical Department of the United States Army in the World War*, ed. M. W. Ireland (Washington, DC: GPO, 1927), 39. The navy experienced tremendous growth during World War I, expanding from 67,000 in service in April 1917 to nearly 500,000 in November 1918. John Lehman, *On Seas of Glory: Heroic Men, Great Ships, and Epic Battles of the American Navy* (New York: Free Press, 2001). The Coast Guard contributed 15 cruising cutters, 5,000 enlisted men, and 200 officers to the navy during the war. Thomas P. Ostrom, *The United States Coast Guard and National Defense: A History from World War I to the Present* (Jefferson, NC: McFarland, 2012), 14. Between April and August 1917, the ranks of the National Guard swelled with incoming volunteers, from 177,000 members to 377,000. On August 5, 1917, President Wilson drafted the guardsmen into service, at which point they became members of the US Army. John K. Mahon, *History of the Militia and the National Guard* (New York: Macmillan, 1983), 156. Eventually, veterans of all branches were eligible for government-sponsored medical care.

22. Albert G. Love, "A Brief Summary of the Vital Statistics of the U.S. Army during the

World War," *Military Surgeon* 51, no. 2 (1922): 147–48. A great majority of the soldiers discharged due to disease had never left the United States; see chapter 2 for a discussion of this issue, and a further description of wounded and ill soldiers.

23. Ibid., 148. Diagnoses and classifications of psychological conditions varied greatly throughout the war. "Mental deficiency" fell under the general category of "mental alienation," which also included diagnoses such as "psychoneurosis," for which approximately 2,000 service members were discharged, and "constitutional psychopathic states," which constituted approximately 3,700 discharges (166–89).

24. Ibid., 147–48.

25. Ibid., 144–45.

26. The establishment of the veterans' health system demonstrated that "organizational interests have a high probability of affecting policy outcomes . . . when they lobby on issues that are highly technical or complex." Anthony J. Nownes, *Pressure and Power: Organized Interests in American Politics* (Boston: Houghton Mifflin, 2001), 202–5.

27. For helpful perspective, see Ruth Clifford Engs, *The Progressive Era's Health Reform Movement: A Historical Dictionary* (Westport, CT: Praeger, 2003). Seminal work on the well-trod subject of Progressivism in the United States includes Elizabeth Sanders, *Roots of Reform: Farmers, Workers, and the American State 1877–1917* (Chicago: University of Chicago Press, 1999), and Michael McGerr, *A Fierce Discontent: The Rise and Fall of the Progressive Movement in America* (Oxford: Oxford University Press, 2005). On international connections between Progressive movements, see Daniel T. Rodgers, *Atlantic Crossings: Social Politics in a Progressive Age* (Cambridge, MA: Belknap Press of Harvard University Press, 1998).

28. Various scholars have brought to light the main components of the War Risk Insurance Act (discussed in chapter 1) and pointed out its historical relevance. William H. Glasson, *Federal Military Pensions in the United States* (New York: Oxford University Press, American Branch, 1918), called it a "radical departure from the existing pension system" (283). Beth Linker concurs, pointing out that the act was written by prominent anti-pension Progressives who "saw medical rehabilitation as a means of conservation, a way to preserve the nation's economic and human resources" (*War's Waste*, 35). K. Walter Hickel, "Entitling Citizens: World War I, Progressivism, and the American Welfare State, 1917–1928" (PhD diss., Columbia University, 1999), argues that it was not only a "crucial step in the codification, institutionalization and reification of (a) medical conception of disability" but also served as an antecedent to "formative steps in welfare state building" (107). Hickel also points out that the War Risk Insurance Act was geared toward "the family unit . . . not the individual man" (118). Rosemary Stevens, too, argues that the framers of the WRIA believed pensions were "unscientific," but she notes that the act also signified a trend of the times—the growing popularity of life insurance policies; there were 49 million private life insurance policies in effect in the United States by 1917, Stevens notes, up from 25 million in 1907. US Bureau of the Census, *Statistical Abstract of the United States, 1919* (Washington, DC: GPO, 1920), 645, cited in Stevens, "The Invention, Stumbling, and Re-Invention of the Modern U.S. Veterans Health Care System, 1918–1924," in *Veterans' Policies, Veterans' Politics: New Perspectives on Veterans in the Modern United States*, ed. Stephen R. Ortiz (Gainesville: University Press of Florida, 2012). To scholars who focus specifically on the medical care of veterans, the War Risk Insurance Act represents a valiant but ultimately short-sighted effort. "The War Risk Act contained a promise of complete medical and hospital care, including prosthetic appliances and other supplies, to be provided at government expense for veterans with service-connected disabilities; but no provision was made for implementing the promise," notes William Pyrle Dillingham, *Federal Aid to Veterans, 1917–1941* (Gainesville: University of Florida Press, 1952), 58. According to Stephen Ward, the very fact that Congress debated and passed the legislation marked a step forward in terms of pre-

paredness, at least in comparison with efforts surrounding previous wars. But, Ward also notes, laws like the WRIA, which provided for hospitalization and pension benefits, "were often written without knowledge of the types of medical problems likely to arise during the war. What in fact constituted a legitimate basis for hospitalization was thus often vague and ill-defined." *The War Generation: Veterans of the First World War*, ed. Stephen R. Ward (London: Kennikat Press, 1975), 42. Gustavus Weber and Laurence Schmeckebier, *The Veterans' Administration, Its History, Activities and Organization* (Washington, DC: Brookings Institution, 1934), point out that the War Risk Insurance Act's stipulation that medical and surgical hospital services would be provided for ex-servicemen led to "one of the most complicated and difficult tasks ever undertaken by the federal government" (154).

29. On Progressive Era workers' compensation and safety laws in the United States, see Price V. Fishback and Shawn Everett Kantor, *A Prelude to the Welfare State: The Origins of Workers' Compensation* (Chicago: University of Chicago Press, 2000); Edward Berkowitz and Monroe Berkowitz, "The Survival of Workers' Compensation," *Social Service Review* 58, no. 2 (1984); David Rosner and Gerald Markowitz, eds., *Dying for Work: Workers' Safety and Health in Twentieth-Century America* (Bloomington: Indiana University Press, 1989), esp. the introduction; David Rosner and Gerald Markowitz, "The Early Movement for Occupational Safety and Health, 1900–1917," in *Sickness and Health in America: Readings in the History of Medicine and Public Health*, ed. Judith Walzer Leavitt and Ronald L. Numbers (Madison: University of Wisconsin Press, 1997); and Mark Aldrich, *Safety First: Technology, Labor, and Business in the Building of American Work Safety, 1870–1939* (Baltimore: Johns Hopkins University Press, 1997). For a global view of industrial hazards and policies aimed at alleviating them, see Christopher Sellers and Joseph Melling, ed., *Dangerous Trade: Histories of Industrial Hazard across a Globalizing World* (Philadelphia: Temple University Press, 2012).

30. Thomas R. Oliver, "The Politics of Public Health Policy," *Annual Review of Public Health* 27 (2006), notes that "public policy typically develops in small steps . . . because of limited time and information, policy makers . . . tend to build on existing policies and programs rather than attempt system-wide reforms" (204). Perhaps because of the incremental nature of its growth, the early development of the veterans' health system, and its relation to American health policy and the larger welfare state, has received relatively limited attention in literature pertaining to the history of US health policy. Aside from the passage of legislation intended to fund health services for poor women and children, one scholar notes, "the 1920s saw no significant health reform proposals . . . Republican administrations pressed voluntarist solutions." Colin Gordon, *Dead on Arrival: The Politics of Health Care in Twentieth-Century America* (Princeton: Princeton University Press, 2003), 14. (On p. 133, Gordon notes the importance of the veterans' health system.) Carol S. Weissert and William G. Weissert, *Governing Health: The Politics of Health Policy*, 3rd ed. (Baltimore: Johns Hopkins University Press, 2006), call Medicare, which went into effect in 1965, "the first major federal health program guaranteeing health care for a large targeted population" (314). Some authors who focus particularly on federal involvement in the health care realm highlight and briefly historicize the importance of the veterans' health system. See, e.g., Ronald Hamowy, *Government and Public Health in America* (Northampton, MA: Edward Elgar, 2007), and William Shonick, *Government and Health Services: Government's Role in the Development of U.S. Health Services, 1930–1980* (New York: Oxford University Press, 1995).

31. Daniel P. Carpenter, *The Forging of Bureaucratic Autonomy: Reputations, Networks, and Policy Innovation in Executive Agencies, 1862–1928* (Princeton: Princeton University Press, 2001), 11. Francis E. Rourke, "Bureaucracy in the American Constitutional Order," *Political Science Quarterly* 102, no. 2 (1987), argues that "bureaucracy's unsung role in the evolution of modern American government has been that of an unwitting change agent" (225).

32. The phrase "protected public" is from Paul Starr, *Remedy and Reaction: The Peculiar*

American Struggle over Health Care Reform (New Haven: Yale University Press, 2011), 41. Like Colin Gordon, Starr recognizes the importance and uniqueness of the veterans' health system but does not discuss its origins in the interwar years. Beatrix Hoffman explores the concept of rationing in *Health Care for Some: Rights and Rationing in the United States since 1930* (Chicago: University of Chicago Press, 2012).

33. Edward Berkowitz notes that the Progressive Era witnessed the emergence of an "occupationally oriented bureaucracy providing benefits to particular groups." Edward Berkowitz and Kim McQuaid, *Creating the Welfare State: The Political Economy of Twentieth-Century Reform* (Lawrence: University Press of Kansas, 1992), 8.

34. On the Merchant Marine, see Leon Fink, *Sweatshops at Sea: Merchant Seamen in the World's First Globalized Industry, from 1812 to the Present* (Chapel Hill: University of North Carolina Press, 2011). On the Marine Hospital Service, see Harry S. Mustard, *Government in Public Health* (New York: Commonwealth Fund, 1945), and Bess Furman, *A Profile of the United States Public Health Service, 1798–1948* (Washington, DC: National Institutes of Health, 1973).

35. Jim Downs, *Sick from Freedom: African-American Illness and Suffering during the Civil War and Reconstruction* (Oxford: Oxford University Press, 2012), esp. chap. 6. On other populations who received publicly sponsored institutional care, see Philip M. Ferguson, *Abandoned to Their Fate: Social Policy and Practice toward Severely Retarded People in America, 1820–1920* (Philadelphia: Temple University Press, 1994), and Gerald N. Grob, *The Mad among Us: A History of the Care of America's Mentally Ill* (New York: Free Press, 1994). Between 1884 and 1922, seventy-three hospitals were built to serve American Indians. James P. Rife and Alan J. Dellapenna, *Caring and Curing: A History of the Indian Health Service* ([Landover, MD]: PHS Commissioner Officers Foundation for the Advancement of Public Health, 2009). On the prewar roots of the Indian Health Service, see David H. DeJong, *If You Knew the Conditions: A Chronicle of the Indian Medical Service and American Indian Health Care, 1908–1955* (Lanham, MD: Lexington, 2010) and *Plagues, Politics, and Policy: A Chronicle of the Indian Health Service, 1955–2008* (Lanham, MD: Lexington, 2011).

36. On Medicaid, see Jonathan Engel, *Poor People's Medicine: Medicaid and American Charity Care since 1965* (Durham, NC: Duke University Press, 2006). On Medicare, see Jonathan Oberlander, *The Political Life of Medicare* (Chicago: University of Chicago Press, 2003), and Theodore R. Marmor, *The Politics of Medicare* (Chicago: Aldine, 1973).

37. Various scholars argue that the United States has a "hybrid" welfare state, in which privately funded initiatives have undercut the expansion of a more extensive public provisions. Political scientist Jacob Hacker emphasizes the idea that public and private benefits historically have been "path dependent"; the development of one has reinforced the development of the other. (The fact that Medicare covers only the elderly, for example, was path dependent on the fact that employer-sponsored benefits had been developed to cover workers.) Jacob S. Hacker, *The Divided Welfare State: The Battle over Public and Private Social Benefits in the United States* (Cambridge: Cambridge University Press, 2002). Jennifer Klein, *For All These Rights: Business, Labor, and the Shaping of America's Public-Private Welfare State* (Princeton: Princeton University Press, 2003), argues that the boundaries of the American national welfare system were formally set by the New Deal years: the private programs of the 1910s and 1920s would provide benefits alongside public ones, forming a cooperative arrangement between business and government. In contrast, Colin D. Moore, "Innovation without Reputation: How Bureaucrats Saved the Veterans' Health Care System," *Perspectives on Politics* 13, no. 2 (2015), offers examples of moments after World War II when the VA's private-public partnerships actually reinforced the strength of government-sponsored benefits. On the growth of private health insurance, see Christy Ford Chapin, *Ensuring America's Health: The Public Creation of the Corporate Health Care System* (Cambridge: Cambridge University Press, 2015). William J. Novak and Gary Gerstle's

debate about the American welfare state illuminates some key areas of concern for historians of US social policy. See William J. Novak, "The Myth of the 'Weak' American State," *American Historical Review* 113, no. 3 (2008), and Gary Gerstle, "A State Both Strong and Weak," *American Historical Review* 115, no. 3 (2010).

38. Michael B. Katz, *In the Shadow of the Poorhouse: A Social History of Welfare in America* (New York: Basic Books, 1996), ix. According to Katz, veterans—like the elderly, workers disabled in accidents, and the unemployed—have "always" been considered a "special category" of individuals who "could claim help as a right through social insurance" (8).

39. The quote is from Robin Rogers-Dillon, *The Welfare Experiments: Politics and Policy Evaluation* (Stanford, CA: Stanford University Press, 2004), 61.

40. Like other twentieth-century federal entitlement and welfare programs, the veterans' health system was shaped in part by ideology and social norms, and, in many instances, it reinforced societal racial and gender hierarchies. A variety of scholars have described the unequal impact of social policies on particular groups and discussed conceptions of social insurance programs versus welfare programs. See Margot Canaday, *The Straight State: Sexuality and Citizenship in Twentieth-Century America* (Princeton: Princeton University Press, 2009); Walter Hickel, "'Justice and the Highest Kind of Equality Require Discrimination': Citizenship, Dependency, and Conscription in the South, 1917–1919," *Journal of Southern History* 66, no. 4 (2000); Ira Katznelson and Suzanne Mettler, "On Race and Policy History: A Dialogue about the G.I. Bill," *Perspectives on Politics* 6, no. 3 (2008); Eileen Boris, "On the Importance of Naming: Gender, Race, and the Writing of Policy History," *Journal of Policy History* 17, no. 1 (2005); Suzanne Mettler, *The Submerged State: How Invisible Government Policies Undermine American Democracy* (Chicago: University of Chicago Press, 2011); Jennifer Mittlestadt, *From Welfare to Workfare* (Chapel Hill: University of North Carolina Press, 2005); Michael K. Brown, *Race, Money, and the American Welfare State* (Ithaca, NY: Cornell University Press, 1999); Jill Quadagno, *The Color of Welfare: How Racism Undermined the War on Poverty* (New York: Oxford University Press, 1996); Alice Kessler-Harris, *In Pursuit of Equity: Women, Men and the Quest for Economic Citizenship in Twentieth-Century America* (Oxford: Oxford University Press, 2001); Ira Katznelson, *When Affirmative Action Was White: An Untold History of Racial Inequality* (New York: Norton, 2005); and Linda Gordon, *Pitied but Not Entitled: Single Mothers and the History of Welfare 1890–1935* (Cambridge, MA: Harvard University Press, 1998).

41. I argue in this book—as others have—that minorities in the United States viewed military service as a means of enhancing their citizenship rights and fought to expand limited post-service access to veterans' benefits. On African American World War I–era service members, see, e.g., W. Douglas Fisher, *African American Doctors of World War I: The Lives of 104 Volunteers* (North Carolina: McFarland & Company, Inc., 2015); Chad Williams, *Torchbearers of Democracy: African American Soldiers in the World War I Era* (Chapel Hill: University of North Carolina Press, 2010); and Adriane Danette Lentz-Smith, *Freedom Struggles: African Americans and World War I* (Cambridge, MA: Harvard University Press, 2009). On the activism of African American veterans in this period, see Jennifer D. Keene, "Protest and Disability: A New Look at African American Soldiers During the First World War," in *Warfare and Belligerence: Perspectives in First World War Studies*, ed. Pierre Purseigle (London: Brill, 2005); Keene, "Long Journey Home"; Pete Daniel, "Black Power in the 1920s: The Case of Tuskegee Veterans Hospital," *Journal of Southern History* 36, no. 2 (1970); David A. Davis, "Not Only War Is Hell: World War I and African American Lynching Narratives," *African American Review* 42, no. 3 (2008); and Louis Woods, "Virtually 'No Negro Veteran . . . Could Get a Loan': African-American Veterans, the GI Bill, and the NAACP's Relentless Campaign against Residential Segregation, 1914–1960," *Journal of African American History* 98, no. 3 (2013). See the essay on sources for references regarding other minority groups.

42. Regardless of whether scholars view the New Deal as a revolutionary challenge to moneyed power or the product of collusion between government and business, as an example of "top-down" or "bottom-up" change, or as a challenge to or instantiation of prevailing societal inequalities, they invariably represent its measures as landmarks in American social policy making. A standout work on the New Deal is Ira Katznelson, *Fear Itself: The New Deal and the Origins of Our Time* (New York: Liveright, 2013). Arthur Schlesinger's foundational three-volume series proposes that during FDR's presidency, the government moved to protect broad swaths of the public from the ravages of private interests. Schlesinger, *The Age of Roosevelt*, vol. 1, *The Crisis of the Old Order, 1919–1933* (New York: Houghton Mifflin, 1957); vol. 2, *The Coming of the New Deal, 1933–1935* (New York: Houghton Mifflin, 1958); vol. 3, *The Politics of Upheaval, 1935–1936* (New York: Houghton Mifflin, 1960). For less celebratory assessments of the New Deal's implications for American liberalism, see Colin Gordon, *New Deals: Business, Labor, and Politics in America, 1920–1935* (Cambridge: Cambridge University Press, 1994); Alan Brinkley, *The End of Reform: New Deal Liberalism in Recession and War* (New York: Random House, 1995); and James E. Sargent *Roosevelt and the Hundred Days: Struggle for the Early New Deal* (New York: Garland, 1981).

43. Daniel Beland, *Social Security: History and Politics from the New Deal to the Privatization Debate* (Lawrence: University Press of Kansas, 2005), traces arguments for the necessity of Social Security to four main issues in the interwar years: (1) the decline of the traditional family structure, (2) the exclusion of elderly workers from jobs, (3) the "degrading status of elderly people living in poorhouses," and (4) the failures of welfare capitalism to offer total protection in an industrial society (48). Michael B. Katz, *The Price of Citizenship: Redefining the American Welfare State* (New York: Henry Holt, 2001), notes that social security was devised in the wake of a "revolt" in the 1920s "against the institutional care of the elderly" (234). Other important works on social security include Larry DeWitt, Daniel Beland, and Edward D. Berkowitz, *Social Security: A Documentary History* (Washington, DC: CQ Press, 2008); Berkowitz, *Mr. Social Security: The Life of Wilbur J. Cohen* (Lawrence: University Press of Kansas, 1995); Berkowitz, *Robert Ball and the Politics of Social Security* (Madison: University of Wisconsin Press, 2003); Berkowitz and Larry DeWitt, *The Other Welfare: Supplemental Security Income and U.S. Social Policy* (Ithaca, NY: Cornell University Press, 2013); Jill S. Quadagno, *The Transformation of Old Age Security: Class and Politics in the American Welfare State* (Chicago: University of Chicago Press, 1988); and Martha Derthick, *Policymaking for Social Security* (Washington, DC: Brookings Institution, 1979).

44. In 1993, Donald T. Critchlow called for "interactional approaches that integrate institutional history and social history" in "A Prognosis of Policy History: Stunted: Or Deceivingly Vital? A Brief Reply to Hugh Davis Graham" *The Public Historian* 15, no. 4 (1993): 58–59. Important books regarding American political development include Gary Gerstle, *Liberty and Coercion: The Paradox of American Government from the Founding to the Present* (Princeton: Princeton University Press, 2015); Brian Balogh, *A Government out of Sight: The Mystery of National Authority in Nineteenth-Century America* (Cambridge: Cambridge University Press, 2009); Daniel P. Carpenter, *The Forging of Bureaucratic Autonomy: Reputations, Networks, and Policy Innovation in Executive Agencies, 1862–1928* (Princeton: Princeton University Press, 2001); Peter B. Evans, Dietrich Rueschemeyer, and Theda Skocpol, *Bringing the State Back In* (New York: Cambridge University Press, 1985); Paul Pierson, *Politics in Time: History, Institutions, and Social Analysis* (Princeton: Princeton University Press, 2004); Karen Orren and Stephen Skowronek, *The Search for American Political Development* (Cambridge: Cambridge University Press, 2004); Stephen Skowronek, *Building a New American State: The Expansion of National Administrative Capacities, 1877–1920* (Cambridge: Cambridge University Press, 1982); and Brian Balogh, "The State of the State among Historians," *Social Science History* 27, no. 3 (2003).

45. General works on the American Legion and Disabled American Veterans (DAV) include Richard E. Patterson et al., *Wars and Scars: The Story of Compassion and Service for Our Nation's Disabled Veterans: A History of the Disabled American Veterans* (n.p.: Disabled American Veterans, n.d.), accessible at www.dav.org/learn-more/about-dav/history/; William Pencak, *For God and Country: The American Legion 1919–1941* (Boston: Northeastern University Press, 1989); and Thomas A. Rumer, *The American Legion: An Official History 1919–1989* (New York: M. Evans, 1990). Donald J. Lisio, "United States: Bread and Butter Politics," in *The War Generation: Veterans of the First World War*, ed. Stephen R. Ward (Port Washington, NY: Kennikat Press, 1975), argues that the Legion and VFW were not only conservative but also promoted a "narrow, intolerant superpatriotism" (41). The evidence in this book supports the more nuanced view of John Kinder, "Encountering Injury: Modern War and the Problem of the Wounded Soldier" (PhD diss., University of Minnesota, 2007), who writes that the "Legion's early identity and work—particularly on behalf of disabled veterans—belies neat categorization." The group both recognized and worked to counter a "genuine failure on the part of the U.S. government to meet the needs of disabled vets" even as it attempted to spread its "militantly patriotic ideology" (263).

46. On the radical forces the Legion and DAV hoped to quell, see Thai Jones, *More Powerful Than Dynamite: Radicals, Plutocrats, Progressives, and New York's Year of Anarchy* (New York: Walker, 2012); Michael Kazin, *American Dreamers: How the Left Changed a Nation* (New York: Knopf, 2011); Regin Schmidt, *Red Scare: F.B.I. and the Origins of Anticommunism in the United States* (Copenhagen: Museum Tusculanum Press, 2000); Louis Adamic, *Dynamite: The Story of Class Violence in America* (Gloucester, MA: P. Smith, 1963); William Preston, *Aliens and Dissenters: Federal Suppression of Radicals, 1903–1933* (New York: Harper & Row, 1963); Patrick Renshaw, *The Wobblies: The Story of the I.W.W. and Syndicalism in the United States* (Garden City, NY: Doubleday, 1967); Melvyn Dubofsky, *We Shall Be All: A History of the Industrial Workers of the World* (Urbana: University of Illinois Press, 1988); and Paul Buhle and Nicole Schulman, *Wobblies! A Graphic History of the I.W.W.* (New York: Verso, 2005).

47. Katz, *In the Shadow of the Poorhouse*, xi.

48. Michael S. Sherry, *In the Shadow of War: The United States since the 1930s* (New Haven: Yale University Press, 1995).

49. Poirier interview.

CHAPTER 1: An Extra-Hazardous Occupation

1. Patrick W. O'Donnell to National Home for Disabled Volunteer Soldiers, Togus, ME, Aug. 10, 1918, National Homes Service, NHDVS, Eastern Branch, Togus, ME, 1866–1938, Sample Case Files of Members #17298-22499, RG 15 (NARA–Boston, MA), box 5, folder 17108: Patrick W. O'Donnell.

2. "Referral to Surgeon from Eastern Branch, N.H.D.V.S. for Patient, Patrick W. O'Donnell," Aug. 22, 1918, in ibid.

3. "Application for Original Admission to the National Home for Disabled Volunteer Soldiers, Alonzo Nichols," Apr. 19, 1916, National Homes Service, NHDVS, Eastern Branch, Togus, ME, 1866–1938, Sample Case Files of Members #11052-16852, RG 15 (NARA–Boston, MA), box 4, folder 16675: Alonzo H. Nichols.

4. A 1922 medical reference manual identified locomotor ataxia and "tabes dorsalis" as the same disease with common symptoms caused by syphilis: "a loss of the deep reflexes and . . . incoordination, lightning pains and ultimate paralysis." Symptoms of severe cases included headache, nausea, constipation, or diarrhea. Charles Lyman Greene, *Medical Diagnosis for the Student and Practitioner* (Philadelphia: P. Blakiston's Son, 1922), 1254, 905. Another of O'Donnell's conditions, gastritis, was caused by "indiscretion in diet, nervous shock, toxic irritants such as ptomaines, arsenic, alcohol," according to the manual.

5. Some of Nichols's heart conditions were linked at the time with Soldier's Heart, "a medico-psychiatric condition" (Sean Dyde, "The Chief Seat of Mischief: Soldier's Heart in the First World War," *Journal of the History of Medicine and Allied Sciences* 66, no. 2 [2011]: 216) and "one of the earliest post-combat disorders to be identified" (Edgar Jones and Simon Wessely, *Shell Shock to PTSD: Military Psychiatry from 1900 to the Gulf War* [Hove, UK: Psychology Press, 2006], 205). According to contemporary sources, soldiers were "particularly liable" to the condition, though it appeared in civil life as well among "persons recovering from exhausting illness, such as typhoid fever or influenza." Symptoms ranged from depression, irritability, and fatigue to shortness of breath, vertigo, and high pulse rate. Greene, *Medical Diagnosis*, 608–9; "Soldier's Heart," *JAMA* 67, no. 1 (July 1, 1916). See the essay on sources for references relating to mental health and war.

6. In addition to receiving typhoid vaccines and tetanus and diphtheria antitoxins, World War I–era military personnel were also inoculated against smallpox, a practice that began as early as the American Revolution. See John D. Grabenstein et al., "Immunization to Protect the US Armed Forces: Heritage, Current Practice, and Prospects," *Epidemiologic Reviews* 28 (2006).

7. C. Vernoy Davis, "World War I Memoirs of C. Vernoy Davis, as a Member of Battery F of the 7th Field Artillery, First Division of the U.S. Regular Army, from May 17th 1917 to August 30th 1919" (1993), 4–7, National World War I Museum at Liberty Memorial, Kansas City, MO.

8. *An Act to Authorize the Establishment of a Bureau of War Risk Insurance in the Treasury Department*, PL 63-193, S. 6357, 38 Stat. 711 (Sept. 2, 1914).

9. Samuel McCune Lindsay, "Purpose and Scope of War Risk Insurance," *Annals of the American Academy of Political and Social Science* 79 (1918). For background on the War Risk Insurance Act, see the introduction.

10. *An Act to Amend an Act Entitled "an Act to Authorize the Establishment of a Bureau of War Risk Insurance in the Treasury Department," Approved September Second, Nineteen Hundred and Fourteen, and for Other Purposes*, PL 65-90, H.R. 5723, 40 Stat. 398 (Oct. 6, 1917), 406.

11. *To Amend the Bureau of Insurance Act so as to Insure the Men in the Army and Navy, Hearings before the Committee on Interstate and Foreign Commerce*, H.R. 5723, 65th Congress, 1st sess., part 3, Aug. 24, 1917 (Washington, DC: GPO, 1917), 187–90. On the Wage Commission, see *Report of Dallas Survey Committee to the Dallas Wage Commission* (Apr. 25, 1917), 2. The report was requested by Dallas mayor Henry D. Lindsley, an insurance and banking executive who was later appointed director of the Bureau of War Risk Insurance. See chapter 3 for more on his tenure there.

12. See, e.g., Beatrix Hoffman, *The Wages of Sickness: The Politics of Health Insurance in Progressive America* (Chapel Hill: University of North Carolina Press, 2001).

13. The information pertaining to the US Pension Bureau is cited in Theda Skocpol, *Protecting Soldiers and Mothers: The Political Origins of Social Policy in the United States* (Cambridge, MA: Belknap Press of Harvard University Press, 1992), 1.

14. *Hearings*, H.R. 5723, part 1, Aug. 11, 1917, 14.

15. Ibid., 23.

16. *Hearings*, H.R. 5723, part 2, Aug. 17, 1917, 73.

17. The first quote is from "Julian W. Mack, 1866–1943," *Social Service Review* 17, no. 4 (1943): 507; the second is from Julian W. Mack, "The Juvenile Court," *Harvard Law Review* 23, no. 2 (1909): 120. Also see Harry Barnard, *The Forging of an American Jew: The Life and Times of Judge Julian W. Mack* (New York: Herzl Press, 1974).

18. Mack, "The Juvenile Court," 120.

19. *Report of the Board of Managers of the National Home for Disabled Volunteer Soldiers for the Fiscal Year Ended June 30, 1917* (Washington, DC: GPO, 1918), 52.

20. Julia C. Lathrop, "Provision for the Care of the Families and Dependents of Soldiers and Sailors," *Proceedings of the Academy of Political Science in the City of New York* 7, no. 4 (1918): 146–49. Lathrop pointed out that, "experts in Europe" were "studying the hospitals for re-education of injured men, and the War Department has large plans under way for putting into operation the best methods of dealing with injuries of varying character."

21. The number of hospitals is cited in Charles E. Rosenberg, *The Care of Strangers: The Rise of America's Hospital System* (New York: Basic Books, 1987), 121, 5. On the history of hospitals, see the introduction.

22. Gerald Markowitz and David Rosner provide a useful overview of worker safety laws in the United States, and government involvement in workers' health in the introduction to *Dying for Work: Workers' Safety and Health in Twentieth-Century America* (Bloomington: Indiana University Press, 1989).

23. Scholars have referred to workers' compensation as "arguably the first widespread social insurance program in U.S. history." Price V. Fishback and Shawn Everett Kantor, *A Prelude to the Welfare State: The Origins of Workers' Compensation* (Chicago: University of Chicago Press, 2000), 1. The number of states comes from Peter M. Lencsis, *Workers Compensation: A Reference and Guide* (Westport, CT: Qurorum, 1998), 13.

24. J. H. Woodward, "Disability Benefits in Life Insurance Policies," *Proceedings of the Casualty Actuarial and Statistical Society of America* 7 part 1, no. 15 (Nov. 17, 1920).

25. Carl Hookstadt, *Comparison of Workmen's Compensation Laws of the United States and Canada up to January 1, 1920*, Bulletin of the United States Bureau of Labor Statistics No. 275, Workmen's Insurance and Compensation Series (Washington, DC: GPO, 1920), 18, 59.

26. Lindsay, "Purpose and Scope of War Risk Insurance," 60–61.

27. Sharon Ann Murphy, *Investing in Life: Insurance in Antebellum America* (Baltimore: Johns Hopkins University Press, 2010), 3–6, 300.

28. *Hearings*, H.R. 5723, part 1, 16.

29. *Hearings*, H.R. 5723, part 2, 85.

30. Lindsay, "Purpose and Scope of War Risk Insurance," 58.

31. *Act to Amend an Act to Authorize the Establishment of a Bureau of War Risk Insurance*, PL 65-90, 40 Stat. 398, 405.

32. On women service members and veterans, see chapters 2 and 6.

33. *Hearings*, H.R. 5723, part 3, 183–85.

34. Ibid., 166. During the war, Sherman served as a member of the Labor Committee of the Advisory Commission of the Council of National Defense, which also shied away from the question of how to structure veterans' medical care. The son of famed Civil War Union Army general William Tecumseh Sherman, P. Tecumseh Sherman served on the New York Board of Aldermen (1888–1889) and as New York State Commissioner of Labor (1905–1907). According to one obituary, "his advice on compensation and insurance problems was sought by many states." "P. T. Sherman Dies; Son of General, 74," *New York Times*, Dec. 7, 1941.

35. Lathrop, "Provision for the Care," 149.

36. "Protection Better than Pensions," *Outlook*, Dec. 12, 1917.

37. Davis, "World War I Memoirs," 8–14.

38. Ibid.

39. Ibid.

40. Ibid. On Fort Sam Houston during the war, Frank W. Weed, *Military Hospitals in the United States*, vol. 5 of *Medical Department of the United States Army in the World War*, ed. M. W. Ireland (Washington, DC: GPO, 1923), 741–44.

41. Davis, "World War I Memoirs," 17–19.

42. "First Annual Report of the Council of National Defense for the Fiscal Year Ended June 30, 1917," S. Doc. 65-156 (Nov. 20, 1917).

43. The council's work was "a brief experiment in state management of the economy, according to Alan Brinkley, *Liberalism and Its Discontents* (Cambridge, MA: Harvard University Press, 1998), 80.

44. Rosemary A. Stevens, *Medicine and the Public Interest: A History of Specialization* (Berkeley: University of California Press, 1998), 149. See also John S. O'Shea, "Responding to Crisis: Franklin H. Martin, the A.C.S., and the Great War," *Bulletin of the American College of Surgeons* 89, no. 6 (2004), and John E. Jennings, "Franklin H. Martin, 1857–1935: A Retrospect and an Appreciation," *Annals of Surgery* 101, no. 4 (1935).

45. "Information Regarding the Correlated Activities of the Council of National Defense and the Advisory Commission, the Medical Departments of Government, and the Committee of American Physicians for Medical Preparedness," RG 62, box 417, Medicine and Sanitation Committee.

46. "Correspondence, April 1917–June 1918," in ibid. For an analysis, see James A. Schafer Jr., "Fighting for Business: The Limits of Professional Cooperation among American Doctors during the First World War," *Journal of the History of Medicine and Allied Sciences* 70, no. 2 (2015).

47. See, e.g., Minutes, CND General Medical Board Meeting, Dec. 9, 1917, RG 62, box 426, General Medical Board, Secretary's Office.

48. Minutes, CND General Medical Board Meeting, Apr. 22, 1917, in ibid., 29–31.

49. Minutes, CND General Medical Board Meeting, May 13, 1917, in ibid., 21–22.

50. Minutes, CND General Medical Board, Dec. 9, 1917, 29. For background on Goldwater, who began managing New York City's Mount Sinai Hospital in 1902, see Stanley M. Aronson, *Perilous Encounters: Commentaries on the Evolution, Art and Science of Medicine from Ancient to Modern Times* (Bloomington, IN: Author House, 2009), 67–71.

51. The magazine was "devoted to the building, equipment, and administration of hospitals, sanatoriums, and allied institutions, and to their medical, surgical, and nursing services." "Magazine Slogan, Noted on Title Page," *Modern Hospital Magazine* 8, no. 1 (1917).

52. Winford Smith, "Relation of the Hospital to the Community," *JAMA* 65, no. 18 (Oct. 30, 1915): 1498.

53. S. S. Goldwater, "Soldiers and the Civil Hospitals," *Modern Hospital Magazine* 10, no. 4 (1918).

54. Earl D. Bond, *Thomas W. Salmon, Psychiatrist* (New York: Norton, 1950), 90–96. Salmon not only established a hospital for the treatment of war neuroses near the front but, as we will see, was also instrumental in establishing plans for the long-term care of veterans in the 1920s.

55. Minutes, CND General Medical Board, Dec. 9, 1917, 26–29.

56. Minutes, CND General Medical Board Meeting, June 24, 1917, CND, box 426, General Medical Board, Secretary's Office.

57. Minutes, CND General Medical Board Meeting, Mar. 10, 1918, in ibid., 15–16.

58. Minutes, CND General Medical Board Meeting, May 5, 1918, in ibid.

59. Minutes, CND General Medical Board Meeting, Oct. 21, 1917," in ibid., 13–14.

60. F. C. Kinder, "Military Medicine and Surgery: Notes on the Care of the Crippled Soldier in England," *JAMA* 69, no. 14 (1919). Army officials, we will see, commonly worried about this condition.

61. The phrase is from Carol R. Byerly, *Fever of War: The Influenza Epidemic in the U.S. Army during World War I* (New York: New York University, 2005), 42.

62. Davis, "World War I Memoirs," 70–78, 96–108.

63. Ibid., 97–108.

64. Ibid., 108–11.

65. Ibid., 111–12.

66. Bobby A. Wintermute, *Public Health and the U.S. Military: A History of the Army Medical Department, 1818–1917* (New York: Routledge, 2011), 5.

67. Mary C. Gillett, *The Army Medical Department, 1865–1917*, Army Historical Series (Washington, DC: Center of Military History, US Army, 1995), 4.

68. For more on the nature of military hospitals and medicine in the pre–World War I years, see ibid., 51–52; also, see chapter 2.

69. Weed, *Military Hospitals*, 25–28.

70. Ibid., 54, 27.

71. Weed, *Military Hospitals*, 28.

72. Frank W. Weed, Charles Lynch, and Loy McAfee, *The Surgeon General's Office*, vol. 1 of *The Medical Department of the United States Army in the World War*, ed. M. W. Ireland (Washington, DC: GPO, 1923), 330. The report contains a helpful overview of the development of military hospitals in the United States between the colonial era and World War I.

73. The quote is from Mary C. Gillett, *The Army Medical Department, 1917–1941* (Washington, DC: Center of Military History, US Army, 2009), 62–63. By October 1918, 170,000 beds were available. From then on, numbers steadily decreased, reaching just under 30,000 by September 1919. Weed, Lynch, and McAfee, *Surgeon General's Office*, 338–39. For a detailed overview of the activities of the Hospital Division, see 327.

74. Ibid., 130.

75. Crane, *Physical Reconstruction and Vocational Education*, 3.

76. "Noted Doctors Join Medical Corps," *New York Times*, Nov. 30, 1908. The Army Medical Reserve Corps was established, in large part, as a result of the disorganization surrounding mobilization for the Spanish-American War. For a brief summary, see Weed, Lynch, and McAfee, *Surgeon General's Office*, 58.

77. Edwin Frederick Hirsch, *Frank Billings: The Architect of Medical Education, an Apostle of Excellence in Clinical Practice, a Leader in Chicago Medicine* (Chicago: University of Chicago Press, 1966).

78. Weed, Lynch, and McAfee, *Surgeon General's Office*, 138, 54.

79. Frank Billings, "Rehabilitation of the Disabled," in *Contributions to Medical and Biological Research*, vol. 2, ed. Thomas Clifford Allbutt, Sir William Osler, and Charles Loomis Dana (New York: Paul B. Hoeber, 1919).

80. Weed, Lynch, and McAfee, *Surgeon General's Office*, 474.

81. Crane, *Physical Reconstruction and Vocational Education*, 5.

82. Ibid., 8. The army, like the Council of National Defense, considered the impact of war on populations in France and England. For example, a representative of the Surgeon General's Office, Joel E. Goldthwait, attended the Inter-Allied Conference for the study of professional reeducation in May 1917, where experts from various nations discussed topics including physical reeducation and treatment, the employment of disabled men in civilian life, and the economic and social interests of the disabled. For more information on the conference, see A. Griffith Boscawen, *Report on the Inter-Allied Conference for the Study of Professional Re-Education, and Other Questions of Interest to Soldiers and Sailors Disabled by the War, 8th to 12th May 1917* (London: His Majesty's Stationery Office, 1917). See also Douglas Crawford McMurtrie, *A Bibliography of the War Cripple*, series 1, no. 1 (New York: Red Cross Institute for Crippled and Disabled Men, 1918).

83. Crane, *Physical Reconstruction and Vocational Education*, 12, 18.

84. *An Act to Amend an Act to Authorize the Establishment of a Bureau of War Risk Insruance in the Treasury Department, Approved*, PL 65-90, section 304.

85. Crane, *Physical Reconstruction and Vocational Education*, 30–31.

86. Lytle Brown, Brigadier General, Director, War Plans Division, to Chief of Staff, memorandum "Re. Request of Promulgation of General Order," July 2, 1918, CWCD.

87. Surgeon General William C. Gorgas to the Chief of Staff, memorandum "Re. Request of Promulgation of a General Order," June 24, 1918, CWCD.

88. Col. Frank Billings, "Modern Military and Surgical Reconstruction and the Measures of Cooperation Practiced by the Medical Department of the Army and the Federal Board for Vocational Education," *Military Surgeon* 47, no. 1 (1920): 2. The tension was evident on a public level, too. During congressional hearings about pneumonia outbreaks at training camps throughout the country during the winter of 1918, Surgeon General Gorgas argued that mass illness and unsatisfactory conditions at camps could be explained by the fact that his superior officers had been nonresponsive to Medical Department requests for more clothing, space, and medical staff. Secretary of War Newton D. Baker rejected such claims. Individual medical officers, he said, were to blame. Baker went so far as to court-martial two doctors for the deaths of recruits from pneumonia, thus absolving himself and his line command of any responsibility. Byerly, *Fever of War*, 40–42.

89. The quote is from Beth Linker, "For Life and Limb: The Reconstruction of a Nation and Its Disabled Soldiers in World War I America" (PhD diss., Yale University, 2006), 184.

90. E. D. Anderson, Colonel, General Staff, Chairman, Equipment Branch, to Chief of Staff, memorandum "Regarding Reconstruction and Rehabilitation of Officers and Enlisted Men," Apr. 30, 1918, CWCD.

91. Henry Jervey, Brigadier General, Acting Assistant, Chief of Staff, Director of Operations, to Adjutant General of the Army, memorandum "Regarding Reconstruction and Rehabilitation of Officers and Enlisted Men," Apr. 1918, CWCD.

92. Anderson, memo "Regarding Reconstruction and Rehabilitation."

93. Lytle Brown, Brigadier General, Director, War Plans Division, to Chief of Staff, memorandum "Regarding Physical Reconstruction," July 20, 1918, CWCD.

94. Lytle Brown, Brigadier General, Director, War Plans Division, to Chief of Staff, memorandum "Regarding Organization of a Department of Education in the Medical Corps," July 1918, CWCD.

95. Crane, *Physical Reconstruction and Vocational Education*, 45–51.

96. Carol R. Byerly, *Good Tuberculosis Men: The Army Medical Department's Struggle with Tuberculosis* (Fort Sam Houston, TX: Office of the Surgeon General, Borden Institute, US Army Medical Department Center and School, 2013), 107–15. On tuberculosis and warfare, see the essay on sources.

97. Thomas W. Salmon, *The Care and Treatment of Mental Diseases and War Neuroses ("Shell Shock") in the British Army* (New York: War Work Committee of the National Committee for Mental Hygiene, 1917), 28. On mental health and warfare, see the essay on sources.

98. Thomas W. Salmon and Norman Fenton, *Neuropsychiatry*, vol. 10 of *The Medical Department of the United States Army in the World War*, ed. M. W. Ireland (Washington, DC: GPO, 1929), 67–69.

99. William S. Graves, Brigadier General, National Army, Assistant to the Chief of Staff, to Adjutant General of the Army, memorandum, Mar. 7, 1918, CWCD.

100. Salmon and Fenton, *Neuropsychiatry*, 62.

101. Ibid.

102. Salmon, *Care and Treatment of Mental Diseases*, 28.

103. Thomas William Salmon, "The Prevention of Mental Diseases," in *Preventive Medicine and Hygiene*, ed. Milton J. Rosenau (New York: D. Appleton, 1913), 306–7.

104. Salmon and Fenton, *Neuropsychiatry*, 10.

105. Ibid., 276–79.

106. Ibid., 51–52. Hospital services for patients with mental illnesses varied in quality based on institution. Five psychiatric wards at Walter Reed Army General Hospital, for example, were "open . . . without bars or mesh, and were comparable in every way with the general medical wards of the hospital." Therefore, "the patient was not constantly reminded of his situation by the sight of bars . . . at no time was he stung with the humiliation of imprisonment" (92–93).

107. Ibid., 278–79.

108. Wilder D. Bancroft et al., *Medical Aspects of Gas Warfare*, vol. 14 of *The Medical Department of the United States Army in the World War*, ed. M. W. Ireland (Washington, DC: GPO, 1926), 274. On chemical weapons and gas, see the essay on sources.

109. Martin J. Hogan, *The Shamrock Battalion of the Rainbow; A Story of the "Fighting Sixty-Ninth* (New York: D. Appleton, 1919), 87–89.

110. Bancroft et al., *Medical Aspects of Gas Warfare*, esp. chap. 4 and pp. 60–64.

111. "Memorandum for the Adjutant General Regarding Physical Reconstruction, from War Department Chief of Staff," Feb. 1918, CWCD.

112. "Walter Reed Army General Hospital Annual Report for 1918," Jan. 30, 1919, RG 112, box 1, entry 401, folder: Annual Report 1918. Walter Reed's wartime activities are discussed in chapter 2.

113. Weed, *Military Hospitals*, 54, 189.

114. Davis, "World War I Memoirs," 147–48. Davis mistakenly referred to the Bureau of War Risk Insurance as the Veterans Bureau, suggesting he might have edited his entries after they were initially written. The BWRI did not officially become known as the Veterans Bureau until 1921.

115. Phil Ray, "World War I Vet Feels Forgotten," *Altoona Mirror*, Jan. 3, 1993.

CHAPTER 2: A Stupendous Task

1. "He 'Comes Back' by Aiding Folks with Income Tax," *Come-Back*, Jan. 22, 1921. All copies of *The Come-Back* located at NMHM.

2. Numbers are from Albert G. Love, "A Brief Summary of the Vital Statistics of the U.S. Army during the World War," *Military Surgeon* 51, no. 2 (1922): 165. Also see "Medical Branch Handles Task in Capable Manner," *Come-Back*, Dec. 4, 1920.

3. *An Act Making Appropriations for Sundry Civil Expenses of the Government for the Fiscal Year Ending June Thirtieth, Nineteen Hundred and Six, and for Other Purposes*, PL 58-216, H.R. 18969, 33 Stat. 1156 (Mar. 3, 1905), 1197. The institution was designated Walter Reed General Hospital on October 18, 1905, seven months after funding for the institution was approved and well before it served any patients. General Orders No. 172 (Washington, DC, October 18, 1905). Following World War I, it was renamed Walter Reed Army Medical Center. Herein, I refer to it as Walter Reed General Hospital, Walter Reed Hospital, or Walter Reed.

4. "Hospital up to Date," *Washington Post*, Oct. 18, 1908.

5. 58 Cong. Rec. H1150 (Jan. 25, 1904).

6. Walter Reed Army General Hospital Annual Reports 1911–20, RG 112, box 1. The quote is from the 1913 annual report.

7. Mary C. Gillett, *The Army Medical Department, 1865–1917*, Army Historical Series (Washington, DC: Center of Military History, US Army, 1995), 50–52.

8. Frank W. Weed, *Military Hospitals in the United States*, vol. 5 of *The Medical Department of the United States Army in the World War*, ed. M. W. Ireland (Washington, DC: GPO, 1923), 35.

9. Ibid., 54.

10. Mary C. Gillett, *The Army Medical Department, 1917–1941* (Washington, DC: Center of Military History, US Army, 2009), 417–55.

11. Walter Reed Hospital Annual Report 1917.

12. Walter Reed Hospital Annual Report 1918. According to a postwar report, 13,752 patients were admitted to Walter Reed in 1918, a slightly lower estimate. Weed, *Military Hospitals*, 305.

13. Weed, *Military Hospitals*, 287–88.

14. The term is from T. J. Jackson Lears, *No Place of Grace: Antimodernism and the Transformation of American Culture, 1880–1920* (New York: Pantheon, 1981), 71, 78.

15. *Occupational Therapy: Principles and Practice*, ed. William Rush Dunton and Sidney Licht (Springfield, IL: Charles C. Thomas, 1950), 1.

16. Virginia Anne Metaxas Quiroga, *Occupational Therapy: The First 30 Years, 1900 to 1930* (Bethesda, MD: American Occupational Therapy Association, 1995), 36–41, 115, 52–55.

17. Maj. B. T. Baldwin, "Report of the Department of Occupational Therapy, Walter Reed General Hospital, Takoma Park, DC," Jan. 30, 1919, OHA 245, box 14, folder: Reports; Weed, *Military Hospitals*, 311–12.

18. Quiroga, *Occupational Therapy*, 173.

19. Baldwin, "Report of the Department of Occupational Therapy," 6–7.

20. Herbert J. Hall, "Bedside and Wheel-Chair Occupations," *Publications of the Red Cross Institute for Crippled and Disabled Men* 2, no. 5 (1919): 7–8.

21. "The Growing Use of Occupational Therapy," OHA 245, box 1, folder 5.

22. Charlene Chalaron, "Opportunities in Occupational Therapy," Vocational Information Monographs no. 16 (1932), OHA 245, box 1, folder: Medical History Book Notes.

23. Hall, "Bedside and Wheel-Chair Occupations," 12.

24. For more on women's work during the war, see, e.g., *Out to Work: A History of Wage-Earning Women in the United States* (New York: Oxford University Press, 1982). See also Kimberly Jensen, *Mobilizing Minerva: American Women in the First World War* (Urbana: University of Illinois Press, 2008); Judith Bellafaire and Mercedes Herrera Graf, *Women Doctors in War* (College Station: Texas A&M University Press, 2009); and Mary T. Sarnecky, *A History of the U.S. Army Nurse Corps* (Philadelphia: University of Pennsylvania Press, 1999).

25. Lena Hitchcock, "The Great Adventure" (undated manuscript), ii, OHA 97, box 3.

26. Ibid., xi.

27. Ibid., 51.

28. For information on the career of Alberta Montgomery, see Army Medical Center, "Data Pertaining to Service of Alberta Montgomery" (June 6, 1933), OHA 245, box 9, folder: Misc. Correspondence.

29. Alberta Montgomery, "Class Notebook" (1919), OHA 245, box 6, folder: Class notebooks.

30. Enrollment was highest in "ward occupations"—bedside projects, such as knitting—most likely because patients were bedridden. Baldwin, "Report of the Department of Occupational Therapy," reports 532 patients were enrolled in ward occupations and 142 in commercial work.

31. Jennifer D. Keene, *Doughboys, the Great War, and the Remaking of America* (Baltimore: Johns Hopkins University Press, 2001), 28.

32. Montgomery, "Class Notebook."

33. Grace Harper, "Re-education from the Point of View of the Disabled Soldier," *American Journal of Care for Cripples* 7, no. 2 (1918): 86.

34. James E. Russell, "Occupational Therapy in Military Hospitals," *American Journal of Care for Cripples* 7 no. 2 (1918): 112–14.

35. According to a government report, between June 1917 and February 1918, 28,300 men were accepted by local draft boards but rejected at camps. Another 172,000 were accepted then

later rejected between February 1918 and November 1918. *Hearings before the Committee on Public Buildings and Grounds, House of Representatives, on Additional Hospital Facilities for Discharged Soldiers, Sailors, Marines, and Army and Navy Nurses,* H. Doc. 481, 66th Congress, 2nd sess., Apr. 26, 1920 (Washington, DC: GPO, 1920), 32. A later report, R. E. Adkins, *Medical Care of Veterans,* 90th Congress, 1st sess. (Washington, DC: GPO, Apr. 1967), 92, put the number of inductees rejected at training camps between 1917 and 1918 considerably higher, at more than 740,000.

36. *Annual Report of the Surgeon General of the Public Health Service of the United States for the Fiscal Year 1918* (Washington, DC: GPO, 1918), 19.

37. In addition to those accepted and later turned away at camps, one in three men eligible to serve was rejected for lack of physical fitness by local draft boards between September 1917 and November 1918. After November 1918, standards for entry were loosened and the rejection rate dropped to one in four. Patrick W. Kelley, *Military Preventive Medicine: Mobilization and Deployment,* vol. 1 (Washington, DC: Office of the Surgeon General, Borden Institute, 2003), 149.

38. "Additional Hospital Facilities for Discharged Soldiers, Sailors, Marines, and Army and Navy Nurses," H. Doc. 66-481 (referred to the Committee on Public Buildings and Grounds, Dec. 8, 1919), 34–35.

39. Ibid., 29–30.

40. *An Act to Amend and Modify the War Risk Insurance Act,* PL 66-104, H.R. 8778, 41 Stat. 371 (Dec. 24, 1919). See chap. 1 regarding medical screening procedures.

41. Albert G. Love, *Medical and Casualty Statistics,* vol. 15, pt. 2 of *The Medical Department of the United States Army in the World War,* ed. M. W. Ireland (Washington, DC: GPO, 1925), 15–18.

42. For a breakdown of causes of admissions and discharges, and locations of discharged soldiers, see ibid., 1183; for a detailed description of "discharges by condition," see 166–89.

43. In the United States, patients spent an average of 20 days in the hospital; ill and wounded soldiers treated abroad spent about 27 days in military hospitals (Love, "Brief Summary").

44. US Army Office of the Surgeon General, "Malingering in U.S. Troops, Home Forces, 1917," *Military Surgeon* 42, no. 3 (1918).

45. Ibid.

46. Wilder D. Bancroft et al., *Medical Aspects of Gas Warfare,* vol. 14 of *The Medical Department of the United States Army in the World War,* ed. M. W. Ireland (Washington, DC: GPO, 1926), 65.

47. Thomas W. Salmon and Norman Fenton, *Neuropsychiatry,* vol. 10 of *The Medical Department of the United States Army in the World War,* ed. M. W. Ireland (Washington, DC: GPO, 1929), 95.

48. Albert Love boasted that the comparatively high disease rate among soldiers who never left the United States demonstrated "evidence of the efficiency of preventive medicine" at the front ("Brief Summary," 146–48).

49. *Annual Report of the Surgeon General to the Secretary of War, 1921* (Washington, DC: GPO, 1921), 11.

50. M. W. Ireland, Albert G. Love, and Charles B. Davenport, *Defects Found in Drafted Men: Statistical Information Compiled from the Draft Records,* 66th Congress, 1st sess. (Washington, DC: GPO, 1919).

51. Love, "Brief Summary," 165.

52. Condict Cutler to H. C. Beckman, July 30, 1918, Condict W. Cutler Papers (1918–ca. 1952), box 1, Columbia University Libraries, Rare Book and Manuscript Library Collections, New York, New York.

53. Condict Cutler to H. C. Beckman, Aug. 22, 1918, in ibid.

54. Arthur Purdy Stout, "War Diary," July 24, 1918, Papers of Arthur Purdy Stout (1885–1985), box 3, folder 8: War Diary, July 4–July 25, 1918, Columbia University Medical Center Archives, New York.

55. Nettie Trax to Mother, Sept. 22, 1917, Papers of Nettie Trax, ID 55632, Veterans History Project Collection, American Folklife Center, Library of Congress, Washington, DC.

56. John V. Hawley (Medical Department, Camp Hospital, Field Hospital, General Hospital), "Army Service Experiences Questionnaire, 1914–1921," World War I Veterans' Survey, AHEC. Emphasis in original.

57. Martin J. Hogan, *The Shamrock Battalion of the Rainbow: A Story of the "Fighting Sixty-Ninth"* (New York: D. Appleton, 1919), 90.

58. Joseph W. Bubendorf (Medical Department, Camp Hospital, Field Hospital, General Hospital), "Army Services Experience Questionnaire," World War I Veterans Survey, AHEC. The soldier's suggestion that doctors abroad were more committed than those who served in the United States was seconded by Paul B. Magnuson, an orthopedic surgeon assigned to the surgeon general's office during the war to "get [doctors] and put them in the position in which we thought they would best serve." When Magnuson began his work in the fall of 1917 and tried to find medical professionals to staff domestic hospitals, he found that "most of the best ones had gone into the Army early; some had been ordered overseas at their own request, so the pickings were pretty slim." Paul B. Magnuson, *Ring the Night Bell* (1960; reprint, Birmingham: University of Alabama School of Medicine, 1986), 163.

59. Robert D. Palmer, "Inspector General's Department Investigation as to the Laundering of Clothing by Patients at Walter Reed General Hospital" (Jan. 31, 1919), 1, RG 159, box 1110, folder 12. The underwear referred to by the *Star* was likely somewhat cumbersome for patients to wash. Soldiers serving on the front lines were commonly issued wool pants and wool long-sleeved shirts to wear as undergarments, though some received cotton pants and cotton long-sleeved shirts for wear in warmer weather. Doran Cart, senior curator, National World War I Museum, telephone interview with author, July 10, 2012. Given that most of the Walter Reed patients who took issue with laundry services at the hospital had fought abroad, and some mentioned the idea that their underwear was comparatively warmer than pajamas, they were likely referring to long wool pants and long-sleeved wool shirts.

60. Palmer, "Investigation as to the Laundering of Clothing," 3–8.

61. "Testimony of Individuals Taken at Walter Reed General Hospital" (Jan. 29, 1919), 3, 36, 55, 61, RG 159, box 1110, folder 12.

62. Ibid., 57, 59. Hospital officials were aware of the problem to come. Walter Reed's 1917 annual report had noted that there was a lack of storage space and transportation to provide for the tremendous increase in the amount of washing being done at the institution; approximately 34,000 pieces had been laundered in 1916, compared with almost 87,000 in 1917.

63. Palmer, "Investigation as to the Laundering of Clothing," 4–8.

64. Major Francis Christian, "Investigation as to the Laundering of Clothing by Patients at Walter Reed General Hospital, Reply to Questions" (Jan. 29, 1919), 52, RG 159, box 1110, folder 12.

65. As the logistics were worked out with Camp Meade, he ordered a stock supply of underwear, shirts, socks, and undershirts to be kept at the hospital, for which patients could exchange soiled or worn items. Col. Schreiner, undated order in "Exhibit A," ibid., 74.

66. Ibid., 51.

67. Hospitals offered rare sites of opportunity for the nongovernmental groups: "When men are sick and lonely they are most susceptible to kindness," one YMCA training manual said. "The atmosphere of hurry and bustle is absent and there is ample time to think." National War Work Council of the Young Men's Christian Association of the United States, "Manual of

Camp Work for Army and Navy Young Men's Christian Associations," 5th ed. (1918), 28. See "Morale Support" finding aid, Army Heritage and Education Center. The civilian groups likely helped raise expectations for high-quality treatment among soldiers, their families, and the general public, and contributed to veterans' demands for better aftercare.

68. "The Work of the American Red Cross during the War, a Statement of Finances and Accomomplishments for the Period July 1, 1917–Feb. 28, 1919," AHEC. The Red Cross spearheaded a wide array of aid efforts, including providing supplies, canteens, ambulance companies, base hospitals, nursing staff, and information offices at military hospitals both abroad and in the United States. During the war, more than 8 million workers served in the organization, of whom more than 23,000 were nurses (ibid.). On the Red Cross, see, e.g., Julia F. Irwin, *Making the World Safe: The American Red Cross and a Nation's Humanitarian Awakening* (Oxford: Oxford University Press, 2013), and Marian Moser Jones, *The American Red Cross from Clara Barton to the New Deal* (Baltimore: Johns Hopkins University Press, 2014).

69. See, e.g., "Great Yuletide Is Planned at Walter Reed," *Come-Back*, Dec. 18, 1918; "Biggest Army Christmas Is Held at Walter Reed," *Come-Back*, Dec. 31, 1918. In January 1919, boxing matches were held between various members of the hospital staff of the Quartermaster Corps and the Knights of Columbus—an "evening's entertainment [that] was of a very meritorious character," according to *The Come-Back*; see "First Boxing Match on Post," *Come-Back*, Jan. 29, 1919.

70. "Work of the Red Cross during the War."

71. "Field Director's Comments for Week Ending December 26, 1919" (Dec. 27, 1919), RG 200, box 936, folder 100.8.

72. "Testimony of Individuals Taken at Walter Reed General Hospital," 32–33.

73. Rea is referred to in correspondence and publications as "Mrs. Henry Rea" rather than Edith Oliver Rea. She was an important and instrumental advocate for injured soldiers and is credited with the 1918 founding of the Red Cross "Gray Ladies" volunteer service at Walter Reed. For more on the Gray Ladies, see "Folder Regarding Red Cross Gray Ladies," OHA 355, box 4, folder: PAO File—Red Cross.

74. "Testimony of Individuals Taken at Walter Reed General Hospital," 47–48.

75. *Hearings before Subcommittee No. 2 (Camps) of the Select Committee on Expenditures in the War Department*, House of Representatives, 66th Congress, 1st sess., July 11–October 31, 1919 (Washington, DC: GPO, 1919), 364.

76. Ibid., 363.

77. Ibid., 364.

78. Here the accounts of the doctor and the patient diverged. Parks alleged that he remained confined for thirty hours; MacArten maintained he was bound for eleven hours. The doctor reported that when he ordered that Parks be placed in a straitjacket, he had "moderately advanced tuberculosis" but was monitored closely during punishment and suffered no severe aftereffects. Roy Parks, by contrast, reported that a fellow patient had to carry him to the bathroom for ten days following the incident, and that, soon afterward, "he spit up about one-half sputum cup of blood." MacArten denied these allegations, arguing that Parks's condition was no worse after his detention than it had been prior to it. MacArten finally noted that new hospital policies forbid placing soldiers in straitjackets unless they were deemed a physical danger to themselves or others. Ibid., 184–86, 192. The "strapping six-footer" quote is from Alex Jay Kimmelman, "Pastime Park: Tucson's First Veterans' Hospital," *Journal of Arizona History* 31, no. 1 (1990): 19.

79. About 380,000 black soldiers served in the wartime army. Eleven percent were assigned to two segregated combat units and 89 percent to labor divisions. John Sibley Butler, "African

Americans in the Military," in *The Oxford Companion to American Military History*, ed. John Whiteclay Chambers and Fred Anderson (Oxford: Oxford University Press, 1999), 8. Black soldiers represented about 8.7 percent of the 3,893,340 soldiers who served in the army during the war. On the total fighting force, see Jennifer D. Keene, *World War I* (Westport, CT: Greenwood, 2006), 33. On African American service members and World War I, see introduction.

80. Cited in Keene, *Doughboys*, 90.

81. On the composition of photographs like figure 2.4, see Beth Linker, "Shooting Disabled Soldiers: Medicine and Photography in World War I America," *Journal of the History of Medicine and Allied Sciences* 66, no. 3 (2011).

82. On the controversy surrounding such a law in Alabama, see Jennifer D. Keene, "The Long Journey Home: Federal Veterans' Policy and African-American Veterans of World War I," in *Veterans' Policies, Veterans' Politics: New Perspectives on Veterans in the Modern United States*, ed. Stephen Ortiz (Gainesville: University Press of Florida, 2012).

83. "Oral History Interview with Alice (Mikel) Duffield. Interviewer: Linda Barnickel," Mar. 4, 2002, Papers of Alice Duffield, ID 1747, Veterans History Project Collection, American Folklife Center, Library of Congress, Washington, DC.

84. Aileen Cole Stewart, "Ready to Serve," *American Journal of Nursing* 63, no. 9 (1963). All nurses served without military rank—as civilian "contract nurses"—until February 1901, when the Army Nurse Corps was created. Black women were not eligible to serve as army nurses until late 1918 when the flu epidemic and the demands of demobilization led the Army Surgeon General's Office to reconsider the whites-only policy.

85. Aileen Cole Stewart (Army Nurse Corps, Continental), interview transcript, n.d., World War I Veterans Survey, AHEC. "Colored nurses' quarters" at Camp Grant in Illinois were, according to army reports, "excellent" and "met all requirements." Weed, *Military Hospitals*, 200. For more on Stewart and African American nurses in the World War, see Lettie Gavin, *American Women in World War I: They Also Served* (Boulder Springs: University Press of Colorado, 1997), 59–61.

86. James Cunningham to Mrs. B. R. Russell, July 7, 1918, RG 159, box 1109, folder 6.

87. Throughout the United States (in the North as well as the South), at least three "architectural patterns" existed for hospitals that admitted black patients in the early twentieth century: the first was the all-black hospital; the second was the "mixed-race hospital," where African Americans were separated from other patients, often in basements, attics, or additional wings. The third model, "rare even in the north," was the integrated hospital, where all patients were treated in the same building. Black patients commonly endured inferior conditions in the latter institutions. P. Preston Reynolds, "Professional and Hospital Discrimination and the U.S. Court of Appeals Fourth Circuit, 1956–1967," *American Journal of Public Health* 94, no. 5 (May 2004).

88. C. S. Hamilton, "Inspector General's Department Report of the Alleged Mistreatment of Private James Cunningham, Company G" (1918), RG 159, box 1109, folder 6.

89. "Wounded Soldiers Are Segregated," *Baltimore Afro-American*, Jan. 17, 1919.

90. Cited in Carol R. Byerly, *Good Tuberculosis Men: The Army Medical Department's Struggle with Tuberculosis* (Fort Sam Houston, TX: Office of the Surgeon General, Borden Institute, U.S. Army Medical Department Center and School, 2013), 129.

91. The quote is from Jennifer Keene, *Doughboys, the Great War, and the Remaking of America*, 85.

92. "Soldiers Unmercifully Clubbed by Southerners at Hospital," *Chicago Defender*, Nov. 2, 1918.

93. "Soldier Complains of Inhuman Treatment," *Chicago Defender*, Aug. 2, 1919.

94. Susan L. Smith, *Sick and Tired of Being Sick and Tired: Black Women's Health Activism in America, 1890–1950* (Philadelphia: University of Pennsylvania Press, 1995), esp. chap. 2; Alondra Nelson, *Body and Soul: The Black Panther Party and the Fight against Medical Discrimination* (Minneapolis: University of Minnesota Press, 2011), esp. chap. 1.

95. Alice Dunbar-Nelson, "Negro Women in War Work," chap. 27 of *Scott's Official History of the American Negro in the World War*, ed. Emmett J. Scott (1919; reprint, New York: Arno Press, 1969). See, e.g., "Church Sends Care Pacakages to Soldiers in Drexel Ave Hospital," *Chicago Defender*, Jan. 3, 1920.

96. By 1920, Circle of War Relief leaders were attempting to ensure that the group was understood as more than just a wartime organization. They lobbied for an official affiliation with the Red Cross that would allow Circle member groups to assist with the "public health work among the colored people of the Country." "Conference between Mrs. Noyes, Miss Fox, Miss Vande Verde and Miss Holmes of the Public Health Service, American Red Cross, and Mrs. Boutte and Mrs. Thoms of the Circle of Negro Relief, New York City," Feb. 18, 1920, RG 200, box 45, folder: 041, Circle for Negro War Relief, Inc.

97. "St. Mary's Hall Secured for Colored Soldiers When Visiting the City," *Afro-American*, July 19, 1918.

98. "Soldiers Overcrowd 'Hotel' at St. Mary's," *Afro-American*, Aug. 9, 1918.

99. "War Mothers of Baltimore Meet Thursday at War Camp Community Services Club," *Afro-American*, Oct. 25, 1918; "Community Club Crowded with Soldiers," *Afro-American*, Nov. 8, 1918. The enthusiastic support for troops had evidently calmed by 1922, when one newspaper article declared that troops at Fort McHenry were "lonely . . . and wish that colored men and women living in the city would come down frequently and give them an entertainment of some kind." "Wounded Men Still at Fort McHenry," *Baltimore Afro-American*, Apr. 21, 1922.

100. "Colored Soldiers' Club Opens in Rockford Near Camp Grant," *Chicago Defender*, Aug. 17, 1918. On Hall, see "George Cleveland Hall, 1864–1930," *Journal of the National Medical Association* 46, no. 3 (1954).

101. William J. Breen, "Black Women and the Great War: Mobilization and Reform in the South," *Journal of Southern History* 44, no. 3 (1978). Also, on African American women during and after the war and Alice Dunbar Nelson, see Nikki L. Brown, "War Work, Social Work, Community Work: Alice Dunbar-Nelson, Federal War Work Agencies, and Southern African American Women," in *Post-bellum, Pre-Harlem: African American Literature and Culture, 1877–1919*, ed. Barbara McCaskill and Caroline Gebhard (New York: New York University Press, 2006); Alice Dunbar Nelson, *Give Us Each Day: The Diary of Alice Dunbar-Nelson*, ed. Gloria T. Hull (New York: Norton, 1984); and Charissa J. Threat, *Nursing Civil Rights: Gender and Race in the Army Nurse Corps* (Urbana: University of Illinois Press, 2015).

102. George McAdie to Col. Henry L. Stimson, July 13, 1920, DF, box 78, folder 15.073: "Investigation of Complaints 1917–1921."

103. A. G. Crane, *Physical Reconstruction and Vocational Education*, vol. 13, part 1 of *The Medical Department of the United States Army in the World War*, ed. M. W. Ireland (Washington, DC: GPO, 1927), 30–31. For a discussion of this term, see chapter 1.

104. Ralph L. Williams, "The Luck of a Buck" (1984), World War I Veterans Survey, folders 2 and 3, AHEC. Private Lilley Cornett, who was receiving treatment at Walter Reed after being injured during training, similarly waived his rights to disability compensation in the future. *Hearings before Subcommittee No. 2 (Camps)*, 332.

105. *Hearings before Subcommittee No. 2 (Camps)*, 364.

106. D. W. Ketcham, Colonel, General Staff, to Chief of Staff, memorandum "Regarding Physical Reconstruction," n.d. [ca. Jan. 1918], CWCD, microfilm 1024, roll 346.

107. War Department Chief of Staff to Adjutant General, memorandum "Regarding Physical Reconstruction," Feb. 1918, in ibid.

108. Henry Jervey, Major General, Assistant Chief of Staff, Director of Operations, to the Adjutant General, memorandum "Regarding Discharge of Disabled Soldiers," Dec. 17, 1918, in ibid. On December 31, 1918, the War Department approved a policy to release disabled soldiers from service who applied to be discharged, if they furnished documents from relatives or friends guaranteeing the necessary specialist treatment after discharge and if they released the War Department from further responsibility for their treatment. See Crane, *Physical Reconstruction and Vocational Education*, 49. As chapter 3 of this book notes, those who requested "waivers" were eventually made eligible for care as veterans.

109. Jervey to Adjutant General, Dec. 17, 1918, 2.

110. Weston P. Chamberlain, "Decisions as to Whether or Not Disabilities Were in Line of Duty," chap. 22 of *Communicable and Other Diseases*, vol. 9 of *The Medical Department of the United States Army in the World War*, ed. M. W. Ireland (Washington, DC: GPO, 1928).

111. Cited in ibid., 590.

112. *Hearings before the Committee on Interstate and Foreign Commerce of the House of Representatives on H.R. 11659*, 65th Congress, 2nd sess., May 1, 1918 (Washington, DC: GPO, 1918), 8.

113. Chamberlain, "Decisions," 590.

114. Ibid., 593, 601.

115. At least twenty-four conditions listed as leading to discharge from Walter Reed Hospital in 1918 pertained to mental illness, including "mental deficiency, imbecile" (seven discharges total, none incurred in the line of duty) and "constitutional psychopathic state, emotional instability" (eight cases discharged, none incurred in line of duty). In order to deal with "nervous and mental cases," the hospital in early 1918 set aside five wards with a total capacity of approximately 150 patients. "Mental patients are no longer kept in the prison ward under observation," the hospital's annual report noted. "The chief features" in the care of such patients, "absence of restraint," were "employment on the wards and in the reconstruction shops [and] hydro and electro-therapy in the Department of Physio-therapy." As such, hospital officials boasted that the care offered at Walter Reed to patients with mental illness was "fully up to that given in the best civil hospitals." Still, of the 696 patients admitted to the hospital's psychiatric wards throughout 1918, 42 were discharged as "recovered," 178 as "improved," and 245 as "unimproved." Influenza posed a major challenge at the hospital in 1918. More than 2,300 patients were treated for the disease in 1918, and 153 of the institution's 299 deaths were due to "broncho-pneumonia." Walter Reed Annual Report 1918, 7–13 (on causes of disability), 13 (on care for patients with mental illnesses), 54 (on influenza).

116. Bancroft et al., *Medical Aspects of Gas Warfare*, 274. These statistics do not reveal the percentage of gas-related disabilities deemed to have occurred in the line of duty.

117. D. W. Ketcham, Colonel, General Staff, to Chief of Staff, memorandum "Regarding Physical Disability in Line of Duty," Apr. 17, 1917, CWCD, microfilm 1024, roll 275.

118. Lytle Brown to the Chief of Staff, memorandum "Regarding Physical Disability in Line of Duty, from Lytle Brown," May 8, 1918, in ibid.

119. "Sworn Testimony of Lucius L. Hopwood, Major, Medical Corps, Taken at Walter Reed General Hospital by Lieut. Colonel C.C. Kinney, I.G.D.," Aug. 5, 1920, RG 159, box 1110, folder 18.

120. Ibid.

121. Walter Reed Army General Hospital Medical Board, "Board Proceedings (Re. The Case of George B. Russo)," May 3, May 7, June 1, 1920, RG 159, box 1110, folder 18.

122. "Sworn Testimony of Lucius L. Hopwood."

123. According to the War Risk Insurance Act, a discharged soldier could receive one of four possible disability ratings: total temporary, total permanent, partial temporary, or partial permanent. In the case of the latter two ratings, the veteran was assessed with a certain percentage of disability. *Hearings before the Subcommittee of the Committee on Appropriations*, Senate, H.R. 13870, 66th Congress, 2nd sess., May 14, 1920 (Washington, DC: GPO, 1920), 5–8. For more on ratings, see chapter 3. The quotes are from Arthur L. Chamberlain, 1st Lt. Engrs., Ward 23, to Lucius Hopwood, Supervisor of Clinical Records, Walter Reed Army General Hospital, Mar. 13, 1920, RG 159, box 1110, folder 18. Also see "History of the Case, Obtained from the Officer, Lieut. Arthur L. Chamberlain," in ibid.

124. Arthur L. Chamberlain to Maj. C. C. Kinney, Insepctor General's Department "Re. Treatment at Walter Reed Hospital," July 16, 1920, RG 159, box 1110, folder 18. For details about medical care under the Bureau of War Risk Insurance and Public Health Service, as well as rules about compensation and discharge, see chapter 4.

125. "Testimony of William H. Vail . . . Taken in Office of Department Inspector, Central Department, Chicago, Ill., Sworn to Captain W.M. Robertson, Inspector General," July 29, 1920, RG 159, box 1110, folder 18.

126. "Sworn Testimony of William L. Keller, Medical Corps (Continued)," 4, in ibid.

127. "Testimony of William H. Vail."

128. Inspector General of the Army, "Report of Investigation into Alleged Premature Discharge of Patients from the Walter Reed General Hospital and to the Alleged Failure of the Bureau of War Risk Insurance to Care for These Patients" (Nov. 23, 1920), RG 159, box 1110, folder 15.

129. "Sworn Testimony of William L. Keller," 3.

130. M. W. Ireland to Hon. C. S. Thomas, US Senate, July 29, 1920, RG 159, box 1110, folder 18. For a discussion of changing discharge rules, see chapter 1.

131. "Sworn Testimony of James D. Glennan, Colonel, Medical Corps, Taken at Walter Reed General Hospital by Colenel C.C. Kinney, I.G.D.," Aug. 5, 1920, 4, RG 159, box 1110, folder 18.

132. Ibid.

133. "Sworn Testimony of William L. Keller," 3.

134. "Sworn Testimony of Private Jeremiah J. Hurley . . . Taken at Walter Reed U.S.A. General Hospital, by Major C. C. Kinney," June 6, 1920, RG 159, box 1110, folder 18.

135. C. C. Kinney, "Report of Investigation Concerning the Treatment and Discharge of Patients at Walter Reed General Hospital," Nov. 15, 1920, 12, in ibid.

136. "Sworn Testimony of Private Jeremiah J. Hurley." Hurley argued that government assistance for veterans was a form of "justice" and not charity. In this, he was hardly alone. At a June 1921 convention of the Disabled American Veterans (an organization discussed in detail in chapter 4), a veteran from California voiced his support for government provision of land and home loans by saying: "I do not feel that the government of the U.S. owes me a permanent living, but I do feel that the government owes me a lasting duty to stand behind me as long as I endeavor to help myself and that duty ceases only when I have demonstrated that I have returned to that state of independence I previously enjoyed. We ask not for coddling but for justice. We request not alms, but that which by the grace of god is rightfully our due, namely assistance." At the convention, the remarks received applause. "Proceedings of the First National Convention of the Disabled American Veterans of the World War, at the Chamber of Commerce, Detroit, Michigan," June 28–30, 1921, Proceedings of National Conventions, DAVNH.

137. "Rehabilitation of Disabled Vets Subject of Careful Analysis," *Come-Back*, Oct. 2, 1920.

138. "President Wilson's Message on Healing the Hurts of Our Wounded," *Come-Back*, Dec. 24, 1918.

139. The cartoon reads: "Ain't it a grand and glorious feeling . . . after you've been wounded and you stay in a hospital in France several long and weary months . . . and when you land in the USA you can't join the hurrah crowds . . . and you go to another hospital here not caring what happens because you'll never be able to earn a living without your right arm . . . and the government tells you it will teach you a new trade without charge . . . and finally you are all fixed and get a better job than you ever had—also your compensation and insurance and everything . . . oh-h-h boy!!! Ain't it a gr-r-r-rand and glor-r-rious feelin'" "Ain't It a Grand and Glorious Feeling," *Come-Back*, Jan. 8, 1919.

140. "Summary of Provisions Made for Disabled Men," *Come-Back*, May 8, 1920.

141. "Free Treatment Available for Ex-servicemen," *Come-Back*, Dec. 24, 1919.

142. "Grab Off Right Dope; You'll Find It Here," *Come-Back*, Mar. 19, 1919.

143. "Compensation under War Risk Act," *Come-Back*, Dec. 31, 1919.

144. "U.S. Will Put Disabled Men in Good Jobs," *Come-Back*, Dec. 4, 1918; "Gotta Be Real to Pass Muster," *Come-Back*, May 21, 1919.

145. "Gotta Be Real to Pass Muster."

146. "Health Service Chiefs Gather," *Come-Back*, Feb. 12, 1921.

147. "American Legion Officials to Parley Soon in Washington," *Come-Back*, Jan. 8, 1921.

148. "Vets Aid Seems Certain Despite Rush," *Come-Back*, Mar. 5, 1921.

149. The quote is from "Reviews Rehabilitation Activities at Fox Hills," *Come-Back*, July 17, 1920.

150. NC State Board of Health, "George Mcadie Standard Certificate of Death, Issued in U.S. Veterans' Hospital, Oteen, North Carolina" (Apr. 23, 1930), Ancestry.com, North Carolina, Deaths, 1906–1930 [database on-line] (Provo, UT: Ancestry.com Operations, 2014).

151. "Photograph of Tombstone of George Mcadie, Riverside Cemetery, Asheville, Buncombe County, North Carolina," Ancestry.com, United States, Find a Grave Index, 1600s–Current [database on-line] (Provo, UT: Ancestry.com Operations, 2012).

152. *Annual Report of the Surgeon General of the Public Health Service of the United States for the Fiscal Year 1920* (Washington, DC: GPO, 1920), 274.

153. Census of the State of New York, County of Monroe, Town of Irondequoit, pp. 35, June 1, 1925; Fifteenth Census of the United States, 1930.

CHAPTER 3: War Is Hell but after Is "Heller"

1. Mother Marianne of Jesus to Lt. Col. A. E. Anderson, July 12, 1920, DF, box 78, folder 15.073: "Investigation of Complaints 1917–1921."

2. Ibid.

3. Newton D. Baker, Secretary of War, General March, memorandum, Apr. 17, 1920, CWCD, microfilm 1024, roll 346.

4. Ibid.

5. "Newton Baker, War Secrtary, Called the 'Little Giant' of National Administration," *Washington Post*, Apr. 23, 1916.

6. Jessica L. Adler, "Baker, Newton D.," in *1914–1918 Online: International Encyclopedia of the First World War*, ed. Ute Daniel et al. (Berlin: Freie Universität Berlin, 2014), http://dx.doi.org/10.15463/ie1418.10118; Daniel R. Beaver, *Newton D. Baker and the American War Effort, 1917–1919* (Lincoln: University of Nebraska Press, 1966); Newton D. Baker, *Why We Went to War* (New York: Harper & Brothers for the Council on Foreign Relations, 1936).

7. On the Council of National Defense, see chapter 1.

8. Henry Jervey, Major General, General Staff, to Chief of Staff, memorandum, Apr. 23, 1920, CWCD, microfilm 1024, roll 346.

9. Henry Jervey, Brigadier General, Gen. Staff, to Chief of Staff, memorandum, May 5, 1920, in ibid.

10. Frank W. Weed, *Military Hospitals in the United States*, vol. 5 of *Medical Department of the United States Army in the World War*, ed. M. W. Ireland (Washington, DC: GPO, 1923), 54.

11. *An Act to Authorize the Establishment of a Bureau of War Risk Insurance in the Treasury Department*, PL 63-193, S. 6357, 38 Stat. 711 (Sept. 2, 1914).

12. *An Act to Amend an Act Entitled "an Act to Authorize the Establishment of a Bureau of War Risk Insruance in the Treasury Department*," Approved September Second, Nineteen Hundred and Fourteen, and for Other Purposes, PL 65-90, H.R. 5723, 40 Stat. 398 (Oct. 6, 1917), 406. On the act, see chapter 1.

13. "The Immense Bureau of 'War Risk,'" *American Review of Reviews* 60 (July 1919).

14. Albert Shaw, "Uncle Sam, Underwriter," *American Review of Reviews* 60 (Nov. 1919).

15. "Glass Takes Oath as Treasury Head," *New York Times*, Dec. 17, 1918.

16. Ibid.; "War Risk Bureau Inquiry Is Halted," *New York Times*, Jan. 11, 1919.

17. "Defends War Risk Bureau," *New York Times*, Mar. 21, 1919.

18. "War Risk Chief out after Break," *New York Times*, May 19, 1919. On the founding and importance of the American Legion, see chapter 4.

19. James B. Morrow, "The Risks of Peace," *Nation's Business*, Aug. 1919; "Cholmeley-Jones in War Risk Bureau," *New York Times*, May 29, 1919.

20. "Immense Bureau of 'War Risk.'"

21. Morrow, "Risks of Peace."

22. Richard G. Cholmeley-Jones, *Every Day Philosophy: A Companion Volume to School-Day Philosophy* (New York: John Lane, 1918).

23. *Annual Report of the Director of the Bureau of War Risk Insurance for the Fiscal Year Ended June 30, 1920* (Washington, DC: GPO, 1920), 100.

24. Ibid., 66.

25. L. B. Rogers, "The War Risk Act and the Medical Services Created under It," *JAMA* 26, no. 16 (Apr. 16, 1921).

26. *Annual Report of the Director of the BWRI for FY1920*, 66.

27. William C. Delanoy to the Secretary of the Treasury, July 30, 1918, CWRIB, box 7. Delanoy served as the first BWRI director, from the time of its establishment in 1914 until October 1918.

28. See notes to the introduction for references on the Public Health Service.

29. The quote is from Bess Furman, *A Profile of the United States Public Health Service, 1798–1948* (Washington, DC: National Institutes of Health, 1973), 314.

30. As the issue gained increasing attention from policy makers and medical professionals, Blue predicted in 1916, "health insurance will constitute the next great step in social legislation." The quote is cited in Forrest A. Walker, "Compulsory Health Insurance: 'The Next Great Step in Social Legislation,'" *Journal of American History* 56, no. 2 (1969).

31. Rupert Blue, "Some of the Larger Problems in the Medical Profession," *Medical Record: A Weekly Journal of Medicine and Surgery* 89, no. 25 (1916).

32. Rupert Blue, "Conserving the Nation's Man Power," *National Geographic*, Sept. 1917, 255.

33. Ibid., 278.

34. *Annual Report of the Surgeon General of the Public Health Service of the United States for the Fiscal Year 1917* (Washington, DC: GPO, 1917), 309–10, 50–65.

35. Hugh S. Cumming, "The Work of the Public Health Service in the Care of Disabled Veterans of the World War," *Military Surgeon* 49, no. 1 (1921): 6.

36. Surgeon General Rupert Blue to Secretary of the Treasury, Sept. 17, 1918, CWRIB, box 7.

37. *Annual Report of the Surgeon General of the PHS for FY1918*, 318.

38. *An Act to Authorize the Secretary of the Treasury to Provide Hospital and Sanatorium Facilities for Discharged Sick and Disabled Soldiers, Sailors, and Marines*, PL 65-326, H.R. 13026, 40 Stat. 1302 (Mar. 3, 1919). Also see "New Tuberculosis Sanatorium Dedicated," *JAMA* 78, no. 8 (1922). When Dawson Springs finally opened in 1922, it was placed under the auspices of the Veterans Bureau, which had begun overseeing care for former service members. The total cost to the government for the institution was $2.3 million.

39. *Hearings before the Committee on Public Buildings and Grounds, House of Representatives, on H.R. 12917, Providing for the Establishment of Sanitoriums for the Treatment of Persons Discharged from the Military and Naval Forces of the United States*, H.R. 8828, H.R. 12881, 65th Congress, 1st sess., Sept. 18, 1918 (Washington, DC: GPO, 1918), 7.

40. Ibid., 5, 13.

41. *Hearings before the Committee on Public Buildings and Grounds, House of Representatives, on the Need of Additional Funds for the Housing Corporation, a Bill to Authorize the Secretary of the Treasury to Provide Hosptial and Sanitorium Facilities for Discharged Sick and Disabled Soldiers and Sailors*, H.R. 13026, Sept. 26 and Oct. 8, 1918 (Washington, DC: GPO, 1918), 30.

42. *Hearings on H.R. 12917*, 6.

43. *Hearings*, H.R. 13026, 31–39.

44. *Hearings on H.R. 12917*, 12.

45. "Hospital and Sanatorium Facilities for Discharged Sick and Disabled Soldiers and Sailors," H. Rep. 65-879, part 2 (Jan. 22, 1919), 5.

46. PL 326 passed with 272 yeas, 7 nays, and 148 representatives not voting. See 65 Cong. Rec. H13026 (Jan. 27, 1919): 2153 (Dyer and Elliott quotes), 2171–72 (vote tally).

47. On the emergence of state workers' compensation laws, see chapter 1.

48. Carl Hookstadt, *Comparison of Workmen's Compensation Laws of the United States and Canada up to January 1, 1920*, Bulletin of the United States Bureau of Labor Statistics No. 275, Workmen's Insurance and Compensation Series (Washington, DC: GPO, 1920), 18, 59.

49. "Disability Rating Schedule of the Neuro-Psychiatric Section, Bureau of War Risk Insurance," 2, ODF, box 103, folder: Rating Section.

50. *Hearings before the Subcommittee of the Committee on Appropriations*, H.R. 13870, Senate, 66th Congress, 2nd sess., May 14, 1920 (Washington, DC: GPO, 1920), 8.

51. "Rating" (1920), 2, ODF, box 100, folder: 758, Rating Tables—1921.

52. *Hearings*, H.R. 13870, Senate, 8.

53. Ibid., 5–15.

54. At the beginning of FY1919, the BWRI reimbursed private hospitals directly, but over the course of the year, as more contract relationships were established, the BWRI reimbursed the PHS, and the PHS reimbursed private hospitals. *Annual Report of the Director of the BWRI for FY1920*, 69–70.

55. "Report of the Medical Division for the Quarter Ending September 30, 1919," 6, CWRIB, box 10.

56. "Report of Referred Cases and Hospital Standings, Medical Division, for the Week Ending Feb. 26, 1920," 4, CWRIB, box 8.

57. *Annual Report of the Director of the BWRI for FY1920*, 69–73.

58. Ibid., 74.

59. Bureau of War Risk Insurance, Treasury Department, "Medical and Surgical Relief for War Heroes" (Nov. 16, 1919), CWRIB, box 7.

60. "Additional Hospital Facilities for Discharged Soldiers, Sailors, Marines, and Army and Navy Nurses," H. Doc. 66-481 (Dec. 8, 1919), 1–8.

61. Ibid., 3–7.

62. Ibid., 10.

63. Ibid., 11–15.

64. Ibid., 17.

65. Ibid., 28–30.

66. Ibid., 45–47.

67. Caldwell's question is restated in Rucker's reply. See W. C. Rucker, Chief Medical Advisor, Bureau of War Risk Insurance, to Senior Surgeon Bert W. Caldwell, US Public Health Service, Supervisor of District No. 8, Chicago, Aug. 25, 1919, CWRIB, box 7.

68. Ibid.

69. C. B. Ames, Acting Attorney General, to Honorary Carter Glass, Secretary of the Treasury, Sept. 2, 1919, CWRIB, box 7.

70. BWRI Chief Medical Adviser, "Report of Investigations of Marine Hospital, Chicago" (Feb. 28, 1920), DF, box 78, folder 15.073: "Investigation of Complaints 1917–1921."

71. "Chasing the Cure: The Tragedy of Service Men Who Must Look to Army for Care," *New York Tribune*, July 29, 1920.

72. Allegations of neglect were made regarding care received circa December 1920. "Declare Veterans Beaten in Hospital," *New York Times*, Dec. 1922.

73. Frank W. Bruhn [BWRI Representative, California], "Report of Dr. Seymour's Sanitarium at Banning, Calif." (June 10, 1920), DF, box 78, folder 15.073: "Investigation of Complaints 1917–1921."

74. "U.S. Public Health Service Hospital, New York" (Apr. 24, 1920), ibid.

75. Minutes, Conference between the Public Health Service and the Bureau of War Risk Insurance, Apr. 13, 1920, 1–2, CWRIB, box 11.

76. Memorandum for the Surgeon General, U.S. Public Health Service, on a Survey of the Organization and Administration of the Office of the Chief Medical Advisor of the Bureau of War Risk Insurance, with Reference to Its Relations to the Public Health Service, Apr. 21, 1919, CWRIB, box 7.

77. Minutes, PHS-BWRI Conference, Apr. 13, 1920, 29–30.

78. Ibid., 36.

79. Cora G. Irvine, Executive Secretary, Home Service Section, ARC, to Bradley Fowlkes, Representative, BWRI, Seattle, Jan. 15, 1920, CWRIB, box 9.

80. "Low Pay Hurts Health Service; Doctors Inadequate to Care for 12,000 Soldiers at U.S. Hospitals," *Washington Post*, Mar. 17, 1920.

81. *Annual Report of the Surgeon General of the Public Health Service of the United States for the Fiscal Year 1920* (Washington, DC: GPO, 1920), 290–91 (on physicians), 262–63 (on nurses), 252–53 (on reconstruction aids)

82. For samples of timelines of various patients' transfers in the spring of 1920, see Memorandum for Dr. Lavinder: Delay Incident to the Transfer of Patients through War Risk Bureau, June 18, 1920, CWRIB, box 6. Regarding the BWRI's accusations that the PHS failed to pass on patients' claims for compensation in a timely manner, see W. C. Rucker, Assistant Surgeon General, USPHS, Chief Medical Advisor, BWRI, to Surgeon General, USPHS, Apr. 21, 1920, CWRIB, box 8.

83. W. C. Rucker, Assistant Surgeon General, USPHS, Chief Medical Advisor, BWRI, to Surgeon General, USPHS, Dec. 2, 1919, CWRIB, box 7.

84. Minutes, PHS-BWRI Conference, Apr. 13, 1920, 12. This portion of the meeting minutes is not directly transcribed but written up as a report of proceedings. The direct quote from the minutes is: "The Director stated that this was one of those unpleasant things which had to be borne with as patiently as possible, and that everything must be done to keep the patient satisfied. If a patient wanted to be transferred to another hospital and if there was an available bed, transfer him; if not, explain matters to him and tell him as soon as there was a vacancy he would be transferred."

85. H. S. Cumming, Surgeon General, PHS, to Director of BWRI, Oct. 20, 1920, CWRIB, box 8.

86. Assistant Surgeon General C. H. Lavinder to Assistant Director in Charge of Medical Division, BWRI, Mar. 17, 1921, CWRIB, box 10, folder: BWRI carbons Jan. 1st to Mar. 31st, 1921.

87. C. A. Knowles, Commanding Officer of US Army General Hospital No. 21, Denver, Colorado, to Surgeon General, US Army, memorandum "Re. Discipline of Civilian Patients," Feb. 17, 1920, RG 407, Central Decimal Files 1917–1925, box 1097, folder 705.15: (3-20-20) to (3-6-18).

88. Minutes, PHS-BWRI Conference, Apr. 13, 1920, 12.

89. "Proceedings of the First National Convention of the Disabled American Veterans of the World War, at the Chamber of Commerce, Detroit, Michigan," June 28–30, 1921, 57, Proceedings of National Conventions, DAVNH.

90. Minutes, PHS-BWRI Conference, Apr. 13, 1920, 15–16.

91. Senior Surgeon, USPHS, Inspector, to Surgeon General USPHS, Sept. 20, 1919, CWRIB, box 7.

92. J. W. Kime, to R. G. Cholmeley-Jones, Director, BWRI, July 24, 1920, CWRIB, box 8.

93. *Hearings*, H.R. 13870, Senate, 5–15. The $80 rate was hard fought in 1919 by veterans' advocates who pointed out that former service members in hospitals were receiving only $30 per month, far too little to support themselves and their families. *American Legion War Risk Insurance Conference, Held at Washington, DC, December 15, 16, 17, 1919* (1919), 38; *An Act to Amend and Modify the War Risk Insurance Act*, PL 66-104, H.R. 8778, 41 Stat. 371 (Dec. 24, 1919).

94. There are various examples of the PHS rejecting institutions as contract facilities, especially for use by psychiatric patients. A sanitarium in St. Joseph, Missouri, for example, was said to be "not well equipped and not up to the standard required for the care and treatment of neuro-psychiatric beneficiaries of the Public Health Service." Office of the Surgeon General, USPHS, Section of Neuropsychiatry, to Assistant Director, Medical Division, BWRI, "Re. C.R. Woodson Sanitarium," Feb. 12, 1921, CWRIB, box 10, folder: BWRI carbons Jan. 1st to Mar. 31st, 1921. Treadway also rejected a contract for the Highland Hospital in North Carolina; although it was a "high-class private institution," he said, "the Superintendent . . . is not in good standing with the local medical profession." W. L. Treadway, Chief Neuropsychiatric Section, USPHS, to Assistant Director in Charge of Medical Division, BWRI, Feb. 8, 1921, CWRIB, box 10, folder: BWRI carbons Jan. 1st to Mar. 31st, 1921.

95. W. L. Treadway, Chief, Neuropsychiatric Section, USPHS, to Assistant Director, Medical Division, BWRI, Jan. 19, 1921, CWRIB, box 10, folder: BWRI carbons Jan. 1st to Mar. 31st, 1921; "Finds 21 Heroes in Place He Calls 'Not Fit for a Dog,'" *Chicago Daily Tribune*, Dec. 7, 1920.

96. Office of the Surgeon General, USPHS, Section of Neuropsychiatry, to Assistant Director, Medical Division, BWRI, "Re. Massillon State Hospital," Feb. 12, 1921, CWRIB, box 10, folder: BWRI carbons Jan. 1st to Mar. 31st, 1921.

97. W. L. Treadway, Chief, Neuropsychiatric Section, USPHS, to Assistant Director, Med-

ical Division, BWRI "Re. Augusta Georgia," June 22, 1921, CWRIB, box 10, folder: BWRI carbons Jan. 1st to Mar. 31st, 1921.

98. W. L. Treadway, Chief Neuropsychiatric Section, USPHS, to Assistant Director in Charge of Medical Division, BWRI, "Re. Central State Hospital, Nashville, Tennessee," Feb. 14, 1921, CWRIB, box 10, folder: BWRI carbons Jan. 1st to Mar. 31st, 1921.

99. W. L. Treadway, Chief Neuropsychiatric Section, USPHS, to Assistant Director in Charge of Medical Division, BWRI, "Re. Crownsville State Hospital, Crownsville, Maryland," Feb. 12, 1921, CWRIB, box 10, folder: BWRI carbons Jan. 1st to Mar. 31st, 1921. Crownsville had multiple missions in the pre–World War I years, including "relieving the county homes of their charges" and "utilizing the patients' labor" to clear grounds and erect buildings. Henry M. Hurd, ed., *The Institutional Care of the Insane in the United States and Canada* (Baltimore: Johns Hopkins Press, 1916), 541–47.

100. The title is as per Clifford's own description: "Reports Prejudice in War Risk Work," *Chicago Defender*, Nov. 6, 1920. Clifford served in the 367th Infantry Regiment of the 92nd Division, which had enlisted ranks made up entirely of African American soldiers. The 367th Infantry was considered by many to be "the most notable unit of the 92nd Division." For more on both bodies, see Emmett J. Scott, *Scott's Official History of the American Negro in the World War* (Chicago: Homewood, 1919), 190 (quote), 130–96 (on the 92nd and 367th).

101. "Reports Prejudice in War Risk Work."

102. Ibid.

103. "Soldiers Cannot Get Insurance," *Afro-American*, Apr. 8, 1921.

104. "Wounded Men Still at Fort McHenry," *Baltimore Afro-American*, Apr. 21, 1922.

105. Leroy J. Knox et al., "Lest We Forget," *Chicago Defender*, Nov. 6, 1920.

106. J. Blaine Poindexter, "U.S. Probes Hospital Fight: Soldiers Discharged after Riot," *Chicago Defender*, Feb. 11, 1922.

107. "Protest Mixing Soldiers Sick in Army Hospital," *Chicago Defender*, Mar. 6, 1920.

108. "Investigation of Conditions at Walter Reed Demanded: Resolution Offered in House after Disabled Veterans Complain Whites and Negroes Are Treated in Same Wards," *Washington Post*, Jan. 23, 1924. The broader intention of the DAV's congressional testimony was to voice opposition to the expenditure of $900,000 of a $6.5 million Veterans Bureau appropriation to improve hospital facilities at Walter Reed. Since the appropriation was intended for the bureau, advocates said, it should be spent only on bureau facilities. The congressional hearings signify how jealously Veterans Bureau funding was guarded in the organization's early years.

109. *Report of the Board of Managers of the National Home for Disabled Volunteer Soldiers for the Fiscal Year Ended June 30, 1919* (Washington, DC: GPO, 1920). On Soldiers' Homes, see introduction.

110. Ibid., 5–6.

111. Ibid., 32.

112. "Analysis of Replies of Various Governors of States Relative to Use of State Soldiers' Homes by World War Veterans" (n.d. [likely composed 1922]), BCH, box 12.

113. *Hearings*, H.R. 13870, Senate, 16–17.

114. Robert Jones to Dr. Foltz, Medical Division, BWRI, Sept. 3, 1919, CWRIB, box 6.

115. William C. Rucker to the PHS Hospital Board, July 28, 1919, CWRIB, box 10, folder: War Risk 1919–1920.

116. Chief Medical Advisor to the Director, National Soldiers' Homes, Apr. 7, 1920, ODF, box 94, folder: National Home for Disabled Volunteer Soldiers, 1920–1921.

117. *Hearings before the Committee on Public Buildings and Grounds, House of Representatives, on Additional Hospital Facilities for Discharged Soldiers, Sailors, Marines, and Army and Navy Nurses*, H. Doc. 481, 66th Congress, 2nd sess., Apr. 26, 1920 (Washington, DC: GPO, 1920), 6.

118. Ibid., 11–13.

119. Ibid., 13.

120. Ibid., 15–16.

121. "Clash over Order to Shift Soldiers," *Boston Daily Globe*, July 31, 1920; Charles S. Groves, "Tells Government War Risk Program: Jones Explains Transfer of Disabled Men," *Boston Daily Globe*, July 30, 1920.

122. Groves, "Tells Government War Risk Program."

123. President, Board of Managers, National Home for Disabled Volunteer Soldiers to Dr. Haven Emerson, Medical Adviser, Veterans Bureau, Washington DC, Aug. 23, 1921, ODF, box 94, folder: National Home for Disabled Volunteer Soldiers, 1920–1921. Soldiers' Home residents had also experienced displacement during the war. The Southern Branch Soldiers' Home in Hampton, Virginia, was transferred to the secretary of war from October 1918 through June 1920, so it could serve soldiers disembarking at the nearby port of Newport News. Due to army needs, veterans were hastily transferred from Hampton to other Soldiers' Home branches, resulting in hardship and trauma for the elderly men. Judith Gladys Cetina, "A History of Veterans' Homes in the United States, 1811–1930" (PhD diss. Case Western Reserve University, 1977), 373–75.

124. *An Act Making Appropriations for Sundry Civil Expenses of the Government for the Fiscal Year Ending June 30, 1921, and for Other Purposes*, PL 66-246, H.R. 13870, 41 Stat. 874 (June 5, 1920), 881.

125. *Hearing before the Subcommittee of the House Committee on Appropriations*, Senate, part 2, H.R. 13820, 66th Congress, 2nd sess., Mar. 12, 1920 (Washington, DC: GPO, 1920), 2546–52.

126. *Hearing before the Subcommittee of the Committee on Appropriations*, H.R. 13870, House, part 1, 66th Congress, 2nd sess., Feb. 16, 1920 (Washington, DC: GPO, 1920), 251–54.

127. Ibid., 241–50.

128. *Hearings*, H.R. 13870, Senate, 86.

129. In fact, the report's authors favored the passage of Public Law 246, not least of all because it allocated $46 million, as opposed to the full $85 million originally requested by William C. Rucker and Rupert Blue in H. Doc. 481 of December 1919. In this way, PL 246 would actually allow Congress to "avoid an expenditure," though there was a distinct possibility that "additional hospitals may be required at a later date." "Hospital for Bureau of War Risk Insurance," H. Rep. 66-1098 (June 3, 1920), 2–3.

130. William S. Terriberry, Senior Surgeon, USPHS, to Surgeon Hugh De Valin, Supervisor, District 13, USPHS, Sept. 18, 1920, CWRIB, box 8.

131. William A. Robinson, Special Representative, B.W.R.I., to Major Grover Sexton, Chief, Investigative Field Service, Sept. 20, 1920, CWRIB, box 8.

132. J. H. Widerman, Representative, BWRI, to Ruth Symonds, American Red Cross, Camp Sevier, SC, July 19, 1920, CWRIB, box 8. During the previous summer, the BWRI had requested that various improvements be made to the Greenville institution, and the PHS had fulfilled the request: plans were made to replace window screens; social workers were hired; proposals were being accepted for the installation of a refrigeration unit; cars and china were supplied to the hospital. Widerman's request for a confidential report suggests that the improvements had not been completed to the satisfaction of patients or the BWRI. See Assistant Surgeon General to Chief Medical Advisor, BWRI, June 28, 1919, CWRIB, box 7. In September 1920, a PHS senior surgeon on duty at the South Carolina hospital wrote to the director of the BWRI to report that he had "conferred with . . . the entire staff of workers" there, and none of them had any complaints about the institution. C. C. Thurber, Hospital Director, to Col. James E. Dedman, USPHS Service Hospital 26, Greenville, SC, Sept. 7, 1920, CWRIB, box 8. By 1921, the Greenville hospital was one of a few scattered across the country that the PHS reported was full to capacity or overcrowded. Surgeon General H. S. Cumming, to Di-

rector, BWRI, "Re. Service Hospitals Practically Filled," June 4, 1921, CWRIB, box 10, folder: War Risk, Jan. 1–June 30, 1921.

133. Grover F. Sexton, Investigative Field Service, to Special Representative, Investigation Field Service, BWRI, Aug. 25, 1920, CWRIB, box 8.

134. R. G. Cholmeley-Jones, Director, BWRI, to Surgeon General Cumming, PHS, Oct. 23, 1920, CWRIB, box 8.

135. H. S. Cumming, Surgeon General, PHS, to Director, BWRI, Oct. 30, 1920, CWRIB, box 8.

136. Terriberry to De Valin, Sept. 18, 1920.

137. Cumming, "Work of the Public Health Service in the Care of Disabled Veterans," 6.

138. H. S. Cumming, Surgeon General, to the Director of the Bureau of War Risk Insurance, July 16, 1920, CWRIB, box 8.

139. Cumming, "Work of the Public Health Service in the Care of Disabled Veterans," 10.

140. "Proceedings of the First National Convention of the Disabled American Veterans," 70. Robert D. Leigh points out that Cholmeley-Jones took a stance similar to that of Cumming and Brown and defended his organization. Congressional representatives, not bureaucrats, were to blame for dysfunctions in the system, Leigh argues. They had failed to fulfill the requests of experts familiar with the extent of the need for medical care. In April 1922, Senator David Walsh issued a report acknowledging as much and placing the blame on Congress, not the BWRI or PHS. As Leigh puts it, between 1919 and 1921 government administrators were "the heroes" and congressional representatives "the villains." Robert D. Leigh, *Federal Health Administration in the United States* (New York: Harper & Bros., 1927), 188–89, 214–15.

141. "Peak Attained in War Risk Men under Army Care," *Come-Back*, Sept. 18, 1920.

142. *Annual Report of the Director of the BWRI for FY1920*, 104–7.

143. Ibid, 107.

144. "R. Cholmeley-Jones Dies in Hospital," *New York Times*, Feb. 22, 1922.

145. Morrow, "Risks of Peace."

CHAPTER 4: The Debt We Owe Them

1. Minutes, Meeting of the National Executive Committee of the American Legion, Washington, DC, Mar. 22–24, 1920, 331–33, National Executive Committee Minutes, ALL. These discussions had to do with a "four-fold" plan, which was not passed but would have provided land settlement aid, home aid, vocational training, and adjusted compensation. The weather was reported in the *Washington Post*, Mar. 22, 1920.

2. *Hearings before the Committee on Ways and Means, House of Representatives, on Several Bills Providing Beneficial Legislation for Soldiers and Sailors in the World War (Soldiers' Adjusted Compensation)*, 66th Congress, 2nd sess., Mar. 2–5, 8–13, 24, 1920 (Washington, DC: GPO, 1920), 592; "Say I.W.W. Attempt to Win Service Men," *New York Times*, Mar. 25, 1920.

3. David Gerber argues that an overemphasis on political motives and advocacy "misconstrues" the goals of individual veterans. David A. Gerber, "Disabled Veterans, the State, and the Experience of Disability in Western Societies, 1914–1950," *Journal of Social History* 36, no. 4 (2003). Theda Skocpol similarly argues against a myopic "pressure group thesis" that overstates the political influence of advocacy organizations. Theda Skocpol, *Protecting Soldiers and Mothers: The Political Origins of Social Policy in the United States* (Cambridge, MA: Belknap Press of Harvard University Press, 1992), esp. 111–15.

4. The membership high point of the period—of approximately 1 million—was reached in 1931. Membership and Post Activities Section, "The American Legion National Membership Record, 1920–2006" (2006), ALL.

5. Society of American Legion Founders, "Proceedings and Committees Caucus of the American Legion, St. Louis Missouri, May 8, 9, 10, 1919," 146, Reports of National Officers, ALL.

6. "Committee Reports and Resolutions Adopted at the First National Convention of the American Legion, Nov. 10, 11, 12, 1919, Minneapolis, Minnesota (Unofficial Summary)," 29, ALL.

7. Minutes, National Executive Committee of the American Legion, Minneapolis, MN, Nov. 13, 1919, 78–85, National Executive Committee Minutes, ALL.

8. Ibid.

9. "Report of the Committee of the American Legion on Hospitalization and Care of Sick and Disabled Ex-Service Men and Women" (undated, probably c. 1920), 3–5, Rehabilitation reports 1920–1930, ALL.

10. Ibid, 2.

11. Caroline Cox, "Invisible Wounds: The American Legion, Shell-Shocked Veterans, and American Society, 1919–1924," in *Traumatic Pasts: History, Psychiatry, and Trauma in the Modern Age, 1870–1930*, ed. Mark S. Micale and Paul Lerner (Cambridge: Cambridge University Press, 2010), 281.

12. Minutes, Committee Meeting, June 9, 1919, American Legion Complete Minutes of National Conventions, ALL.

13. Minutes, National Executive Committee, Mar. 22–24, 1920, 52.

14. Ibid., 52–62.

15. Ibid., 61–62.

16. Ibid., 55–60.

17. "Proceedings of the First National Convention of the Disabled American Veterans of the World War, at the Chamber of Commerce, Detroit, Michigan," June 28–30, 1921, 22, Proceedings of National Conventions, DAVNH.

18. 61 Cong. Rec. H6403 (Oct. 17, 1921).

19. "Proceedings of the First National Convention," 22.

20. Membership in the DAV ranged from about 23,000 to approximately 48,000 throughout the 1920s and 1930s before jumping to more than 100,000 after World War II. See "Membership by National Commander Terms," DAVNH. Special thanks to Rojean Long, secretary in the DAV membership department, for providing access to this document.

21. For correspondence related to no fault auto insurance, see "No Fault Auto Insurance Correspondence and Clippings," MSS 903, box 2, folder 13. Marx referred to the Ford case in a 1926 letter to Franklin D. Roosevelt: Marx to Roosevelt "Re. Ford Case," June 21, 1926, MSS 903, box 1, folder 21. Marx's involvement in the case is also mentioned in Charles L. Westheimer, "Biography of Robert S. Marx" (Oct. 1974), 23–24, MSS 903, box 1, folder 1.

22. In February 1917 Marx declared, "I am too passionately American but I cannot comprehend the advantage of a Jewish state in Palestine to an American Jew. No government is so capable and none so willing to protect its citizens regardless of creed as our own. . . . America is my legally secured home . . . it is my own—my native land." "Extract from Address in Opposition to Zionism, Delivered by Robert S. Marx, before the Cincinnati Zionist Society" (clipping from *The Jewish Community* 1, no. 3), Feb. 7, 1917, MSS 903, box 6, vol. 11. Also see Robert S. Marx, "Speech Regarding Contribution of American Jews to U.S. Wars," 1928, MSS 903, box 2, folder 11.

23. "Collection of *Strength and Health* Magazines and Pamphlets on Hand Balancing," MSS 903, box 3, folder 3.

24. "Last Will and Testament of Robert S. Marx," 1955, MSS 903, box 1, folder 3.

25. William Marx's political savvy and connections may have influenced his decision to reach out to a local congressman to help guarantee the safety of his son, who was in Europe when war broke out in 1914. Rep. Alfred G. Allen assured the elder Marx that he would attempt to secure a spot for Robert Marx on one of two army transports bringing Americans back to the United States in the summer of 1914. Congressman Alfred G. Allen to William Marx, Aug. 14, 1914, MSS 903, box 1, folder 10. Correspondence to and from William Marx reveals his political involvement. In 1905, he was invited to the Conference of Democratic Candidates and to serve on the Democratic Campaign Committee of Hamilton County. In the same year, he was also the Cincinnati candidate of the Citizen's Municipal Party and nominated for the Board of Public Service. "Letters to William Marx," 1905, MSS 903, box 1, folder 12. Also see William Marx's obituary, *Cincinnati Enquirer*, Mar. 3, 1915.

26. Quoted in Westheimer, "Biography of Robert S. Marx," 11.

27. "Biographical Sketches of Robert S. Marx" (1959–1960), MSS 903, box 1, folder 2. For further reference to Marx's involvement in Americanization programs, see "Something about Citizen Marx," *Cincinnati Post*, Oct. 31, 1919, clipping in MSS 903, box 6, vol. 11.

28. On Marx's involvement with the enrollment committee, see "Concerted Effort Being Made to Secure Adequate Representation" (Feb. 25, 1916), MSS 903, box 1, folder 12.

29. Conrad H. Marshall, *History of "M" Company, 357th Infantry—1917–1919* ([Carnegie, OK]: [Carnegie Herald], 1919), available at https://catalog.hathitrust.org/Record/009577196. On Marx see p. 38. See also Sgt. George von Roeder, "Short History of the 357th Infantry," www.90thdivisionassoc.org/90thdivisionfolders/Mervinbooks/357/35701.pdf.

30. Robert S. Marx, "Autobiography," 85–86, MSS 903, box 4, vol. 1.

31. See chapter 2 for accounts from army doctors and nurses serving abroad regarding the heroism of front line soldiers.

32. The quote is from a letter Marx wrote to his mother on October 24, 1918, contained in Marx, "Autobiography," appendix 2, 24–25.

33. Ibid., 210–14.

34. "The Story of Robert Marx," *Cincinnati Post*, Oct. 29, 1919, clipping in MSS 903, box 6, vol. 11.

35. Marx, "Autobiography," foreword, 5.

36. Robert Marx to his mother, Paris, France, Dec. 18, 1918, in ibid., appendix 2, 24–25.

37. Ibid., foreword, 5. For more details regarding Marx's whereabouts during service and following his injury, see "Discharge Certificate for Robert S. Marx," MSS 903, box 7, vol. 13.

38. Robert S. Marx, "Memorial Address, Armistice Day, Delivered at Emery Auditorium," Nov. 11, 1920, 16, MSS 903, box 2, folder 11.

39. According to one editorial, Marx's "gallant military record, his able leadership in civic affairs and his recognized ability as a lawyer say more for him than any words of ours can." *Cincinnati Post* editorial endorsement, 1919, clipping in MSS 903, box 6, vol. 11.

40. Dan Morgan Smith to Editors of Cincinnati Newspapers, Apr. 4, 1919, MSS 903, box 7, vols. 13–14.

41. *Cincinnati Post* editorial endorsement, 1919. According to a newspaper advertisement, "Judge Chas. J, Hunt, former Republican City Solicitor and a Judge of the common pleas court wrote of (the Democrat) Marx: 'the zeal, patriotism and bravery shown by you in behalf of your country in the American army in France, in which service you were so severely wounded, exemplify qualities which are needed on the bench and should not be forgotten by your fellow citizens,'" "Robert S. Marx Indorsed by Republicans and Democrats," 1919, MSS 903, box 6, vol. 11.

42. The group announced that it would have a "noonday meeting . . . to further the candi-

dacy of Robert S. Marx." Newspaper advertisement from Soldiers and Sailors Committee, 1919, MSS 903, box 6, vol. 11.

43. "Marx's victory over Gibson," a local newspaper reported, "was attributed to the soldier voters standing by a comrade. Marx had a splendid military record and was seriously wounded when fighting in France. His race largely was made upon this record, and the soldier boys responded to the call by overcoming Republican majorities of more than 20,000 . . . and pushing him over the goal by a small but sufficient majority." "Gibson Defeated by Marx," *Cincinnati Enquirer*, Nov. 5, 1919.

44. "First Commander Recalls Early Years," Documents regarding DAV History, box 54, undated clipping from *DAV Magazine*, DAVNH. For a similar account, see "History of the Beginning of the Disabled Veterans," in ibid. Marx's memory differed slightly from the account he shared at the DAV's first annual convention, when he told attendees that the organization came about when "a group of wounded and disabled men" who "felt the need for an association of their own" met in Cincinnati in March 1920. Simultaneously, "similar organizations were formed in disconnected parts of the country." In September 1920, the groups came together for a caucus and formed a "temporary national organization." "Proceedings of the First National Convention," 22–24.

45. Charles C. Quitman, "History of the Formation of the Disabled American Veterans, Sworn Affidavit," Jan. 23, 1926, Documents regarding DAV History, box 54, DAVNH. In 1954, Quitman reiterated his claim that he and others had established the group but that Marx was "responsible in a large measure for the rapid development of the organization." A recent history of the DAV seconds Quitman's account: frustrated with the government's lack of services, it says, a group of disabled Cincinnati veterans sought help from "better-known disabled soldiers" in order to "make their voices heard." Richard E. Patterson et al., *Wars and Scars: The Story of Compassion and Service for Our Nation's Disabled Veterans: A History of the Disabled American Veterans* (Disabled American Veterans, n.d.), accessible at www.dav.org/learn-more/about-dav/history/. Charles Quitman enlisted in June 1916 and was discharged in April 1919. During the war, he served as a stretcher-bearer in battles at Meuse-Argonne and Ypres-lys. On Quitman's war record, see "Ohio Soldiers, Sailors and Marines, World War, 1917–1918," 13821. Quitman lived with his father and mother in Cincinnati upon returning from the war. By 1930, he had moved to San Diego and become an attorney. Fourteenth Census of the United States, Hamilton County, OH, Enumeration District 29, Sheet 13, 1920; Fifteenth Census of the United States, San Diego County, CA, Enumeration District 37–126, Sheet 5B, 1930.

46. Cox's assessment was contained in a personal letter to Joe Tumulty, President Woodrow Wilson's personal secretary, requesting that Tumulty see to it that Wilson transmit a message to the DAV Convention. James M. Cox to Robert Marx, containing correspondence with Joe Tumulty, Jan. 10, 1921, MSS 903, box 1, folder 17.

47. Franklin D. Roosevelt to Robert S. Marx, telegram, June 27, 1921, MSS 903, box 1, folder 17.

48. Robert S. Marx to Franklin D. Roosevelt, "Re. Endorsement at National Convention," June 14, 1921, MSS 903, box 1, folder 17.

49. On FDR's cuts to benefits in the 1930s, see chapter 7.

50. "National Commander Issues First Message to Disabled Comrades," *Disabled American Veterans Weekly Magazine*, July 22, 1922.

51. "Disabled Veterans Form Organization," clipping, Sept. 5, 1920, MSS 903, box 7, vol. 13.

52. Westheimer, "Biography of Robert S. Marx," 53, notes that Marx maintained a friendship with Bernarr McFadden. Marx's personal papers contain a collection of health and fitness magazines. See MSS 903, box 3.

53. "Disabled Vets to 'Come Back,'" *Chattanooga News*, June 28, 1921.

54. "Heroes' Session" and "Disabled Veterans to Convene," undated clippings, MSS 903, box 7, vol. 13.

55. "Proceedings of the First National Convention," 22.

56. Ibid., 76.

57. Michael Aaronsohn, *Broken Lights* (Cincinnati: Johnson & Hardin, 1946), esp. 284–92.

58. "Disabled Group Names Detroit for Convention," *Stars and Stripes*, Apr. 16, 1921, clipping in MSS 903, box 7, vol. 13.

59. "Disabled Veterans," *Vallejo Chronicle*, June 24, 1922, clipping in MSS 903, box 8, vol. 16.

60. "Veterans Will Try to Unravel Red Tape in Federal Bureau's Work When They Hold Meeting," *Tuscon Arizona Star*, June 22, 1922, clipping in MSS 903, box 8, vol. 16.

61. "Four Disabled Veterans Leave Tacoma for National Meeting," *Tacoma Washington Ledger*, June 22, 1922, clipping in MSS 903, box 8, vol. 16.

62. "Texas Veteran Hops into City on Long Hike," *Santa Barbara News*, June 23, 1922, clipping in MSS 903, box 8, vol. 16.

63. "Wards of the Nation," *San Francisco Examiner*, June 26, 1922, clipping in MSS 903, box 8, vol. 16.

64. "The Most American Thing in America . . . ," *San Francisco Bulletin*, June 26, 1922, clipping in MSS 903, box 8, vol. 16.

65. "Convention of the Disabled Veterans of the World War, San Francisco, California, 1922," MSS 903, box 8, vol. 16.

66. *Incorporation of the Disabled American Veterans, Sub-committee of the Committee on the Judiciary, House Unpublished Hearings*, 67th Congress, 1st sess., June 15, 1921, 5–6, 8.

67. The first quote is from Joseph Walsh (R-MA), the second from Richard Yates (R-IL), *Incorporation of the Disabled American Veterans, Committee on the Judiciary, House Hearings*, H.R. 216, 67th Congress, 1st sess., July 7, 1921 (Washington, DC: GPO, 1921).

68. *Incorporating the Disabled American Veterans of the World War, House Report No. 263*, 67th Congress, 1st sess., July 13, 1921 (Washington, DC: GPO, 1921), 2. In spite of Marx's efforts in 1921, the DAV was finally incorporated nationally in June 1932: "To Incorporate the Disabled American Veterans of the World War," S. Rep. 72-823 (June 13, 1932).

69. Aaronsohn, *Broken Lights*, 313–17.

70. Minutes, National Executive Committee of the American Legion, Washington DC, May 18–19, 1920, National Executive Committee Minutes, ALL, 129–63.

71. "Real Bonus Issue Is Based on Whether Disabled or Healthy Veterans Get First Thought, Say Stimson," *Come-Back*, Mar. 12, 1921.

72. "Legion Leader Visits Hospital; Commander D'Olier's Speech Proved Legion Is Back of Wounded Veterans," *Come-Back*, Dec. 17, 1919.

73. Regarding, e.g., the establishment of a post of the Disabled Emergency Officers of the World War, see "Officer Patients Organize at Reed," *Come-Back*, Mar. 16, 1920. On the establishment of "the disabled men's bureau of service and legislative relief," see "Reed Patients Band Together in Unique Body," *Come-Back*, Apr. 3, 1920.

74. "Legion Members, Alive or Dead?," *Come-Back*, Feb. 28, 1920.

75. "Legion Notes," *Come-Back*, Mar. 13, 1920.

76. Joel E. Goldthwait, *The Division of Orthopaedic Surgery in the A.E.F.* (Norwood, MA: Privately printed at the Plimpton Press, 1941), 7.

77. Minutes, National Executive Committee, Mar. 22–24, 1920, 248, 254.

78. Ibid., 258.

79. Thai Jones, *More Powerful than Dynamite: Radicals, Plutocrats, Progressives, and New York's Year of Anarchy* (New York: Walker, 2012).

80. Vincent St. John, *The I.W.W.—Its History, Structure, and Methods* (Chicago: IWW Publishing Bureau, 1917).

81. Minutes, National Executive Committee, Mar. 22–24, 1920, 258–59. On postwar tensions in the Pacific Northwest, see, e.g., Tom Copeland, *The Centralia Tragedy of 1919: Elmer Smith and the Wobblies* (Seattle: University of Washington Press, 1993).

82. *Hearings on Several Bills*, 616–19.

83. Ibid.

84. "Regarding Radicals," *Come-Back*, Apr. 3, 1920. The following week the newspaper called "the lone effort to spread radical literature among the patients of Walter Reed Army General Hospital . . . a fiasco." It reiterated the lofty ideal that "wholesome, virile Americanism saturates the very fiber of the men who made the greatest sacrifices excepting death itself." "We Stood for It! We Stand for It! Can You Beat It!," *Come-Back*, Apr. 10, 1920.

85. *Hearings on Several Bills*, 603.

86. 66 Cong. Rec. S2734 (Feb. 7, 1921).

87. *The American Legion War Risk Insurance Conference Held at Washington, D.C., December 15, 16, 17, 1919, by Invitation of R. G. Cholmeley-Jones, Director of the Bureau of War Risk Insurance* (1919), held by University of California Libraries. Quotes are from remarks made during dinner and reception, Dec. 16, 1919, 54–60.

88. Ibid., 33–36.

89. Ibid., 49.

90. Minutes, National Executive Committee, May 18–19, 1920, 30–80.

91. Ibid., 71–72.

92. Private Soldiers and Sailors Legion, "Compulsory Military Training," Feb. 13, 1920, American Civil Liberties Union Records, Subgroup 1: Roger Baldwin Years, reel 16, vol. 118, p. 154, Princeton University Library, Department of Rare Books and Special Collections.

93. The Private Soldiers' Legion sought to organize only noncommissioned officers to demand that military higher-ups be held accountable for their supposed errors during the war and that all veterans be granted jobs or land. "Declaration of Principles and Constitution of the Private Soldiers and Sailors Legion," Mar. 1919, ibid. By its own account, in the immediate postwar years the Private Soldiers' and Sailors' Legion attracted as many as 700,000 members. William Pencak, *For God and Country: The American Legion 1919–1941* (Boston: Northeastern University Press, 1989), 51. The group was vocal in debates regarding soldiers' bonuses and other pertinent issues; its president, Marvin Gates Sperry, was called to testify before Congress on such matters. In early 1922, however, Sperry was accused of embezzlement. Though the charges were later dismissed as being unfounded, internal conflicts among the Private Soldiers' and Sailors' Legion leaders rendered the organization all but defunct. "Ex-Soldier Organizer Is Held as Embezzler; Lobbied for Bonus and Started Buddies' Club," *New York Times*, May 23, 1922; "Buddies' Club Head Faces Court Today: M.G. Sperry Brought from Washington on Embezzlement Charge," *Baltimore Sun*, May 23, 1922; "Sperry Charges Dismissed: Baltimore Magistrate Says He Was 'Fooled' into Issuing Warrant," *New York Times*, May 24, 1922; "Evidence Lacking: Sperry Dismissed . . . Magistrate Apologizes," *Baltimore Sun*, May 24, 1922; "Charges Clerks Sold Everything in Office; Only Wallpaper Left," *Washington Post*, Aug. 30, 1922.

94. Albert Desilver to Scott Nearing, Oct. 29, 1920, ACLU Records, Subgroup 1: Roger Baldwin Years, reel 16, vol. 118, p. 258.

95. "World War Veterans, Inc. (Northwest Division)," n.d., in ibid., 267. The WWVA was among the first proposed advocacy organizations to represent former service members who had served in the World War; in February 1919, Rep. George K. Denton (D-IN) sought federal

recognition for incorporation of the group. Denton argued that the WWVA should be based in Indiana because, he said, the first American killed after the United States declared war was from that state. In 1923, one newspaper referred to the organization as "highly radical . . . and in reality a subsidiary of the Communist party of America." The negative publicity surrounding the political leanings of the Private Soldiers' and Sailors' Legion and the World War Veterans of America undercut membership and helped the American Legion to assume a position as the primary veterans' advocacy group of the time. "An Unfair Scheme," *Atlanta Constitution*, Nov. 6, 1923. "To counteract the loyal and patriotic actions of the American Legion," the *Los Angeles Times* reported, "the Communists have secured control (if they did not inspire its formation in the first place) of the World War Veterans." "Reds Plot to Destroy All Police Protection," *Los Angeles Times*, July 23, 1923.

96. "Proceedings of the First National Convention," 80–83.

97. *Hearings*, H.R. 216. In 1922, rumors surfaced that Horr was attempting to organize several chapters to break away from the DAV and form their own organization. He vehemently denied the charges, but he nonetheless played a more muted role in the DAV thereafter. "Proceedings at the Second Annual Convention of the Disabled American Veterans of the World War, Held at the St. Francis Hotel, San Francisco, California," June 26–June 30, 1922, Documents Regarding DAV History, DAVNH, 196. Horr eventually ran for various political offices (to serve as a Republican congressman, senator, and mayor), winning a post only once, a seat in the 72nd Congress (1931–1933). For more on Horr, see "Ralph Horr Congressional Biography," http://bioguide.congress.gov/scripts/biodisplay.pl?index=H000793.

98. "Proceedings of the First National Convention," 80–83.

99. Marx urged veterans to acknowledge the good work of the federal board, in addition to recognizing its shortfalls. "Marx Backs up Federal Board for Veterans," newspaper clipping, May 21, 1921, MSS 903, box 7, vol. 13. Regarding the confrontation with Bodine, see "Injured Soldiers Clash in Meeting," newspaper clipping, May 16, 1921; "Soldiers' League Called Bolshevist . . . Assailed by Disabled American Veterans at Lively Meeting in Y.M.C.A.," newspaper clipping, n.d.; "Rival Organizations of Disabled Heroes of World War Clash," newspaper clipping, n.d., all in ibid.

100. "Disabled War Veterans' Convention," clipping from the *Albany (NY) Evening Journal*, July 21, 1921, MSS 903, box 7, vol. 13.

101. "Call on All States to Check Red Flag," *New York Times*, July 1, 1921.

102. Marx noted that his organization had "no axes to grind," though he did occasionally tailor his language to particular political situations. The quote is from "Disabled Vets Turn to Talk," newspaper clipping, June 26, 1921, MSS 903, box 7, vol. 13. When justifying the necessity of issuing the DAV a charter, Marx appealed to legislators by saying the organization could serve as a means of unifying disabled veterans in a group that Congress could be sure was "under the right leadership." *Hearings*, H.R. 216.

103. The first quote is from George Steinmetz, *Regulating the Social: The Welfare State and Local Politics in Imperial Germany* (Princeton: Princeton University Press, 1993), 205. The second is from Ann Shola Orloff, *The Politics of Pensions: A Comparative Analysis of Britain, Canada, and the United States* (Madison: University of Wisconsin Press, 1993), 286.

104. The quote is from "Many Important Bills Die with 66th Congress," *Baltimore Sun*, Mar. 5, 1921.

105. *An Act Providing Additional Hospital Facilities for Patients of the Bureau of War Risk Insurance and of the Federal Board for Vocational Education, Division of Rehabilitation, and for Other Purposes*, PL 67-384, H.R. 15894, 41 Stat. 1364 (Mar. 4, 1921).

106. "Measures for Aid of Vets Are Facing Congressional Jam," *Come-Back*, Feb. 5, 1921.

107. See chapter 3 for a further description of PL 246, which allocated $46 million to the Bureau of War Risk Insurance and brought about a storm of protest from PHS officials.

108. 66 Cong. Rec. H2708-10 (Feb. 7, 1921). For the series of requests from senators to locate facilities in their own states, see 2711–14.

109. Ibid., 2709.

110. Ibid., 2734.

111. Ibid., 2731–33.

112. "Freak Bills in Congress," *New York Times*, Dec. 16, 1923; "Urges $600,000,000 Loan for Buildings," *New York Times*, Apr. 22, 1923.

113. 66 Cong. Rec. S2715-18 (Feb. 7, 1921).

114. Ibid., 2732, 2736 (vote tally).

115. Many concerns raised by Democrats in the House were alleviated following further discussions in the Senate. In its final form, the Langley Bill contained few specific recommendations regarding where the appropriation should be spent, with the exception of three military forts, which were transferred to the Treasury Department via the law. *Act Providing Additional Hospital Facilities*, PL 67-384, 41 Stat. 1364.

116. "Harding Will Help Disabled War Vets . . . President Elect Discusses Problem with Judge Robert S. Marx," *Cincinnati Enquirer*, Dec. 23, 1920.

117. "Pershing Lauds Plan Extending Aid to Wounded," *Come-Back*, Feb. 12, 1921.

118. "Delays in Hospital Construction, Conclusions," Aug. 22, 1922, BCH, box 27.

119. Quoted in Rosemary Stevens, *American Medicine and the Public Interest* (New Haven: Yale University Press, 1972), 129.

120. "Meeting of the American Conference on Hospital Service," *Public Health Reports* 36, no. 36 (Sept. 9, 1921): 2222–23.

121. On Billings and Salmon, see chapter 1 and the note on sources.

122. The committee assumed, for example, that more beds in Soldiers' Homes would eventually come in handy "to take care of their necessarily increased work at a later period." It also noted that it was "trying to place the institutions in such a way as to fit in with the plans suggested for a new department of welfare," which is discussed later in this chapter. See memorandum, Advisory Committee to the Chairman, Committee on Hospitalization, Treasury Department, "Preliminary Reports," Apr. 18, 1921, BCH, box 25.

123. "To Mention to the President," June 11, 1921, BCH, box 27.

124. The term "crisis expansion" is used in a letter to the secretary of the Treasury quoted in *Report of the Consultants on Hospitalization Appointed by the Secretary of the Treasury to Provide Additional Hospital Facilities under Public Act 384* (Washington, DC: GPO, Jan. 25, 1922).

125. Austin T. Walden and Chas A. Shaw to the American Legion, Sept. 25, 1919, Georgia —History File—Department—History, ALL.

126. C. Baxter Jones to Franklin D'Olier, Sept. 16, 1919, ibid.

127. "An Open Letter from the Colored Delegation of Louisiana to the National Executive Committee of the American Legion," July 3, 1919, ibid.; Jones to D'Olier, Sept. 16, 1919.

128. Louis H. Bell, Member from Georgia, National Executive Committee, to Col. Henry D. Lindsley, Chairman, National Executive Committee, July 18, 1919, Georgia—History File— Department—History, ALL.

129. "Extract of Letter Written by James M. Parker," Apr. 24, 1919, ibid.

130. Irvine F. Belser, State Adjutant of South Carolina, to Henry D. Lindsley, Chairman, American Legion, Aug. 30, 1919, ibid.

131. W. L. Price, Department Commander, Virginia, to Lemuel Bolles, Sept. 18, 1920, Administration & Organization Files—Membership—Black—folder 1, ALL.

132. Henry D. Lindsley to Irvine F. Belser, Sept. 15, 1919, Georgia—History File—Department—History, ALL.

133. Minutes, National Executive Committee, June 9, 1919, 135–45, National Executive Committee Minutes, ALL.

134. Ibid, 140. John Inzer had long been candid about his segregationist views. In 1917, he wrote to his senator to share his belief that if military camps were integrated, as the secretary of War was proposing, "there will be blood shed and much of it . . . if Secretary Baker thinks he can have both races trained in the same camp, he will find out his mistake when it is too late." John W. Inzer, Ashville, Alabama, to John H. Bankhead, Washington, DC, Sept. 6, 1917, John Hollis Bankhead Papers, LPR49, box 31, folder: European War, 1914–1918—Military officers—Universal service, 1917 August–1918 January, Alabama Department of Archives and History, Montgomery, available through the Alabama History Education Initiative, http://digital.archives.alabama.gov/cdm/singleitem/collection/voices/id/3805/rec/8.

135. Pencak, *For God and Country*, 68–69.

136. Aaronsohn, *Broken Lights*, 321.

137. "Proceedings of the First National Convention," 65. For references on Asian American veterans, see the essay on sources.

138. Ibid.; "Negroes from Texas Rejected Because Charter Revoked," clipping from *San Francisco Call*, June 28, 1922, MSS 903, box 8, vol. 16. Although veterans of color were discriminated against and the DAV was not wholly egalitarian, it was more accepting in many ways than some other groups of its time. By 1933, the DAV had created a "national chapter of colored members"; state and local chapters were urged to send membership requests from eligible African Americans to national headquarters, so they could be referred to that unit. "Proceedings of the First National Convention," 49. Occasionally, Marx used his perch as national commander to promote the idea that—contrary to the beliefs of some—American Jews were proud patriots. *The Disabled American Veterans of the World War, Manual*, 1934–1935, 14–16, Documents Regarding DAV History, Unsorted Files, DAVNH. In the late 1920s, he connected the disproportionate part played by American Jews in the war effort with an attack on the anti-Semitic stories being printed in Henry Ford's *Dearborn Independent*. "The American Jew is but three per cent of the American population, and yet we furnished from four to five per cent of the Army, Navy and Marine Corps," he said. "Jewish War Hero and Head of the Disabled American Veterans of the World War Thrills Audience," clipping from *Temple Emanu-El Newsletter*, July 7, 1922, MSS 903, box 7, vol. 13.

139. "Proceedings of the First National Convention," 49.

140. "Report of Conference Held in Offices of Consultants on Hospitalization," May 9, 1921, 63, BCH, box 35.

141. Ibid., 63–64.

142. Ibid., 65. The data would have come as no surprise to activists who had long recognized that African Americans had higher mortality and sickness rates because of socioeconomic conditions and unequal access to quality facilities and doctors. See, e.g., W. E. B. Du Bois, *The Health and Physique of the Negro American: Report of a Social Study Made under the Direction of Atlanta University* (Atlanta, GA: University of Atlanta Press, 1906), and W. Montague Cobb, *Medical Care and the Plight of the Negro* (New York: National Association for the Advancement of Colored People, 1947). On stigma regarding mental illness, see Martin Summers, "Diagnosing the Ailments of Black Citizenship: African American Physicians and the Politics of Mental Illness, 1895–1940," in *Precarious Prescriptions: Contested Histories of Race and Health in North America*, ed. Laurie B. Green, John Mckiernan-González, and Martin Summers (Minneapolis: University of Minnesota Press, 2014). See also Anne C. Rose, *Psychology and Selfhood in the Segregated South* (Chapel Hill: University of North Carolina Press, 2009).

143. Ibid., 66.

144. Alice Dunbar-Nelson, "Negro Women in War Work," chap. 27 of *Scott's Official History of the American Negro in the World War*, ed. Emmett J. Scott (Chicago: Homewood Press, 1919). On efforts and debates surrounding the creation of all-black hospitals, see Vanessa Northington Gamble, *Making a Place for Ourselves: The Black Hospital Movement, 1920–1945* (New York: Oxford University Press, 1995), which includes a discussion of Tuskegee (183–86).

145. Adam Fairclough, foreword to *Long is the Way and Hard: One Hundred Years of the NAACP*, ed. Kevern Verney and Lee Sartain (Fayetteville: University of Arkansas Press, 2009), xi.

146. "Forum: Does Not Want to Go South for Hospital Treatment Says Wounded Soldier," *Baltimore Afro-American*, Aug. 5, 1921.

147. "Ex-Service Men Want Hospital Located North," *Baltimore Afro-American*, Nov. 4, 1921.

148. On Tuskegee Veterans' Hospital, see, e.g., Jennifer D. Keene, "The Long Journey Home: Federal Veterans' Policy and African American Veterans of World War I," in *Veterans' Policies, Veterans' Politics: New Perspectives on Veterans in the Modern United States*, ed. Stephen Ortiz (Gainesville: University Press of Florida, 2012); and Pete Daniel, "Black Power in the 1920s: The Case of Tuskegee Veterans Hospital," *Journal of Southern History* 36, no. 2 (Aug. 1970).

CHAPTER 5: Administrative Geometry

1. Charles R. Forbes, speech delivered at Conference of Officers in Charge of Government Hospitals, Jan. 20, 1922, DF, box 126, folder 060: "Speeches, 1922."

2. Available at www.presidency.ucsb.edu/ws/?pid=25833.

3. *Annual Report of the Director of the Bureau of War Risk Insurance for the Fiscal Year Ended June 30, 1920* (Washington, DC: GPO, 1920), 107.

4. *Annual Report of the Surgeon General of the Public Health Service of the United States for the Fiscal Year 1920* (Washington, DC: GPO, 1920), 240.

5. "John Jacob Rogers, Bay State Member of Congress Dead," *Washington Post*, Mar. 29, 1925.

6. "Goes to Inspect Hospitals," *Washington Post*, Apr. 21, 1922.

7. "New Englanders in the Globe Spotlight: The Angel of Walter Reed," *Washington Post*, Nov. 16, 1921.

8. "Edith Nourse Rogers Mourned by Nation," *Boston Globe*, Sept. 11, 1960; Victoria Schuck, "Rogers, Edith Nourse, March 19, 1881–Sept. 10, 1960," in *Notable American Women: The Modern Period* (Cambridge, MA: Harvard University Press, 1980).

9. The quote is from "Consolidation of U.S. Bureaus Plan of Legion's Proposed Bill," *Come-Back*, Dec. 4, 1920. Also see "For One Soldier Bureau; Bill Backed by American Legion Is Introduced in the House," *New York Times*, Dec. 12, 1920.

10. *Bureau of Veteran Reestablishment, Hearing before the Committee on Interstate and Foreign Commerce of the House of Representatives, on H.R. 14961*, 66th Congress, 3rd sess., Jan. 7, 1921 (Washington, DC: GPO, 1921), 69.

11. Ibid., 8–15.

12. Ibid., 80.

13. Ibid., 8–15.

14. *Hearings before the Subcommittee of the Committee on Appropriations*, H.R. 13870, Senate, 66th Congress, 2nd sess., May 14, 1920 (Washington, DC: GPO, 1920), 23–24.

15. *Hearing on H.R. 14961*, 41–45.

16. Ibid., 27–40.

17. Ibid.

18. Ibid., 21–26. Sherburne, a brigadier general, was referred to as a "principal founder of the Legion" in Edward D. Sirois and William McGinnis, *Smashing through the "World War"* (Salem, MA: Meek, 1919), 175.

19. *Hearing on H.R. 14961*, 53–57.

20. Ibid., 60.

21. Ibid., 84–88.

22. Ibid., 88.

23. Ibid., 89–92.

24. Ibid., 9–10.

25. Ibid., 81.

26. As Madeleine Edison Sloane, daughter of Thomas Edison, told the *New York Times*, the Rogers Bill was "killed in subcommittee, presumably because of the unwillingness of the officials of the existing boards to work under one director." Sloane lamented that there was "no coordination" among the government bureaus overseeing care for disabled soldiers, and now Congress had failed to pass the bill that represented the one viable solution to the problem. Sloane and others focused on the emotional issue of veterans' neglect and the crisis at hand rather than the complex and arcane concerns brought up by PHS and other officials regarding the issue of consolidation. "Public Help Asked for Veterans' Bill: Plan for Federal Bureau of Rehabilitation Would Concentrate Relief Activities," *New York Times*, Mar. 20, 1921.

27. "Proceedings of Committee Appointed by the President of the United States to Investigate the Administration of Law in Caring for the Crippled and Impaired Soldiers of the Late World War," Apr. 5, 1921, in *Hearings before a Subcommittee of the Committee on Interstate and Foreign Commerce of the House of Representatives*, H.R. 3, part I, 67th Congress, 1st sess., Apr. 29, 1921 (Washington, DC: GPO, 1921); see "Exhibit 2," letter from President Warren G. Harding to "General Dawes and members of the Committee," 44.

28. Dawes would later serve as director of the Bureau of the Budget under Harding and as Calvin Coolidge's vice president. He also won a Nobel Peace Prize for conceiving of the 1924 Dawes Plan, which was intended to stabilize Germany's economy. On Dawes, see John Erwin Pixton, "The Early Career of Charles G. Dawes [to 1905]" (PhD diss., University of Chicago, 1952); Bascom N. Timmons, *Portrait of an American: Charles G. Dawes* (New York: Henry Holt, 1953); and Paul Roscoe Leach, *That Man Dawes* (Chicago: Reilly & Lee, 1930).

29. "Proceedings of Committee to Investigate the Administration of Law," 45 (regarding corporations versus investigative committees).

30. Ibid., 116–17.

31. Ibid., 70.

32. Ibid., 66.

33. Carl Sferrazza Anthony, *Florence Harding: The First Lady, the Jazz Age, and the Death of America's Most Scandalous President* (New York: William Morrow, 1998), 86.

34. Admiral Joel T. Boone, oral history interview by Raymond Henle, July 22, 1967, 16, Scripps Library, Miller Center, University of Virginia, Charlottesville.

35. Eugene P. Trani and David L. Wilson, *The Presidency of Warren G. Harding* (Lawrence: Regents Press of Kansas, 1977), 45.

36. When Sawyer was nominated, he was 62 years old—two years past the maximum age for commissioned, active duty personnel. But Harding's attorney general Harry M. Daugherty argued that the age limitations did not apply in times of war, and the United States was technically still at war with Germany in March 1921. "Sawyer Nomination Goes to the Senate," *New York Times*, Mar. 9, 1921.

37. "The Drive on Doctor Sawyer," *Peoria Transcript*, Oct. 22, 1922, Microfilms, Rehabili-

tation—Veterans' Administration Hospitals—Hospitalization (con't) Rehab—VA—Hospitals—Survey 1929 Library 92–1012, ALL.

38. White House statement, quoted in "Sawyer Nomination Goes to the Senate."

39. *Department of Public Welfare, Joint Hearings before the Committees on Education, on S. 1607 and H.R. 5837*, 67th Congress, 1st sess., May 11, 12, 13, 18, 20, 1921 (Washington, DC: GPO, 1921), 5, 11.

40. Ibid., 4–18. For a description of the proposed department, see "Report of Brigadier Gen. C. E. Sawyer to the President Relative to the Creation of a Department of Public Welfare," May 4, 1922, RFBH, box 1.

41. See chapter 3 for details about controversies surrounding placing veterans in Soldiers' Homes in 1920 and 1921.

42. *Joint Hearings on S. 1607 and H.R. 5837*, 5, 10.

43. Ibid., 17. Towner's sentiment was representative of the feelings of many education advocates; see Hugh S. Magill, "Education and the Federal Government," *Today's Education* 10–11 (Nov. 1921).

44. On the Shepperd-Towner Act, see, e.g. Nancy F. Cott, *The Grounding of Modern Feminism* (New Haven: Yale University Press, 1987).

45. "Proceedings of Committee to Investigate the Administration of Law," 83–85.

46. "To Mention to the President," June 11, 1921, BCH, box 27.

47. "Proceedings of Committee to Investigate the Administration of Law," 130.

48. Ibid., 49 ("Bird's eye" quote), 127–30 (general recommendations). See chapter 4 for a description of the White Committee.

49. "Tells of U.S. Army Driving Back Huns," *Washington Post*, Feb. 8, 1920.

50. "Burton E. Sweet," *New York Times*, Jan. 5, 1957. Sweet ran as a state senator in a crowded field in 1922 rather than running to retain his House seat. In spite of his efforts on behalf of veterans, he lost the election to Republican progressive Smith W. Brookhart, who was known to "attack . . . the Interests, the Railroads, the Wets" and possess a "pugnacious cowhide radicalism" that "nettled patrician senators." See "Iowa: Again, Brookhart," *Time*, Apr. 20, 1936, and "Iowa Victory Aids Cause of Progressives," *New York Tribune*, June 7, 1922.

51. *Hearing on H.R. 14961*, 33, 80.

52. "Proceedings of Committee to Investigate the Administration of Law," 10; "Veterans' Bureau, to Accompany H.R. 6611," H. Rep. 67-104 (May 27, 1921), 1.

53. *Hearing on H.R. 14961*, 105–6.

54. *Hearings before a Subcommittee of the Committee on Finance, United States Senate, on H.R. 6611, an Act to Establish in the Treasury Department a Veterans' Bureau and to Improve the Facilities and Service of Such Bureau, and Further to Amend and Modify the War Risk Insurance Act*, 67th Congress, 1st sess., July 11, 1921 (Washington, DC: GPO, 1921), 60–61.

55. Ibid., 17–20.

56. At this point, all ex-soldiers, whether they had incurred tuberculosis in the line of duty or were reported to have it upon entrance into the service, had to prove the condition arose within two years of discharge. As the next chapter notes, the World War Veterans' Act of 1924 expanded eligibility for benefits and hospital care to any and all veterans, regardless of service connection or time elapsed since discharge.

57. *Hearings on H.R. 6611*, 32.

58. "Investigation of Incapacitated Soldiers' Relief Bureaus," S. Rpt. 67-233 (July 20, 1921). The report was published the same day the Senate voted on the VB Bill.

59. 67 Cong. Rec. S4106 (July 20, 1921). No roll call vote was recorded.

60. Although ninety-six House representatives (who hailed from both parties and all re-

gions) did miss the roll call vote (some because they were "unavoidably absent"), no policy maker took a stand against the Bill. See 67 Cong. Rec. H2428 (June 10, 1921). Two of the representatives who missed the vote on the VB were Royal C. Johnson (R-SD) and John W. Langley (R-KY), who appear in this book as strong advocates for veterans. Their absence suggests that at least some of those who abstained from voting did not oppose the expansion of veterans' benefits. The official vote tally was 335 yeas, 0 noes. Immediately following the House vote, Burton Sweet paid tribute to Col. Frederick W. Galbraith, the national commander of the American Legion, who had "taken an active and enthusiastic part in the framing" of the VB legislation. Killed in a car crash just a few weeks before the House vote on the bill, Galbraith was "well and favorably known by a large number of the Members of the House and Senate," according to Sweet, and was constantly "discussing and setting forth the needs of his comrades." Sweet's heartfelt tribute to Galbraith on the congressional floor was a testament to the respect offered by legislators to the American Legion and its representatives (ibid., 2428–29). Galbraith was highly revered and deeply mourned by many. "Our faith in our country is strengthened in that it can breed such men," Theodore Roosevelt said in a eulogy offered at Galbraith's funeral. "Good citizen, tender husband and father, valiant soldier, splendid idealist—his death has left us poorer but his life has left us richer." "Thousands Mourn at Galbraith Bier," *New York Times*, June 12, 1921.

61. 67 Cong. Rec. S4474 (Aug. 1, 1921).

62. *An Act to Establish a Veterans' Bureau and to Improve the Facilities and Services of Such Bureau, and Further to Amend and Modify the War Risk Insurance Act*, PL 67-47, H.R. 6611, 42 Stat. 147 (Aug. 9, 1921).

63. Ibid.

64. A useful summary of this transition period can be found in *Annual Report of the Director, United States Veterans' Bureau for the Fiscal Year Ended June 30, 1922* (Washington, DC: GPO, 1922), 1–24.

65. On Cholmeley-Jones's resignation, see "Cholmeley-Jones Resigns; Quits War Risk Bureau to Enter Corporation in New York," *New York Times*, Mar. 6, 1921. On April 9, Treasury secretary Andrew Mellon reappointed Cholmeley-Jones, who noted that he only planned to stay briefly, in order "to render emergency services." "Cholmeley-Jones to Stay," *New York Times*, Apr. 10, 1921. About two weeks later, Charles Forbes took his place as director. "Takes War Insurance Job; Colonel C. R. Forbes Named to Succeed R. G. Cholmeley-Jones," *New York Times*, Apr. 28, 1921.

66. "Col. C. Forbes Dies; Led Veterans' Unit," *New York Times*, Apr. 12, 1952.

67. "F. M. Goodwin Named for Assistant Interior Post," *New York Tribune*, Apr. 26, 1921.

68. Rosemary A. Stevens, "The Invention, Stumbling, and Re-invention of the Modern U.S. Veterans Health Care System, 1918–1924," in *Veterans' Policies, Veterans' Politics: New Perspectives on Veterans in the Modern United States*, ed. Stephen R. Ortiz (Gainesville: University Press of Florida, 2012).

69. *Hearings on H.R. 6611*, 15.

70. *Report of the Consultants on Hospitalization Appointed by the Secretary of the Treasury to Provide Additional Hospital Facilities under Public Act 384* (Washington, DC: GPO, 1923), 41–55.

71. "Report of Conference Held in Offices of Consultants on Hospitalization, Room 271, Treasury Building, Washington, D.C.; Meeting of Consultants with Representatives from Veterans' Bureau," Sept. 29, 1921, 40, 50, ODF, box 95, folder 654.

72. Robert U. Patterson, Assistant Director, Veterans Bureau, to Dr. William C. White, Chairman, Committee of Hospital Consultants, memorandum, Sept. 16, 1921, RFBH, box 1, folder: Treasury Dept. Consultants on Hospitalization (White Committee). Emphasis in original.

73. Federal Board of Hospitalization, Annual Report 1924 (June 1924), 1, RFBH, box 15, folder: 97. Also see "Draft of Circular No. 44: Federal Board of Hospitalization," Nov. 1, 1921, RFBH, box 2, folder: Federal Board of Hospitalization Organizations, Functions, and Membership.

74. See chapter 6 for a discussion of the first Langley Bill.

75. Letter from Charles Forbes, Nov. 29, 1921, CWRIB, box 7.

76. *Hearings before the Subcommittee of the Committee on Appropriations, United States Senate, on H.R. 9237, a Bill Making Appropriations to Supply Deficiencies in Appropriations for the Fiscal Year Ending June 30, 1922,* 67th Congress, 2nd sess., Dec. 6, 1921 (Washington, DC: GPO, 1921). The January 10, 1922, meeting minutes of the Federal Board of Hospitalization contain the FBH's approval of Forbes's request to oversee hospital building. The board unanimously decided that the Veterans Bureau would determine "the locations and kind of hospitals to be built and operated for the care of world war veterans." See Proceedings of the Federal Board of Hospitalization (Addendum to Minutes of Eleventh Meeting of the Federal Board of Hospitalization), Jan. 10, 1922, CWRIB, box 6.

77. Robert U. Patterson to General Sawyer, memorandum, Sept. 12, 1921, RFBH, box 1.

78. *Hearings on H.R. 9237,* 8.

79. *Hearings before the Committee on Public Buildings and Grounds, House of Representatives, on H.R. 8791, Additional Hospital Facilities,* 67th Congress, 2nd sess., Feb. 8, 1922 (Washington, DC: GPO, 1922), 4.

80. Exec. Order No. 3669 (Apr. 29, 1922).

81. *An Act Making an Appropriation for Additional Hospital Facilities for Patients of the United States Veterans' Bureau,* PL 67-216, H.R. 11547, 42 Stat. 507 (May 11, 1922).

82. *Hearings on H.R. 8791,* 6.

83. *An Act to Authorize an Appropriation to Enable the Director of the United States Veterans' Bureau to Provide for the Construction of Additional Hospital Facilities and to Provide Medical, Surgical, and Hospital Services and Supplies for Persons Who Served in the World War, the Spanish-American War, the Philippine Insurrection, and the Boxer Rebellion, and Are Patients of the United States Veterans' Bureau,* PL 67-194, H.R. 10864, 42 Stat. 496 (Apr. 20, 1922).

84. The largest of these institutions were planned at Tupper Lake, NY, and Camp Custer, MI. Brigadier General C. E. Sawyer, "Annual Report, Federal Board of Hospitalization, 1922," Sept. 5, 1922, RFBH, box 15.

85. The largest of these institutions were to be located at Palo Alto, CA, the Bronx, NY, and Milwaukee, WI (ibid.). While the capacity of the VB continued to grow, the agency faced a challenge in fulfilling its own mandate to locate all hospitalized veterans in VB facilities—as opposed to other government owned or government contracted hospitals—not least of all because many former soldiers resisted being moved to institutions that were far from their homes (ibid.). According to the 1922 annual report of the Veterans Bureau: "consistent effort was made to remove patients from contract hospitals to Veterans Bureau hospitals where vacant beds were available. Because of objection on the part of the patients to being transferred away from their home localities, this program has been considerably handicapped." *VB Annual Report FY1922,* 16–17. While more than 5,400 bureau beds remained vacant, no fewer than 6,000 veteran-patients were being treated in Public Health Service, army, and navy hospitals, Soldiers' Homes, and at St. Elizabeths, the Washington, DC–based federal hospital for neuropsychiatric patients (ibid. 86–88). An additional 2,248 patients underwent treatment in 1922 in more than 1,200 civil hospitals under contract with the Veterans Bureau. Although 1,255 hospitals were under contract with the VB in June 1922, the bureau only used 648 of them. 113 civil hospitals not under contract were also housing VB patients (ibid., 78–79).

86. *VB Annual Report FY1922,* 6.

87. *Report of the Consultants on Hospitalization*, 29–30. For more on the controversy over supplies, see *Equipment of Hospitals Transferred to Veterans' Bureau, Decisions of the Comptroller General of the United States*, vol. 1 (Washington, DC: GPO, May 12, 1922), 650–52, and "Allotments of Appropriations to United States Public Health Service, Letter from the Director of the Veterans' Bureau, Transmitting, for the Consideration of the Senate, a Draft of Legislation Providing for the Making of Allotments of Appropriations by the United States Veterans' Bureau to the United States Public Health Service," S. Doc. 67-204 (May 18, 1922).

88. Charles Forbes to A. A. Sprague, Aug. 24, 1922, Microfilms, Rehabilitation—Veterans' Administration Hospitals—Hospitalization (con't) Rehab—VA—Hospitals—Survey 1929 Library 92-1012, ALL.

89. A. A. Sprague to Charles Forbes, Sept. 12, 1922, in ibid.

90. Anthony, *Florence Harding*, 368–71.

91. T. H. Scott to Charles Sawyer, Aug. 31, 1922, RFBH, box 15; Richard Seelye Jones, "Politics and Disabled Soldiers," *Spotlight* 8, no. 5 (Dec. 1, 1923). Carl Sferraza Anthony cites correspondence regarding Sawyer's spying in *Florence Harding*, 368.

92. "Dr. Scott Did Not Resign from Veterans' Bureau," *JAMA* 80, no. 10 (Mar. 10, 1923).

93. Charles Forbes, "Field Notes from Hospital Visits," Apr. 1922, DF, box 126. Allegations of neglect at Sea View Hospital and others would soon become public. See, e.g., "Woman Finds Cruel Neglect at Sea View," *New York Tribune*, Oct. 27, 1922.

94. "Report of Conference Held in Offices of Consultants on Hospitalization," 21.

95. "Summary of Matters Presented at Meeting of Federal Board of Hospitalization," Dec. 4, 1922, CWRIB, box 1; Surgeon General H. S. Cumming to General Sawyer, memorandum, Dec. 18, 1922, CWRIB, box 5.

96. On March 2, 1923, the Senate adopted a resolution providing for a committee of three senators—David Walsh of Massachusetts, David A. Reed of Pennsylvania, and Tasker L. Oddie of Nevada—to oversee an investigation of the Veterans Bureau. On the same day, Forbes resigned as director of the agency. See S. Res. 67-466 (Mar. 2, 1923).

97. "Hines Chosen Head of Veteran Bureau," *New York Times*, Feb. 28, 1923. Around the time Forbes was being investigated, another advocate for veterans' benefits came under fire. John W. Langley, who had sponsored legislation in 1920 and 1921 to fund veterans' hospitals, was convicted of violating prohibition and participating in a "whiskey ring" with some of the same shady characters that colored Forbes's years as VB director. For details on Langley's conviction, parole, and pardon, see "J. W. Langley Dead; Ex-Representative," *New York Times*, Jan. 18. 1932; "Langley Indicted with Five Others in Liquor Plot," *New York Times*, May 28, 1924; and "Langley Pleads Not Guilty," *New York Times*, Apr. 16, 1924.

98. For an insightful account of Forbes, his tenure at the VB, and the emerging scandal, see Rosemary Stevens, *A Time of Scandal: Charles Forbes, Warren G. Harding, and the Making of the Veterans Bureau* (Baltimore: Johns Hopkins University Press, 2016). For contemporary accounts, see "Intrigue, Debauchery, Corruption Are Charged against Former Director of Veterans' Bureau," *Atlanta Constitution*, Oct. 25, 1923; "Claims Forbes Tried to Change Dope into Gold," *Chicago Daily Tribune*, Oct. 30, 1923; "Forbes Accuses Foes of Perjury and Conspiracy," *Chicago Daily Tribune*, Nov. 14, 1923; "Charles Forbes Blames Sawyer and 'Politics,'" *Atlanta Constitution*, Nov. 14, 1923; "Forbes in Grafting Ring, Says O'Ryan," *Baltimore Sun*, Nov. 16, 1923; "Charles Forbes Split Profits with Builders," *Chicago Daily Tribune*, Feb. 8, 1924; "Start Trial of Forbes Here in April, U.S. Plan," *Chicago Daily Tribune*, Mar. 2, 1924; "Mortimer's Story Is Controverted; Stenographer Denies Either Mortimer or Thompson Was in Hotel at Time of Transaction," *Atlanta Constitution*, Dec. 19, 1924; "Forbes Witnesses Assail Mortimer," *New York Times*, Dec. 30, 1924; "Forbes Won over Army Engineers," *Boston Daily Globe*, Jan. 6, 1925; "Forbes Fails to Take Stand; Defense Claims Its Case Complete Without," *Boston Daily Globe*,

Jan. 22, 1925; "Forbes Given Two Years in Prison," *Boston Daily Globe*, Feb. 4, 1925; and "Forbes Looks to High Courts; Will Fight Guilty Verdict 'to Last Ditch,'" *Boston Daily Globe*, Feb. 5, 1925.

99. "Delays in Hospital Construction, Conclusions," Aug. 22, 1922, BCH, box 27.

100. Ibid.

101. *Report of the Consultants on Hospitalization*, 35.

102. "Charge Huge Waste in Hospitalization," *Washington Post*, Mar. 21, 1923.

103. Letter to the secretary of the Treasury, quoted in *Report of the Consultants on Hospitalization*, 34. In 1921, the committee had used as a guideline for its recommended hospital program H. Doc. 481, which estimated that more than thirty thousand beds would be necessary in order to provide for veteran-patients in the years to come. For more on H. Doc. 481, see chapter 4.

104. *Report of the Consultants on Hospitalization*.

105. *VB Annual Report FY1922*, 75.

106. Sawyer, "Annual Report, Federal Board of Hospitalization, 1922." The FBH report noted that St. Elizabeths was the only hospital to be operating at full capacity; each of its 878 beds was filled in late summer 1922—a testament to the extent of need for beds for patients suffering from mental illness.

107. Daniel P. Carpenter, *The Forging of Bureaucratic Autonomy: Reputations, Networks, and Policy Innovation in Executive Agencies, 1862–1928* (Princeton: Princeton University Press, 2001).

108. Reed Smoot, "Bureaus and More Bureaus," *Nation's Business*, Oct. 1929, 44.

109. Silas Bent, "Veteran Problems Seen by General Hines," *New York Times*, Mar. 11, 1923; "Hospitalization Plan to Stand, Hines Says," *Washington Post*, Mar. 22, 1923.

110. "Six Months of Director Hines," *New York Times*, Oct. 16, 1923.

111. Bent, "Veteran Problems Seen by General Hines."

112. Ibid.

113. "Hines Cuts Red Tape in Veterans' Bureau," *New York Times*, Mar. 11, 1923; "Hines Bans Hard-Boiled Tactics in Veterans' Bureau," *Chicago Daily Tribune*, Mar. 11, 1923.

114. "To Oust Squabblers in Veterans' Bureau," *New York Times*, Apr. 24, 1923.

115. Ibid.

116. "Detour between Ex-soldiers and Their Money Will Be Cut," *Christian Science Monitor*, Apr. 3, 1923.

117. "General Hines Saves $750,000," *New York Times*, June 2, 1923. By October 1923, thirty-three subdistrict offices had been closed ("Six Months of Director Hines").

118. "Hines Drops 2,025 Clerks," *New York Times*, Sept. 29, 1923.

119. "Six Months of Director Hines."

120. "Investigating Hospitals," *New York Times*, Apr. 1, 1923.

121. "Hines to Ask for Millions," *Los Angeles Times*, Dec. 27, 1923.

122. *An Act to Consolidate, Codify, Revise, and Reenact the Laws Affecting the Establishment of the U.S. Veterans Bureau and the Administration of the War Risk Insurance Act, as Amended, and the Vocational Rehabilitation Act, as Amended*, PL 68-242, S. 2273, 43 Stat. 607 (June 7, 1924).

123. A legislative history of veterans' benefits maintains that 1923 amendments to the War Risk Insurance Act began "to lay the groundwork for a body of law that eventually would lead to presuming a service-connection that associated specific diseases and disorders with specific historic episodes of military service." Economic Systems Inc., *V.A. Disability Compensation Program: Legislative History* (Washington, DC: VA Office of Policy, Planning, and Preparedness, Dec. 2004), 37.

124. *Hearings before the Committee on World War Veterans' Legislation, House of Representatives, on Proposed Legislation as Recommended by the Director of the United States Veterans' Bureau and American Legion, Disabled American Veterans, and Veterans of Foreign Wars*, 68th Congress, 1st sess.,

Feb. 20, 1924 (Washington, DC: GPO, 1924), 12–23. According to one newspaper article, the VB was mailing checks to veterans in more than eighty-one countries in early 1924. "Veterans' Bureau Mails Checks to 81 Countries," *Washington Post*, June 2, 1924.

125. *Hearings on Proposed Legislation*, 12. For more on VB hospitals in 1924, see *Annual Report of the Director, United States Veterans' Bureau, for the Fiscal Year Ended June 30, 1924* (Washington, DC: GPO, 1924), 44–45.

126. Statements of General George H. Wood, President, Board of Managers, in *Hearings Conducted by the Subcommittee of the Committee on Appropriations, House of Representatives, in Charge of the Third Deficiency Appropriation Bill for the Fiscal Year 1923*, 67th Congress, 4th sess., Feb. 9, 1923 (Washington, DC: GPO, 1923).

127. Hearings *on Proposed Legislation*, 12–14.

128. *VB Annual Report FY1922*, 24–46, esp. 31, 35; *VB Annual Report FY1924*, 44.

129. *Hearings on Proposed Legislation*, 47.

130. Ibid.

131. The quote is from Stephen R. Ortiz, *Beyond the Bonus March and G.I. Bill* (New York: New York University Press, 2010), 30.

132. *Hearings before the Committee on World War Legislation, House of Representatives, on Proposed Legislation as Recommended by the Director of the United States Veterans' Bureau, the Amerian Legion, Disabled American Veterans, and Veterans of Foreign Wars, and H.R. 7320*, 68th Congress, 1st sess., part 2, Mar. 3, 1924 (Washington, DC: GPO, 1924), 553–56.

133. Ibid.

134. *Hearings on Proposed Legislation*, 46–47.

135. Ibid., 45–46.

136. *Hearings on H.R. 7320*, part 2, 549.

137. *Hearings on Proposed Legislation*, 48.

138. *Hearings on H.R. 7320*, part 2, 556.

139. Ibid., 553.

140. Ibid., 558–61.

141. *Hearings on Proposed Legislation*, 47.

142. Some political scientists have deemed the idea of subgovernments and iron triangles—wherein advocates work with members of Congress and bureaucrats to create and ensure the passage of legislation—"simplistic and wrong" (Carol S. Weissert and William G. Weissert, *Governing Health: The Politics of Health Policy*, 3rd ed. [Baltimore: Johns Hopkins University Press, 2006], 147–49), but the concept effectively illuminates the influence of veterans' groups in the interwar period. On subgovernments, congressional committees, and interest groups, see the essay on sources.

143. 68 Cong. Rec. H945–50 (Jan. 14, 1924).

144. Jeffrey M. Berry and Clyde Wilcox, *The Interest Group Society*, 5th ed. (New York: Pearson, 2009), 138.

145. The quote is from Thomas A. Rumer, *The American Legion: An Official History, 1919–1989* (New York: M. Evans, 1990), 154–55.

146. 68 Cong. Rec. H10171–74 (June 2, 1924).

147. See chapter 7 for a discussion of contemporary research on costs of medical care.

148. "League of Veterans Plans to Kill Bonus," *New York Times*, June 3, 1924; "Seek Injunction to Block Bonus," *Atlanta Journal-Constitution*, June 5, 1924.

149. "First Annual Message of President Calvin Coolidge," www.presidency.ucsb.edu/ws/index.php?pid=29564#axzz1XqMJjKaq.

150. For an example of the relatively favorable coverage received by the World War Veterans' Act, see "Better Care for Ex-Service Men to Be Provided," *Sun*, June 11, 1924.

151. 68 Cong. Rec. H10171-72(June 2, 1924).

152. Senator David Walsh, "Investigation of the United States Veterans' Bureau, Third Preliminary Report, Pursuant to S. Res. 466, 67th Cong., 4th Sess.," S. Rep. 68-103, parts 1–3 (1924), 5. Various newspaper articles regarding mismanagement at the VB were published the day the WWVA became law. See, e.g., "Oddie, Adding Data, Pushes His Charges upon Veteran 'Ring,'" *Washington Post*, June 7, 1924, and "Jurors in Forbes Case Make Sealed Report," *Washington Post*, June 7, 1924.

153. 68 Cong. Rec. H10174 (June 2, 1924).

154. *Annual Report of the Director of the United States Veterans' Bureau, for the Fiscal Year Ended June 30, 1930* (Washington, DC: GPO, 1930), 7–9.

155. Kathleen J. Frydl, *The G.I. Bill* (New York: Cambridge University Press, 2009), 49.

CHAPTER 6: I Never Did Feel Well Again

1. Elam Shirk to Senator Reed, Dec. 7, 1923, ODF, box 92, Folder: Sen. Inv. Comm. Dec. 1923.

2. Edwin Jackson Algeo to Hon. G.W. Pepper, Nov. 8, 1923, in ibid.

3. Indeed, the Senate report on the investigation contained wide-ranging and damning allegations regarding "maladministration of the Veterans' Bureau." Senator David Walsh, "Investigation of the United States Veterans' Bureau, Third Preliminary Report, Pursuant to S. Res. 466, 67th Cong., 4th Sess.," S. Rep. 68-103, part 1–3 (1924).

4. *Annual Report of the Administrator of Veterans' Affairs for the Year 1932* (Washington, DC: GPO, 1932), 69.

5. Charles A. Beard and William Beard, *The American Leviathan: The Republic in the Machine Age* (New York: Macmillan, 1930), 776–80.

6. *Regulations and Procedure, United States Veterans' Bureau, Active and Obsolete Issues as of December 31, 1928* (Washington, DC: GPO, 1930). For an overview of fifty-five statutes related to veterans' entitlements passed between the end of the war and the late 1920s, see *Laws Governing the Organization and Administration of the Bureau of War Risk Insurance and the U.S. Veterans' Bureau and the Federal Board for Vocational Education in Its Relation to Veterans of the World War* (Washington, DC: GPO, 1927).

7. John J. O'Brien to C. R. Forbes, Mar. 9, 1922, DF, box 126, folder 054: Statement of What the VB is Doing. Emphasis in original circular.

8. Ibid.

9. George B. Norton, Commander American Legion Post No. 154, Nappanee, IN, to C. R. Forbes, Mar. 15, 1922, DF, box 126, folder 054: Statement of What the VB is Doing.

10. Letter from "an Ex-Soldier," 1922, in ibid.

11. Edgar A. Sentman to Bureau of War Risk Insurance, Mar. 4, 1922, in ibid.

12. Orley A. Rhodes to Veterans Bureau, Mar. 28, 1922, in ibid.

13. R. B. Snyder to Veterans Bureau, n.d., in ibid.

14. Omer Ginn Platt to Veterans Bureau, Apr. 27, 1922, in ibid.

15. Anonymous letter to the Veterans Bureau, Mar. 29, 1922, in ibid.

16. Paul M. Prugh to C. R. Forbes, Mar. 18, 1922, in ibid.

17. Edward N. Reedy to C. R. Forbes, Mar. 18, 1922, in ibid.

18. C. R. Forbes to George B. Norton, Mar. 17, 1922, in ibid.

19. Laurence Stallings, *Plumes* (Columbia: University of South Carolina Press, 1924), 290–91.

20. *An Act to Consolidate, Codify, Revise, and Reenact the Laws Affecting the Establishment of the United States Veterans' Bureau and the Administration of the War Risk Insurance Act, as Amended, and the Vocational Rehabilitation Act, as Amended*, PL 68-242, S. 2237, 43 Stat. 607 (June 7, 1924), 620–21. On the World War Veterans' Act, see chapter 5.

21. "Correspondence Re. Donald J. McDaniel," ODF, box 92, folder: Sen. Inv. Comm. Dec. 1923.

22. "Correspondence between Bartley J. O'Reilly and John F. O'Ryan," in ibid.

23. Dr. Edville G. Abbott "to Whom It May Concern," Mar. 27, 1923, ODF, box 79, folder #3: Dist. Manager—Dist #1 July–Dec. 1922.

24. Letter from Willard L. Ellsworth, Mar. 27, 1923, in ibid.

25. L. B. Rogers to Honorable Medill Mccormick, Apr. 10, 1923, in ibid.

26. Frank T. Hines to Honorable William J. Harris, May 18, 1923, ODF, box 94, folder #38: "H" Congressional.

27. "Correspondence Re. Donald J. McDaniel."

28. Ibid.

29. Ibid.

30. Charles A. Strickel to Veterans Bureau, DF, box 126, folder 054: Statement of What the VB is Doing.

31. John J. Murphy to George H. Moses, July 8, 1924, ODF, box 95, folder 639: Board of Appeals.

32. Peter Echo to John F. O'Ryan, Nov. 18, 1923, ODF, box 92, folder: Senate Investigative Committee, December 1923.

33. "Correspondence between Bartley J. O'Reilly and John F. O'Ryan."

34. *Annual Report of the Director, United States Veterans' Bureau for the Fiscal Year Ended June 30, 1922* (Washington, DC: GPO, 1922), 29; *Annual Report of the Director, United States Veterans' Bureau for the Fiscal Year Ended June 30, 1923* (Washington, DC: GPO, 1923), 28.

35. *VB Annual Report FY1924*, 3, 37.

36. *Hearings before the Committee on World War Veterans' Legislation, House of Representatives, on Proposed Legislation as Recommended by the Director of the United States Veterans' Bureau and American Legion, Disabled American Veterans, and Veterans of Foreign Wars*, 68th Congress, 1st sess., Feb. 20, 1924 (Washington, DC: GPO, 1924), 32. On the World War Veterans' Act, see chapter 5.

37. "Medical and Hospital Care of Beneficiaries of the United States Veterans Bureau, Haven Emerson," in *Transactions of the American Hospital Association, Twenty-Third Annual Conference, Held at West Baden, Indiana, September 12th to 16th, 1921* (Chicago: American Hospital Association, 1921), 127, 138.

38. "Accuses Veterans of Faking Illness," *New York Times*, Sept. 13, 1921.

39. *Manual for Medical Examiners of the United States Veterans Bureau* (Washington, DC: GPO, 1929), 6.

40. *Regulations and Procedure, Active and Obsolete Issues*, 1824.

41. L. B. Rogers to Honorable Frederick Hale, July 11, 1922, ODF, box 79, folder #3: Dist. Manager—Dist #1 July–Dec. 1922.

42. L. B. Rogers to Frank Hines, Jan. 2, 1924, ODF, box 100, folder: Ratings Tables, 1924.

43. See chapter 3 for a description of the BWRI's rating process.

44. See, e.g., Watson B. Miller, American Legion, to George Brown, Director of Compensation, Veterans Administration, July 21, 1933, and George Brown, reply to Watson Miller, Sept. 28, 1933, PGAF, box 256, folder 812: 1933.

45. *VB Annual Report FY1924*, 39. A 1928 schedule for healed gunshot wounds—a work-related disability unique to military veterans—serves as an example. Rather than being classified as total or partial, temporary or permanent, such injuries were rated according to a numerical system corresponding with an individual's occupation and degree of disability: "slight," "moderate," "moderately severe," or "severe." See "Extension No. 5 Schedule of Disability

Ratings, Readjusted Ratings for Disability from Healed Gunshot Wounds and Other Lacerated Wounds of Muscles of the Extremities and Other Skeletal Muscles," June 1928, DF, box 217, folder 10.0: Adjudication.

46. California was one of eighteen states that allowed workers with permanent total disabilities to receive lifelong compensation and one of four states that developed "elaborate schedules for permanent partial disabilities based as far as possible upon the actual loss of earning power." It was also one of four states that allowed compensation for "aggravation of a preexisting disease." California compensated workers at 65 percent of their wages—second only to the federal government's level of compensation of slightly more than 66 percent. Carl Hookstadt, *Comparison of Workmen's Compensation Laws of the United States and Canada up to January 1, 1920*, Bulletin of the United States Bureau of Labor Statistics No. 275, Workmen's Insurance and Compensation Series (Washington, DC: GPO, 1920), 11, 50, 64, 68.

47. *Annual Report of the Director, United States Veterans' Bureau, for the Fiscal Year Ended June 30, 1927* (Washington, DC: GPO, 1927), 1–2.

48. *VB Annual Report FY1924*, 15–17.

49. *Annual Report of the Director, United States Veterans' Bureau for the Fiscal Year Ended June 30, 1925* (Washington, DC: GPO, 1925), 385.

50. *VB Annual Report FY1924*, 39.

51. *VB Annual Report FY1925*, 385.

52. Chief, Rating Section, District 1, F. A. Fearney to Martin Cooley, Medical Division, US Veterans Bureau, Washington, DC, Feb. 13, 1923, ODF, box 79, folder #3: Dist. Manager—Dist #1 July–Dec. 1922.

53. *VB Annual Report FY1924*, 51.

54. *VB Annual Report FY1925*, 136–39.

55. *Annual Report of the Administrator of Veterans' Affairs 1932*, 13–15. The annual report contained no statistical information regarding black women or other minorities in hospitals.

56. *Annual Report of the Administrator of Veterans' Affairs for the Fiscal Year Ended June 30 1941* (Washington, DC: GPO, 1941), 48.

57. Secretary of War John W. Weeks to General George H. Wood, June 27, 1923, PGAF, box 91, folder: Women Beneficiaries 1923. For a gendered history of veterans' policies in the United States, and other secondary sources on the topic, see my chapter in *The Routledge Handbook of Gender, War, and the US Military*, ed. Kara Dixon Vuic (New York: Routledge, forthcoming).

58. "Report Submitted to Director of the Veterans Bureau on Behalf of the Los Angeles Chamber of Commerce," PGAF, box 91, folder: Women Beneficiaries 1924.

59. "Report of the Committee on Rehabilitation to the Third Annual Convention of the American Legion, Kansas City, Missouri," Nov. 1, 1921, Rehabilitation Reports, ALL.

60. Percy Cantwell to Dr. E. O. Crossman, Medical Director, Veterans Bureau, Feb. 11, 1925, PGAF, box 91, folder: Women Beneficiaries 1925.

61. Edwin Bettelheim to Frank T. Hines, Jan. 6, 1925, in ibid.

62. US Veterans' Bureau to Medical Officers in Charge, Veterans' Hospitals, May 2, 1923, PGAF, box 91, folder: Women Beneficiaries 1923.

63. The estimate of beneficiaries was contained in a 1924 report, which noted state-by-state populations of women veterans. New York, Pennsylvania, and Washington, DC, had the highest number of eligible women veterans. George E. Ijams, Veterans Bureau, to Capt, Watson B. Miller, Chairman, National Rehabilitation Committee, the American Legion, "Re. Adequate Facilities for the Care of Women Beneficiaries Afflicted with Neuropsychiatric Disabilities," Aug. 13, 1924, in PGAF, box 91, folder: Women Beneficiaries 1924.

64. "Plan Aid for Disabled Women War Workers," *New York Times*, June 7, 1925; "Women Who Served Overseas Declared in Dire Need of Aid," *New York Herald*, June 30, 1925. For more on the Women's Overseas Service League, see Helene M. Sillia, *Lest We Forget . . . A History of Women's Overseas Service League, Founded in 1921 by Women Who Served Overseas in World War I* (privately printed, 1978).

65. Winthrop Adams to Manager of District 1, Veterans Bureau, Oct. 8, 1924, PGAF, folder: Women Beneficiaries 1925.

66. "Compensation—Active Disability Cases, All Districts, Female Beneficiaries with Four Classes of Major Disability," Sept. 30, 1923, PGAF, box 91, folder: Women Beneficiaries 1923.

67. H. C. Watts, District Medical Officer, San Francisco, Dist. No. 12, to Veterans' Bureau Director, Jan. 23, 1924, PGAF, box 91, folder: Women Beneficiaries 1924.

68. Letter and report from W. W. Verner, Regional Medical Officer, Dist. 2, to Veterans' Bureau Director, July 29, 1925, PGAF, box 91, folder: Women Beneficiaries 1925.

69. *VB Annual Report FY1925*, 109. According to the report, 139 of 425 female patients were admitted to state or civil hospitals, compared with 98 of 667 male patients. About 45 percent of both men and women were admitted to VB hospitals, but men were more likely to be sent to other types of federally operated hospitals (marine, army, navy, and Soldiers' Home) rather than state or civil institutions.

70. Memo and reports from Chief, Construction Division to Assistant Director of Hospital and Rehabilitation Services, "Re. Present Government Facilities for Female Patients," June 10, 1924, PGAF, box 91, folder: 1924 March–June.

71. Watts to VB Director, Jan. 23, 1924.

72. Winthrop Adams, District Medical Officer, to Director, U.S. Veterans' Bureau, May 14, 1924, PGAF, box 91, folder: Women Beneficiaries 1924 March–June.

73. Edith Nourse Rogers to Frank T. Hines, July 31, 1930, PGAF, box 91, folder: Women Beneficiaries 1926–1931.

74. "Compensation—Active Disability Cases."

75. Grace C. Patrick to Dr. M. R. Stewart, May 21, 1924, PGAF, box 91, folder: 1924 March–June.

76. Dr. Stewart to Dr. Crossman, Medical Director, memorandum "Re. Hospitalization of Women Beneficiaries," May 6, 1924, PGAF, box 91, folder: 1924 March–June.

77. Dr. Stewart to the Director, memorandum "Re. Report of Visit to Veterans' Hospital under Construction at Excelsior Springs," May 21, 1924, in ibid.

78. R. L. Cook to Director of the U.S. Veterans' Bureau, May 10, 1923, PGAF, box 91, folder: Women Beneficiaries 1923.

79. O. C. Willihite to Director of U.S. Veterans' Bureau, May 22, 1924, PGAF, box 91, folder: 1924 March–June.

80. James Dedman to District Managers, Sept. 17, 1923, PGAF, box 91, folder: Women Beneficiaries 1923.

81. President, Board of Managers, George H. Wood to Major James W. Wadsworth, July 23, 1923, in ibid. One report refers to the Battle Mountain institutions as "the oldest facility in the VA medical system established solely to provide medical care." "Battle Mountain Sanitarium, National Home for Disabled Volunteer Soldiers" (National Register of Historic Places Registration nomination, Apr. 25, 2008).

82. L. A. Walker to Director, US Veterans' Bureau, May 8, 1923, PGAF, box 91, folder: Women Beneficiaries 1923.

83. Letter from L. H. Sinclair, Acting Regional Mgr., Helena Regional Office, June 13, 1925, PGAF, box 91, folder: Women Beneficiaries 1925.

84. On St. Elizabeths and black patients, see Matthew Gambino, "These Strangers within Our Gates: Race, Psychiatry and Mental Illness among Black Americans at St. Elizabeths Hospital in Washington, DC, 1900–1940," *History of Psychiatry* 19 (2008).

85. *VB Annual Report FY1925*, 136–39.

86. Charles M. Griffith to Medical Director, Jan. 11, 1933, PGAF, box 91, folder: January 1933.

87. "Refuse to Treat Negro Veteran," *New York Amsterdam News*, Feb. 18, 1925.

88. State of Tennessee Local Board for County of Bradley (Cleveland, TN), "Call to Report, Camp Meade, Annapolis Junction, Maryland," Apr. 29, 1918; "Registration Card, Solomon Paul Suddeth, Cleveland, Tennessee," June 5, 1917; Soldiers' Home record of Solomon Suddeth, Battle Mountain Branch, Dec. 26, 1923; Fourteenth Census of the United States, 1920—Population, Bradley County, TN, 4th District, Cleveland City; "Tennessee Obituaries: Cleveland, Tenn., Solomon Suddith [*sic*]," *Chicago Defender*, Feb. 16, 1924. As of July 1924, there were approximately 40 black patients among 560 total VB beneficiaries housed at the Johnson City home (*VB Annual Report FY1924*, 120).

89. The Salvation Army on 7th Street NW was the only post to provide assistance to African Americans. See *Shaw Historic District Brochure* (Washington, DC: District of Columbia Historic Preservation Office of Planning, 2008).

90. "Correspondence Re. Solomon Suddeth," Dec. 1923, ODF, box 91, folder 223: The President of the United States, 1921–24.

91. "Tennessee Obituaries: Cleveland, Tenn., Solomon Suddith [*sic*]"; "Deaths Reported: Solomon P. Suddeth," *Washington Post*, Jan. 24, 1924.

92. "Correspondence Re. Henry H. Davis," 1923, ODF, box 92, folder: Sen. Inv. Comm. Dec. 1923.

93. Ibid.

94. Ibid.

95. In addition to other chapters of this book and sources mentioned in the introduction, see, e.g., "Jim Crow War Veterans in U.S. Hospital: Citizens Angered over Inhuman Treatment," *Chicago Defender*, Mar. 6, 1926.

96. George W. Randall to Charles C. Forbes, Mar. 22, 1922, and anonymous letter to US Veterans Bureau, Mar. 30, 1922, DF, box 126, folder 054: Statement of What the VB is Doing.

97. Harriet H. Baird, "Some Experiences of a Nurse in the United States Veterans' Bureau Nursing Service," *United States Veterans' Bureau Medical Bulletin* 1, no. 5 (1925). For an overview of the Nursing Service, see Mary A. Hickey, "Nursing Service of the U.S. Veterans' Bureau," *American Journal of Nursing* 25, no. 7 (1925).

98. Karen Buhler-Wilkerson, *No Place Like Home: A History of Nursing and Home Care in the United States* (Baltimore: Johns Hopkins University Press, 2001), 18.

99. Baird, "Some Experiences of a Nurse," 53–55.

100. Michael B. Katz, *In the Shadow of the Poorhouse: A Social History in America* (New York: Basic Books, 1996), 216–17.

101. "Correspondence Re. George A. Leazott," 1927–28, National Homes Service, NHDVS, Eastern Branch, Togus, ME, 1866–1938, Sample Case Files of Members, box 5, folder: Togus Home, #19452 George A. Leazott, RG 15, NARA, Boston.

102. *Report of the Board of Managers of the National Home for Disabled Volunteer Soldiers for the Fiscal Year Ended June 30, 1919* (Washington, DC: GPO, 1920). By 1930, there were eleven National Homes (a facility at Bath, New York, was added to the previous list of ten). *Report of the Board of Managers of the National Home for Disabled Volunteer Soldiers* (Washington, DC: GPO, 1913–31).

103. Margaret Bridgman to Keith Ryan, Jan. 30, 1928, National Homes Service, NHDVS,

Eastern Branch, Togus, ME, 1866–1938, Sample Case Files of Members, box 5, folder: Togus Home, #19451 Louis H. Willett, RG 15, NARA, Boston.

104. Keith Ryan to Margaret Bridgman, Associated Charities of Albany, Feb. 2, 1928, in ibid.

105. Ibid.

106. Later in 1935, Roderick was admitted to Togus once again—for upper back pain and rectal bleeding attributed to hemorrhoids. Home officials judged the conditions not worthy of medical treatment. "Correspondence Re. Arthur Roderick," 1930–1935, in ibid.

107. *VB Annual Report FY1924*, 20, 45; *Annual Report of the Director, United States Veterans' Bureau, for the Fiscal Year Ended June 30, 1929* (Washington, DC: GPO, 1929), 13.

108. *Annual Report of the Administrator of Veterans' Affairs for the Year 1933* (Washington, DC: GPO, 1933), 13–14. Those numbers had ballooned again by June 1941, when the agency operated hospital facilities at 91 locations in 45 states with a total bed capacity of more than 61,000 (18,747 of them considered domiciliary). In 1941, the agency was utilizing about 2,570 beds in army, navy, Public Health Service, and other government hospitals. *Annual Report of the Director, United States Veterans' Bureau, for the Fiscal Year Ended June 30, 1941* (Washington, DC: GPO, 1941), 11.

109. *Hearings before the Committee on Public Buildings and Grounds, House of Representatives, on H.R. 12917, Providing for the Establishment of Sanitoriums for the Treatment of Persons Discharged from the Military and Naval Forces of the United States*, H.R. 8828, H.R. 12881, 65th Congress, 1st sess., Sept. 18, 1918 (Washington, DC: GPO, 1918), 3–4.

110. Harry Hardy Post No. 47, American Legion, Burnstead, ND, to Hon. George M. Young, Feb. 15, 1921, RG 233, Petitions and Memorials Referred to Committee on Ways and Means during 66th Congress, box 870, folder: Hospital Facilities for War Veterans.

111. "Resolution from Helen Jean Christie Tent No. 17, Daughters of Union Veterans of the Civil War, Los Angeles, California," 1928, RG 233, Petitions and Memorials Referred to the Committee on Military Affairs during the 70th Congress, box 578, folder HR70A-H9.1.

112. Stanton Post No. 55, Grand Army of the Republic, to Honorable Josef Crail, Dec. 8, 1928, ibid.

113. "The Commonwealth of Massachusetts, An Order," 1922, Records of the US House of Representatives, RG 233, Petitions and Memorials Referred to the Committee on Public Buildings and Grounds, box 490, folder HR67A-H18.1: Hospital for Disabled Veterans.

114. "Concurrent Resolution from the State of Indiana," Feb. 1, 1927, Records of the US House of Representatives, RG 233, Petitions and Memorials Referred to the Committee on World War Veterans during the 69th Congress, box 420, folder HR69A-H19.1: Veterans Hospital.

115. J. R. Collins, to Hon. John Kissel, "Protesting Committee against the Palo Alto Site," Feb. 1, 1922, RG 233, Records of the US House of Representatives, Petitions and Memorials Referred to the Committee on Public Buildings and Grounds during the 67th Congress, box 490, folder HR67A-H18.1: Hospital for Disabled Veterans.

116. On the White Committee and Forbes, see chapters 4 and 5.

117. *Report of the Consultants on Hospitalization Appointed by the Secretary of the Treasury to Provide Additional Hospital Facilities under Public Act 384* (Washington, DC: GPO, 1923), 7.

118. Charles R. Forbes to President Warren G. Harding, May 16, 1922, DF, box 108, folder NM 60E2. According to the *VB Annual Report FY1922*, "an intensive study of hospital plans was begun for the information of the director"—specifically focused on neuropsychiatric beds (32).

119. *VB Annual Report FY1922*, 79.

120. The quote is from "Delays in Hospital Construction, Conclusions," Aug. 22, 1922, BCH, box 27. Regarding projects based on assessment of real need, see "Hospitalization Facilities Required for Disabled Ex-service Men and Women Suffering from Mental Diseases," in

"Preliminary Reports, Memo from the Advisory Committee to the Chairman, Committee on Hospitalization, Treasury Department," Apr. 18, 1921, BCH, box 25, Folder: Preliminary Report, Advisory Committee. See also *Report of the Consultants on Hospitalization*, vii–viii.

121. On the Federal Board of Hospitalization, see chapter 5.

122. Minutes, Twelfth Meeting of the Federal Board of Hospitalization, Feb. 10, 1922, 3, CWRIB, box 6.

123. Rosemary A. Stevens, "Can the Government Govern? Lessons from the Formation of the Veterans Administration," *Journal of Health Politics, Policy, and Law* 16, no. 2 (1991): 296–98.

124. *Hearings before the Subcommittee on the Hospital Building Program*, H.R. 15633, 69th Congress, 2nd sess., Jan. 7, 1927 (Washington, DC: GPO, 1927), 1–5.

125. "Correspondence between Honorable F. A. Sebring and Frank T. Hines," May 1930, DF, box 218, folder 15.076: Hospitalization.

126. "Additional Hospital, Domiciliary, and Out-patient Dispensary Facilities for World War Veterans," H. Rep. 70-1222 (Apr. 11 and 14, 1928), part 1, pp. 6–7.

127. *An Act Making Appropriations for the Executive Office and Sundry Independent Executive Bureaus, Boards, Commissions, and Offices for the Fiscal Year Ending June 30, 1928*, PL 600, 69th Congress, [H.R. 15959] (Washington, DC: GPO, 1928).

128. "Additional Hospital, Domiciliary, and out-Patient Dispensary Facilities," part 2, p. 4.

129. *Annual Report of the Director of the United States Veterans' Bureau, for the Fiscal Year Ended June 30, 1930* (Washington, DC: GPO, 1930), 2.

130. *Independent Offices Appropriation Bill for 1930, Hearing before the Subcommittee of House Committee on Appropriations*, H.R. 16301, 70th Cong, 2nd sess., Dec. 22, 1928 (Washington, DC: GPO, 1928), 520.

131. *Annual Report of the Director, United States Veterans' Bureau for the Fiscal Year Ended June 30, 1928* (Washington, DC: GPO, 1928), 8–9.

132. Of patients remaining in hospitals by the end of the fiscal year, 54 percent were being treated for non-service-connected conditions. *Annual Report of the Administrator of Veterans' Affairs for the Year 1931* (Washington, DC: GPO, 1931), 14.

133. *VB Annual Report FY1928*, 15.

134. *VB Annual Report FY1930*, 2.

135. *Annual Report of the Administrator of Veterans' Affairs 1931*, 2.

136. *VB Annual Report FY1928*, 2. A 1921 Senate report noted that the functions of various government agencies were "so closely interrelated" that they should be overseen by one new government entity. "Investigation of Incapacitated Soldiers' Relief Bureaus," S. Rpt. 67-233 (July 20, 1921).

137. *Annual Report of the Administrator of Veterans' Affairs 1931*, 2–3.

138. *Hearings on H.R. 6141*, 12, 192–94, 24.

139. Ibid., 20–22, 191–92.

140. *Annual Report of the Administrator of Veterans' Affairs*, 1932, p. 11.

CHAPTER 7: State Medicine

1. "Bulletin of the Department of Kansas United Spanish War Veterans," Dec. 1933, Records of the US House of Representatives, RG 233, Petitions and Memorials Referred to the Committee on Appropriations of the 73rd Congress, box 392, folder HR73A-H2.14.

2. Eddie Wells and John Moss, *We're Not Heroes: Cartoons of Life in a Veterans' Hospital* (1933), Book Collection, US Army Heritage and Education Center, Carlisle, PA.

3. Jonathan Engel, *Doctors and Reformers: Discussion and Debate over Health Policy, 1925–1950* (Columbia: University of South Carolina Press, 2002), 25.

4. I. S. Falk, C. Rufus Rorem, and Martha D. Ring, *The Costs of Medical Care: A Summary of*

Investigations on the Economic Aspects of the Prevention and Care of Illness (Chicago: University of Chicago Press, 1933), 525–27.

5. For excerpts of the reports and the names of the physicians who signed each, see "'Final Report' of the Committee on the Costs of Medical Care," *California and Western Medicine* 37, no. 6 (1932). Emphasis in original.

6. "Report of the Ninth Conference of the Medical Council with the Director and the Medical Director of the United States Veterans' Bureau at Washington, D.C.," Nov. 12–13, 1928, 11, DF, box 215, folder 002-002.04.

7. "The Trend of Veterans' Relief Legislation: State Medicine," *JAMA* 86, no. 4 (Jan. 23, 1926).

8. "Wilbur Opposes More Hospitals for Veterans," *New York Herald Tribune*, Feb. 16, 1932.

9. Ray Lyman Wilbur, *The Memoirs of Ray Lyman Wilbur* (Stanford, CA: Stanford University Press, 1960), 643, and "Medicine at the Cross-Roads," *California and Western Medicine* 38, no. 5 (1933).

10. "Conference of Secretaries of Constituent State Medical Associations (Continued)," *American Medical Association Bulletin* 16, no. 1 (1922): 56–57. In 1906, Billings had told a meeting of the Physicians' Club of Chicago that he supported a system of compulsory sickness insurance because he felt it would "have an influence in preventing illness[,] which every physician works for, and the wholesome effect of it on the community will be great." C. S. Bacon, "The Physicians' Club of Chicago," *JAMA* 46, no. 19 (May 12, 1906). Ronald Numbers, *Almost Persuaded: American Physicians and Compulsory Health Insurance, 1912–1920* (Baltimore: Johns Hopkins University Press, 1978), argues that in the considerably more conservative era of the early 1920s, Billings was forced to recant his earlier support of compulsory insurance to maintain his position on the Board of Trustees of the American Medical Association (30, 108).

11. In 1929, doctors working for the VB could earn $3,200 per year. The Civil Service Commission advertised in medical journals about the "diversified and interesting service" they could perform as bureau physicians. See, e.g., "The United States Veterans' Bureau Needs Physicians," *Radiology* 13, no. 3 (1929).

12. *Annual Report of the Director, United States Veterans' Bureau, for the Fiscal Year Ended June 30, 1927* (Washington, DC: GPO, 1927), 8–9.

13. "Medical News, California: Physicians Mobilize to Aid Veterans," *JAMA* 79, no. 3 (July 15, 1922).

14. "The Care of the Veteran," *JAMA* 83, no. 20 (Nov. 15, 1924).

15. "Correspondence Re. The Care of the Veteran," *JAMA* 84, no. 1 (Jan. 3, 1925).

16. "Trend of Veterans' Relief Legislation."

17. "Federalized Medical Treatment Versus the Private Practitioner," *JAMA* 86, no. 24 (June 12, 1926).

18. "The Care of Veterans," *JAMA* 97, no. 12 (Sept. 19, 1931). Also see "The Veteran and the Hospital," *JAMA* 98, no. 24 (June 11, 1932); "Medic Journal Opposes More Vet Hospitals," *Chicago Daily Tribune*, Sept. 17, 1931; and "Doctors Urged to Fight Legion Hospital Plan," *Chicago Daily Tribune*, June 12, 1934.

19. Charles D. Aring and J. Fremont Bateman, "Nurturing a National Neurosis," *JAMA* 109, no. 14 (Oct. 2, 1937).

20. Minutes, American Medical Association House of Delegates, 85th Annual Session, Cleveland, OH, June 11–15, 1934, 32, available through the AMA Archives Digital Collection, at http://ama.nmtvault.com/jsp/viewer.jsp?doc_id=ama_arch%2FHOD00001%2Fooooo025&page_name=44.

21. Wilbur, *Memoirs*, 304.

22. Minutes, American Medical Association House of Delegates, 82nd Annual Session,

Philadelphia, PA, June 8–12, 1931, 32–34, available at http://ama.nmtvault.com/jsp/viewer.jsp?doc_id=ama_arch%2FHOD00001%2F00000022&page_name=40.

23. Peter Marshall Murray, "The President's Column," *Journal of the National Medical Association* 24, no. 2 (1932): 48.

24. "Editorial: The Veterans' Hospital Controversy," *Journal of the National Medical Association* 24, no. 3 (1932): 39.

25. Representatives of the NAACP, the National Negro Publishers Association, the National Association of Colored Graduate Nurses, and the National Medical Association, which represented black physicians, noted during a 1946 meeting with VA officials that "to accept segregation would be a backward step." A. C. Terrence, "The Problem of Veterans' Facilities," *Journal of the National Medical Association* 38, no. 1 (1946). Also see quotes later in this chapter from Charles Houston's congressional testimony regarding the Social Security Act. For more on African American veterans' activism in the context of civil rights and larger struggles for health care access, see Jessica L. Adler, "I Never Did Feel Quite Well Again: African American Veterans and Health Care in the Great War Era" (presented at the Annual Meeting of the American Association for the History of Medicine, Minneapolis, MN, May 1, 2016).

26. "Home-Town Care for Veterans," *Saturday Evening Post*, Jan. 7, 1933.

27. Paul H. Fesler to Hugh Scott, Jan. 18, 1932, RG 15, Policy and Admin. Files, box 99, folder: Cases Feb–March 1932, NAB.

28. Senator George Norris to George Ijams, Jan. 14, 1932, in ibid.

29. *Mortality Statistics, 1931 and 1932, Selected Tables* (Washington, DC: GPO, 1934), 1.

30. *Hearings before the Committee on World War Veterans' Legislation, House of Representatives, Seventy-First Congress, Second Session on H.R. 7825*, Jan. 21, 1930 (Washington, DC: GPO, 1930), 105–14.

31. For references on gas and warfare, see the essay on sources.

32. Hawes was especially concerned with ensuring that physicians did not confuse the symptoms of tuberculosis with those of exposure to gas. John B. Hawes, "Diagnositc Pitfalls: The Late Effects of Gassing vs. Tuburculosis," *Boston Medical and Surgical Journal* 185, no. 1–4 (July 7, 1921), and "Remarks on the Differential Diagnosis between Tuberculosis and Certain Other Chronic Pulmonary Infections with Special Reference to the Late Effects of Gas and Influenza," *Boston Medical and Surgical Journal* 185, no. 10 (Sept. 8, 1921).

33. Edward B. Vedder, *The Medical Aspects of Chemical Warfare with a Chapter on the Naval Medical Aspects of Chemical Warfare* (Baltimore: Williams & Wilkins, 1925), 247–48.

34. John L. Hankins and Walter C. Klotz, "Permanent Effects of Gas in Warfare," in *Transactions of the Eighteenth Annual Meeting of the National Tuberculosis Association, Washington, D.C., May 4, 5, and 6, 1922* (Albany: Hamilton, 1922), 258–60.

35. Harry L. Gilchrist and Phillip B. Matz, *The Residual Effects of Wartime Gases* (Washington, DC: GPO, 1933), 14.

36. Leon A. Fox, "The Residual Effects of War Gases," *JAMA* 101, no. 6 (Aug. 5, 1933).

37. A. P. Francine, "Tuberculosis and Poison Gas," in *Transactions of the Eighteenth Annual Meeting of the National Tuberculosis Association*, 264–65.

38. "Address of Brigadier General Frank T. Hines before the Field Officers Class, Chemical Warfare School, Edgewood Arsenal, Maryland," Aug. 3, 1938, Frank T. Hines Papers, AHEC. Following the 1930 creation of the Veterans Administration, Frank Hines's title changed from "director" to "administrator."

39. The first quote is from Andrew Ede, "The Natural Defense of a Scientific People: The Public Debate over Chemical Warfare in Post-WWI America," *Bulletin for the History of Chemistry* 27, no. 2 (2002), 133. The second is from Amos A. Fries, "Discussion on Papers by Dr. Hankins and Dr. Klotz and by Dr. Francine," in *Transactions of the Eighteenth Annual Meeting of*

the National Tuberculosis Association; Washington, D.C., May 4, 5, and 6, 1922 (Albany, NY: Hamilton Printing, 1922), 266. Also see Wilder D. Bancroft et al., *Medical Aspects of Gas Warfare*, vol. 14 of *The Medical Department of the United States Army in the World War*, ed. M. W. Ireland (Washington, DC: GPO, 1926), 274.

40. See, e.g., Gilbert W. Beebe, "Lung Cancer in World War I Veterans: Possible Relation to Mustard-Gas Injury and 1918 Influenza Epidemic," *Journal of the National Cancer Institute* 25, no. 6 (1960).

41. Constance M. Pechura and David P. Rall, *Veterans at Risk: The Health Effects of Mustard Gas and Lewisite* (Washington, DC: National Academy Press, 1993).

42. Quoted in John M. Kinder, *Paying with Their Bodies: American War and the Problem of the Disabled Veteran* (Chicago: University of Chicago Press, 2015), 181–83.

43. On the Bonus Army, see, e.g., Donald J. Lisio, *The President and Protest: Hoover, MacArthur, and the Bonus March*, 2nd ed. (New York: Fordham University Press, 1994), and Paul Dickson and Thomas B. Allen, *The Bonus Army: An American Epic* (New York: Walker, 2004).

44. Frank T. Hines to Admiral G. E. Riggs, Surgeon General, US Navy, Oct. 10, 1932, FBH, box 19, folder: Policy re. eligibility for care in VA facilities . . . 1932.

45. Letters from government officials to Frank T. Hines, Oct. 1932, in ibid. Emphasis in original.

46. Excerpted from *American Legion Monthly*, quoted in Stephen R. Ortiz, *Beyond the Bonus March and G.I. Bill* (New York: New York University Press, 2010), 73.

47. *An Act to Maintain the Credit of the United States Government*, H.R. 2820, PL 73-2, 48 Stat. 8 (Mar. 20, 1933), 11.

48. Ortiz, *Beyond the Bonus March*, 74. See also Stephen R. Ortiz, "The New Deal for Veterans: The Economy Act, the Veterans of Foreign Wars, and the Origins of New Deal Dissent," *Journal of Military History* 70, no. 2 (2006).

49. *Regulations Relating to Veterans' Relief*, S. Doc. 19, 73rd Congress, 1st sess. (Washington, DC: GPO, Apr. 10, 1933), 45.

50. *Annual Report of the Administrator of Veterans' Affairs for the Year 1933* (Washington, DC: GPO, 1933), 11.

51. Ibid., 1–2.

52. Chris Rasmussen, "'This Thing Has Ceased to Be a Joke': The Veterans of Future Wars and the Meanings of Political Satire in the 1930s," *Journal of American History* 103, no. 1 (2016): 85.

53. L. E. Dowling and Frank Williams to Senator Simeon D. Fess, Mar. 1933, RG 46, Petitions and Memorials of State Legislatures to 73rd Congress, box 164, folder 73A-K2.

54. Ortiz, *Beyond the Bonus March*, 71, 223n12.

55. The January 1935 letter focused on pending bonus legislation, but its sentiments mirrored those contained in FDR's Economy Act regarding medical care—the importance of ensuring that only those with service-connected ailments would receive benefits. American Veterans Association to Members of Congress, Jan. 21, 1935, RG 233, Records of the US House of Representatives, Petitions and Memorials Referred to the Committee on Ways and Means in the 74th Congress, box 487, folder HR74A-H21.2–21.4.

56. Resolution from Associated War Veterans, Birmingham, AL, Jan. 14, 1934, RG 46, Senate Petitions 73rd Cong., box 132, folder 73A-J18: Veterans Legislation.

57. See, e.g., letters from Emmett Evans and Howard W. Romeo, Apr. 22 and May 9, 1934, in ibid. World War I, Butler argued, created "21,000 new millionaires and billionaires." He wondered, "How many of these war millionaires shouldered a rifle? How many of them dug a trench? How many of them knew what it meant to go hungry in a rat-infested dug-out?" Smedley D. Butler, *War Is a Racket* (New York: Round Table Press, 1935). Also see Nancy Beck

Young, *Wright Patman: Populism, Liberalism, and the American Dream* (Dallas: Southern Methodist University Press, 2000).

58. Telegram from Max Adler, Mar. 14, 1934, in RG 46, Senate Petitions 73rd Cong., box 132, folder 73A-J18: Veterans Legislation.

59. Resolution of Gun Hill Post No. 271, Bronx, New York City, Veterans of Foreign Wars, May 9, 1933, in ibid.

60. Letter from Thomas Jefferson Post No. 541, New York City, Jan. 9, 1934, RG 233, House Petitions 73rd Cong., box 392, folder HR73A-H214.

61. Telegram from F. L. Carroll, Department Commander, Phoenix, AZ, Apr. 19, 1934, RG 46, Petitions and Memorials Referred to the Committee on Appropriations during the 72nd Congress, box 124, folder SEN72A-J23.

62. Thomas Donovan, Commander of Col. John Jacob Astor Camp No. 6, United Spanish War Veterans, United States Soldiers' Home, Washington, DC, to Representative Stephen Rudd, Jan. 1934, RG 233, House Petitions 73rd Cong., box 405, folder HR73A-H22.4.

63. Petition to Repeal the Economy Act, n.d., RG 233, House Petitions 73rd Cong., box 392, folder HR73A-H214.

64. Letter from United Spanish War Veterans, Blakesburg, IA, 1934, in ibid.

65. Letter from General Henry W. Lawton Camp, No. 21, United Spanish War Veterans, Brooklyn, NY, to Senator Royal S. Copeland, 1933, RG 46, Senate Petitions 73rd Cong., box 164, folder 73A-K2.

66. John D. Kirchenstein (15th Field Artillery Regiment, Division 1-20),"Army Services Experience Questionnaire, 1914–1921," World War I Veterans' Survey, AHEC.

67. Harold A. Lafferty (149th Field Artillery, Division 26-42), "Army Service Experiences Questionnaire, 1914–1921."

68. Edmond D. Sorenson (7th Sanitary Train, Division 1-20), "Army Services Experience Questionnaire, 1914–1921."

69. Mitchel B. Wallerstein, "Terminating Entitlements: Veterans' Disability Benefits in the Depression," *Policy Sciences* 7, no. 2 (1976): 179.

70. *Annual Report of the Administrator of Veterans' Affairs for the Year 1934* (Washington, DC: GPO, 1934), 9–12.

71. Ibid., 1.

72. *Annual Report of the Administrator of Veterans' Affairs for the Fiscal Year Ended June 30, 1941* (Washington, DC: GPO, 1941), 49. Carol Byerly cites data showing that death rates in the United States due to tuberculosis decreased from about 200 per 100,000 in 1900 to approximately 5 per 100,000 in 1955. Carol R. Byerly, *Good Tuberculosis Men: The Army Medical Department's Struggle with Tuberculosis* (Fort Sam Houston, TX: Office of the Surgeon General, Borden Institute, US Army Medical Department Center and School, 2013), xix.

73. Robert M. Ball, "Social Insurance and the Right to Assistance" (1947), in *Social Insurance and Social Justice: Social Security, Medicare, and the Capaign against Entitlements*, ed. Leah Rogne, Carroll L. Estes, Brian R. Grossman, Brooke A. Hollister, and Erica Solway (New York: Springer, 2009), 16.

74. Rogne et al., *Social Insurance and Social Justice*, xxvi.

75. "Text of President Roosevelt's Message Vetoing the Soldiers' Bonus Bill," *New York Times*, May 23, 1935.

76. For references on social security, see introduction.

77. *Report to the President of the Committee on Economic Security* (Washington, DC: GPO, 1935).

78. The text of the act is in Paul H. Douglas, *Social Security in the United States: An Analysis and Appraisal of the Gederal Social Security Act* (New York: Whittlesey House, 1939), 437.

79. *Hearings before the Committee on Finance, United States Senate, Seventy-Fourth Congress, First Session on S. 1130 a Bill to Alleviate the Hazards of Old Age, Unemployment, Illness, and Dependency,* Jan. 22–Feb. 20, 1935 (Washington, DC: GPO, 1935), 647.

80. 74 Cong. Rec. H5544 (Apr. 12, 1935).

81. 74 Cong. Rec. H5544 (Apr. 17, 1935).

82. 74 Cong. Rec. H6075 (Apr. 19, 1935).

83. *Ernest Lundeen, Late a Senator from Minnesota* (Washington, DC: GPO, 1942), 39.

84. Richard Pearson, "Stephen Young, Former Senator from Ohio, Dies," *Washington Post,* Dec. 2, 1984.

85. In a message to Congress in January 1935, Franklin Roosevelt declared, "To dole out relief… is to administer a narcotic, a subtle destroyer of the human spirit." To these ends, Roosevelt favored not only social security but also "work relief programs" administered in large part at the local level. 74 Cong. Rec. H5544 (Apr. 12, 1935).

86. Originally, social security benefits were not accessible to domestic workers, farm laborers, people who were self-employed or worked for nonprofits, and members of the military, who were covered by a separate system of benefits. The quotes are from Robert M. Ball, "The Nine Guiding Principles of Social Security," in *Straight Talk about Social Security,* ed. Thomas N. Bethell (New York: The Century Foundation Press, 1998).

87. The Social Security Administration's Office provides a variety of historical documents on its website, including unpublished meeting minutes of the Committee on Economic Security relating to health from January 1935: "Volume 7: Health in Relation to Economic Security," www.ssa.gov/history/reports/ces/ces7intro.html.

88. "Medical Advisory Board—Minutes of Meetings, Part 1: Tuesday Morning Session, January 29, 1935," in "Volume 7: Health in Relation to Economic Security," www.ssa.gov /history/reports/ces/ces7minutes.html.

89. During Bierring's 1935 congressional testimony, Rep. John D. Dingell (D-MI), a long-time proponent of improving citizens' health via federal intervention, queried, "You naturally, I assume, are opposed to any interference with the traditional ethical practice of the medical profession, as it is known today, are you not?" "I am, sir; yes, sir," Bierring replied. *Economic Security Act, Hearings before the Committee on Ways and Means, House of Representatives, on H.R. 4120, a Bill to Alleviate the Hazards of Old Age, Unemployment, Illness, and Dependency, to Establish a Social Insurance Board in the Department of Labor, to Raise Revenue, and for Other Purposes,* 74th Congress, 1st sess., Jan.–Feb. 1935 (Washington, DC: GPO, 1935), 649. Isidore Falk, a member of the Committee on Economic Security who believed the AMA supported public health measures as a means of defending against the entrenchment of a more far-reaching federally centered voluntary insurance program, noted in a 1968 interview that AMA "spokesmen" like Bierring "were reflecting the position of the power structure of the medical profession in the United States. Whether they were reflecting the views of individual physicians numerically or not, nobody could know." "Reminiscences of Isidore Sydney Falk; Oral History 1968," 55, Social Security Project, Columbia University Center for Oral History, New York.

90. Beatrix Hoffman, among others, argues that "grassroots movements" are a crucial driver of reform in the United States. "Public opinion has generally run in favor of health care reform," she writes, "but popular approval has not been matched by the rise of a large-scale, activist popular movement for change." Beatrix Hoffman, "Health Care Reform and Social Movements in the United States," *American Journal of Public Health* 93, no. 1 (2003): 75.

91. "Reminiscences of Isidore Sydney Falk; Oral History 1963," 39, Social Security Project, Columbia University.

92. On "categorical" entitlements, see, e.g., Edward D. Berkowitz and Larry DeWitt, *The*

Other Welfare: Supplemental Security Income and U.S. Social Policy (Ithaca, NY: Cornell University Press, 2013), 5.

93. "Reminiscences of Isidore Sydney Falk; Oral History 1968," 39, 170. During discussions in January 1935 about social security's prospective health measures, a doctor called attention to existing infrastructure: "There is a vast number of things, vital statistics, public health, drugs, veterans' bureau, perhaps hundreds of things which pertain to this which it seems to me would be most economically handled by drawing them all together with some central authority" ("Medical Advisory Board—Minutes, Part 1," 12).

94. "By the middle of the twentieth century, advocates of maternal health, children's health, veterans' health, public health, and rural health all claimed administrative beachheads. The progress of national health insurance was slowed not by a poverty of administrative capacity or experience but by the tremendous variety of federal approaches and interests—including the Women's Bureau, the Children's Bureau, the Veterans' Administration." Colin Gordon, *Dead on Arrival: The Politics of Health Care in Twentieth-Century America* (Princeton: Princeton University Press, 2003), 289.

95. Paul Starr, *Remedy and Reaction: The Peculiar American Struggle over Health Care Reform* (New Haven: Yale University Press, 2011), argues that the "protected public" grew in the 1960s, with the creation of Medicare and Medicaid (41).

CONCLUSION: The Legacy of Great War Health Policy

1. *Annual Report of the Administrator of Veterans' Affairs for the Fiscal Year Ended June 30, 1941* (Washington, DC: GPO, 1941).

2. Albert Deutsch, "Neglect of Psychiatric Cases Laid to Vets Bureau," *PM*, Jan. 16, 1945.

3. The quote is from Barry S. Levy and Victor W. Sidel, eds., *War and Public Health*, 2nd ed. (Oxford: Oxford University Press, 2008), 3.

4. *Administrator of Veterans Affairs Annual Report for Fiscal Year Ending June 30, 1946* (Washington, DC: GPO, 1946), 81 (admissions), 1 (veteran population).

5. Albert Deutsch, "Vets' Setup Needs Revamping Now to Avert Scandal," *PM*, Jan. 7, 1945.

6. Albert Deutsch, "Veterans Hospitals Called 'Back Waters of Medicine,'" *PM*, Jan. 9, 1945, and "Patient Just a Case History to Veterans Bureau," *PM*, Jan. 11, 1945.

7. Deutsch, "Patient Just a Case History to Veterans Bureau."

8. Deutsch, "Vets' Setup Needs Revamping."

9. Albert Q. Maisel, *The Wounded Get Back* (New York: Harcourt, Brace, 1944) and *Miracles of Military Medicine* (New York: Duell, Sloan & Pearce, 1943).

10. Albert Q. Maisel, "The Veteran Betrayed," *Reader's Digest*, Apr. 1945; also see Maisel, "Third Rate Medicine for First Rate Men," *Cosmopolitan*, Mar. 1945.

11. 79 Cong. Rec. A2786–87.

12. "Vets' Leaders to See Hines on Hospitalization," *Chicago Daily Tribune*, Mar. 12, 1945; "Washington News," *Los Angeles Times*, Mar. 12, 1945.

13. Alden Whitman, "Gen. Omar N. Bradley Dead at 88; Last of Army's Five-Star Generals," *New York Times*, Apr. 9, 1981.

14. Omar Bradley and Clay Blair, *A General's Life: An Autobiography* (New York: Simon & Schuster, 1983), 446–50.

15. Ibid., 450.

16. Paul B. Magnuson, *Ring the Night Bell* (1960; reprint, Birmingham: University of Alabama School of Medicine, 1986), 278.

17. Ibid., 298, 303, 284. For Magnuson's narrative description of the move away from Civil Service, see 276–305. Omar Bradley recalled that his team established affiliations with sixty-

three of seventy-seven "Class-A medical schools." "We were not able to magically upgrade VA medicine overnight," he wrote, "but I believe it is fair to say that within two years we had launched it on the right track." Bradley and Blair, *A General's Life*, 462. For Bradley's description of the move away from civil service, see 458–462.

18. On Vietnam Era benefits, and literature on the history of the veterans' health system, see the introduction.

19. "Reagan Would Elevate V.A. to Cabinet Level," *New York Times*, Nov. 11, 1987. On the complex legislative maneuvering that led to the change, see Paul C. Light, *Forging Legislation* (New York: Norton, 1991).

20. Michael F. Cannon, "V.H.A. Is Not the Way," *Nationalreview.com*, Mar. 6, 2006.

21. Emily Friedman, "Mitt Romney Floats 'Private Sector Competition' for Vets' Health Care System," *ABCnews.com*, Nov. 11, 2011; Paul Krugman, "Vouchers for Veterans," *New York Times*, Nov. 13, 2011.

22. Joel Kupersmith, "Thoughts on the VA Scandal and the Future," *HealthAffairs Blog*, June 13, 2014, http://healthaffairs.org/blog/2014/06/13/thoughts-on-the-va-scandal-and-the -future/.

23. "Despite $10b 'Fix,' Veterans Are Waiting Even Longer to See Doctors," NPR.org, May 16, 2016.

24. On Paul Starr's conception of the "protected public," see introduction.

25. "Pelosi Floor Speech in Opposition to House G.O.P. Vote to Take Away Health Care Protections for Millions of Americans," press release, July 11, 2012, www.democraticleader .gov/newsroom/pelosi-floor-speech-opposition-house-gop-vote-take-away-health-care-pro tections-millions-americans/.

26. "Remarks by the President at the Annual Conference of the American Medical Association," press release, June 15, 2009, www.whitehouse.gov/the-press-office/remarks-president -annual-conference-american-medical-association.

27. "Transcript: Rep. Paul Ryan's Convention Speech," NPR.org, Aug. 29, 2012.

28. Matt Patterson, "No Free Lunch: The True Cost of Obamacare," *National Policy Analysis* 590 (Oct. 2009).

29. Mark Steyn, "Untangling the Spaghetti," *National Review*, Aug. 11, 2009.

30. "Declaration of Principles and Constitution of the Private Soldiers and Sailors Legion," Mar. 1919, American Civil Liberties Union Records, Subgroup 1: Roger Baldwin Years, reel 16, vol. 118, p. 154, Princeton University Library, Department of Rare Books and Special Collections.

Essay on Sources

This book showcases how government officials, soldiers, veterans, advocacy groups, and caregivers, among others, influenced, viewed, and experienced the creation and growth of the veterans' health system. In this section I describe where I found perspectives from members of those groups, beginning with a discussion of the archives. I also offer an overview of integral scholarly work, which expands on the introduction and its notes, as well as the references contained in subsequent chapters.

Various collections at the National Archives and Records Administration (NARA) contain materials that shed light on the government perspective. NARA records, especially those of the Veterans Bureau and Veterans Administration—(Record Group 15)—were some of the most important for this study, and many of its dusty cardboard boxes remain unopened and unexplored. The massive collection is located at the National Archives Building in Washington, DC, College Park, Maryland, and various regional NARA centers. Government services in the World War I era were under the auspices of a variety of federal agencies, so it is revealing to examine RG 15 in concert with correspondence from other National Archives collections, including the Public Health Service, the War Department, the Adjutant General's Office, and the Federal Board of Hospitalization. Additionally, regional branches of NARA hold records that showcase local experiences with veterans' health services. At the Boston NARA branch, for example, patient case files in the records of the National Soldiers' Home at Togus, Maine, reveal the dynamics of a relationship between the VB and local Soldiers' Home officials.

Official government documents provide perspectives on correspondence from NARA. Annual reports of the army surgeon general, the Bureau of War Risk Insurance, and the Veterans Bureau/Veterans Administration offer consolidated information and hard data that need to be read critically. Additionally, the

Congressional Record is a vital complement to inter- and intra-agency documents. It not only contains the voices of elected officials but also shows which debates, controversies, and issues received public airing, who had the ear of people in power, and what arguments were used to justify ideas for enhanced or limited veterans' services.

Voices of private citizens, service members, veterans, and caregivers can be found in both archival and published sources. At the National Archives Building, the Center for Legislative Archives holds correspondence related to ongoing activities in the House and Senate, which offers perspective on how members of state legislatures, interest groups, and individual constituents perceived federal policy debates. In the files of the Veterans Bureau, some digging is necessary. For example, former service members' accounts of treatment in Public Health Service hospitals—complete with full quotations—may be unearthed in letters sent between officials. The *Congressional Record*, too, boasts testimony from soldiers, veterans, and bureaucrats. Published firsthand accounts of service members, caregivers, and others who actively participated in the Great War—such as Martin J. Hogan, *The Shamrock Battalion of the Rainbow; A Story of the Fighting Sixty-Ninth* (New York: D. Appleton, 1919)—are increasingly available via online archives such as HathiTrust.

Beyond published accounts and government records, researchers can get a sense of the experiences of soldiers, veterans, and caregivers by searching a variety of archives. Since many doctors who served abroad during World War I were affiliated with US medical schools, their personal papers may be found in university archives. The Columbia University Medical Center Archives and Rare Book and Manuscript Library Collections, for example, hold the papers and oral histories of physicians who served during World War I. The Otis Historical Archives at the National Museum of Health and Medicine contains all editions of Walter Reed's hospital newspaper, *The Come-Back*, the personal papers of men and women caregivers who served at Walter Reed, and photographs and documents pertaining to certain medical services offered at the hospital at the beginning of the twentieth century. Hospital newspapers and histories are also available at the US Army Heritage and Education Center (AHEC), where a plethora of sources of interest to scholars of military or veterans' history of any period may be found. A brief note can hardly do justice to the center's varied collections, but for this book, postwar surveys of former service members, organized by unit, were particularly useful—especially if they contained additional materials provided by veterans surveyed, such as memoirs and correspondence.

In addition to boasting useful archival collections, AHEC offers on its website bibliographies that can serve as an orienting point on a variety of topics, from air defense to post-traumatic stress disorder. The Veterans' History Project Collection at the Library of Congress's American Folklife Center makes available oral histories of people who have served, some of them fully transcribed. The National World War I Museum in Kansas City also holds unpublished accounts regarding service; the memoirs of C. Vernoy Davis, cited in chapter 1, are just one example.

The archives of the American Legion in Indianapolis and the Disabled American Veterans in Cold Spring, Kentucky, contain crucial documents related to the dynamics of veterans' social and political activism. Meeting minutes and other files at the American Legion, for example, offer perspective on how legislative and social issues gained attention, and the machinations of political lobbying. Records of prominent members and leaders of the organizations may be housed elsewhere. The personal papers of Robert S. Marx, for example, the first national commander of the Disabled American Veterans, can be found at the Cincinnati Historical Society Library and Archives.

Published contemporary periodicals also provide important perspective. For the viewpoints of veterans' groups, see the *American Legion Weekly* (later, the *American Legion Monthly*) and the *Disabled American Veterans Magazine*. For the perspectives of caregivers and physicians, consult *Military Surgeon, Modern Hospital Magazine, Journal of the American Medical Association, Journal of the National Medical Association*, and the *United States Veterans' Bureau Medical Bulletin*. Minutes from national meetings of the American Medical Association from 1847 through 1941, which provide invaluable insight into the perspectives of physician-leaders, are available online via the AMA Archives Digital Collection at http://ama.nmtvault.com. African American newspapers, such as the *Baltimore Afro-American* and the *Chicago Defender*, offer insight into the experiences and perceptions of black service members and veterans.

In addition to archival materials, this book draws from and builds on secondary sources beyond those already cited. Poison gas, mental illness, and tuberculosis each posed long-term health challenges among soldiers and veterans. General sources on chemical weapons and their use during World War I include Thomas I. Faith, *Behind the Gas Mask: The U.S. Chemical Warfare Service in War and Peace* (Urbana: University of Illinois Press, 2014); Nicholas J. McCamley, *The Secret History of Chemical Warfare* (Barnsley: Pen & Sword, 2006); Jeremy Paxman, *A Higher Form of Killing: The Secret History of Chemical and Biological War-*

fare (New York: Random House, 2002); Robert J. T. Joy, "Historical Aspects of Medical Defense against Chemical Warfare," chap. 3 of *Medical Aspects of Chemical and Biological Warfare*, ed. Frederick R. Sidell, Ernest T. Takafuji, and David R. Franz (Falls Church, VA: Office of the Army Surgeon General, 1997); Marion Girard, *A Strange and Formidable Weapon: British Responses to World War I Poison Gas* (Lincoln: University of Nebraska Press, 2008); Tim Cook, *No Place to Run: The Canadian Corps and Gas Warfare in the First World War* (Vancouver: University of British Columbia Press, 1999); Charles E. Heller, *Chemical Warfare in World War I: The American Experience, 1917–1918* (Fort Leavenworth: Combat Studies Institute, US Army Command and General Staff College, 1984); Donald Richter, *Chemical Soldiers: British Gas Warfare in World War I* (Lawrence: University Press of Kansas, 1992); and Gerald J. Fitzgerald, "Chemical Warfare and Medical Response during World War I," *American Journal of Public Health* 98, no. 4 (2008).

As chapter 7 notes, the notion that chemical weapons had long-term and dire health effects gained credence throughout the twentieth century. Sources on chemical and incendiary weapons and their impacts include Peter Sills, *Toxic War: The Story of Agent Orange* (Nashville: Vanderbilt University Press, 2014); Edwin A. Martini, *Agent Orange: History, Science, and the Politics of Uncertainty* (Amherst: University of Massachusetts Press, 2012); Edmund Russell, *War and Nature: Fighting Humans and Insects with Chemicals from World War I to Silent Spring* (Cambridge: Cambridge University Press, 2001); and Robert M. Neer, *Napalm: An American Biography* (Cambridge, MA: Belknap Press of Harvard University Press, 2013). For an overview of research findings in the 1970s regarding the impact of chemical weapons on US veterans and others around the world, see Stockholm International Peace Research Institute (SIPRI), *Delayed Toxic Effects of Chemical Warfare Agents* (Stockholm: Almqvist & Wiksell International, 1975). On viewpoints in the 1990s, see Constance M. Pechura and David P. Rall, *Veterans at Risk: The Health Effects of Mustard Gas and Lewisite* (Washington, DC: National Academy Press, 1993). A 2007 textbook on the medical impact of gas warfare notes that a variety of studies (including the 1993 report) suggest a correlation between exposure to chemical weapons and an array of chronic conditions but that one should bear in mind "all human studies dealing with chronic mustard disease processes are retrospective and fraught with the problems inherent in retrospective studies." William J. Smith, Matthew G. Clark, Thomas B. Talbot, Patricia Ann Caple, Frederick R. Sidell, and Charles G. Hurst, "Long-Term Health Effects of Chemical Threat Agents," in *Medical As-*

pects of Chemical Warfare, ed. Shirley D. Tuorinsky (Falls Church, VA: Office of Army Surgeon General; Washington, DC: Borden Institute, Walter Reed Army Medical Center, 2008).

There has been a flowering of work on the psychological impact of military service during World War I and beyond. Jay Winter notes that the existence of a Division of Neuro-psychiatry was unique to the American Expeditionary Forces and argues that "Americans were latecomers to the war, but that fact may have helped them develop a more sophisticated approach to the treatment of psychologically or neurologically damaged soldiers." "Shell Shock," chap. 13 of *The Cambridge History of the First World War*, vol. 3, *Civil Society*, ed. Jay Winter (Cambridge: Cambridge University Press, 2014). Also see Jay Winter, "Shell-Shock and the Cultural History of the Great War," *Journal of Contemporary History* 35, no. 1 (2000). Annessa Stagner, "Healing a Soldier, Restoring the Nation: Representations of Shell Shock in the United States During and after the First World War," *Journal of Contemporary History* 49, no. 2 (2014), points out that estimates of those discharged with shell shock ranged from 15,000 to 76,000, which she attributes in part to "the ambiguity regarding the meaning of shell shock." See also Peter Barham, *Forgotten Lunatics of the Great War* (New Haven: Yale University Press, 2004); Michael Roper, *The Secret Battle: Emotional Survival in the Great War* (Manchester: Manchester University Press, 2010); Gregory M. Thomas, *Treating the Trauma of the Great War: Soldiers, Civilians, and Psychiatry in France, 1914–1940* (Baton Rouge: Louisiana State University Press, 2009); Alexander Watson, *Enduring the Great War: Combat, Morale and Collapse in the German and British Armies, 1914–1918* (New York: Cambridge University Press, 2008); Fiona Reid, *Broken Men: Shell Shock, Treatment and Recovery in Britain, 1914–1930* (London: Continuum, 2010); Ben Shepherd, *A War of Nerves: Soldiers and Psychiatrists in the Twentieth Century* (Cambridge, MA: Harvard University Press, 2001); Anthony Babington, *Shell-Shock: A History of the Changing Attitudes to War Neurosis* (London: Leo Cooper, 1997); and Mark O. Humphries and Kellen Kurchinski, "Rest, Relax and Get Well: A Re-conceptualisation of Great War Shell Shock Treatment," *War & Society* 27, no. 2 (2008). Work on other periods includes Eric T. Dean, *Shook over Hell: Post-Traumatic Stress, Vietnam, and the Civil War* (Cambridge, MA: Harvard University Press, 1997); Mark Osborne Humphries and Terry Copp, *Combat Stress in the 20th Century: The Commonwealth Perspective* (Ontario: Canadian Defence Academy Press, 2010); Daryl S. Paulson and Stanley Krippner, *Haunted by Combat: Understanding PTSD in War Veterans* (Lanham, MD: Rowman & Littlefield, 2010); and Edgar Jones and Simon Wessely, *Shell Shock to PTSD: Military Psychiatry from 1900 to the Gulf War* (Hove: Psychology Press, 2006). For a reading of PTSD as a culturally constructed disease, see Jerry Lembcke, *PTSD: Diagnosis and Identity in Post-Empire America* (Lanham, MD: Lexington, 2013), and Allan Young, *The Harmony of Illusions: Inventing Post-Traumatic Stress Disorder* (Princeton: Princeton University Press, 1997).

On the general history of mental illness and psychiatry in the United States in the World War I era and beyond, see Mark S. Micale and Paul Lerner, *Traumatic Pasts: History, Psychiatry, and Trauma in the Modern Age, 1870–1930* (Cambridge: Cambridge University Press, 2010); Gerald N. Grob, *The Mad among Us: A History of the Care of America's Mentally Ill* (New York: Free Press, 1994); Grob, *Mental Illness and American Society, 1875–1940* (Princeton: Princeton University Press, 1983); Walter Bromberg, *Psychiatry between the Wars, 1918–1945: A Recollection* (Westport, CT: Greenwood, 1982); Martin Halliwell, *Therapeutic Revolutions: Medicine, Psychiatry, and American Culture, 1945–1970* (New Brunswick, NJ: Rutgers University Press); and S. D. Lamb, *Pathologist of the Mind: Adolf Meyer and the Origins of American Psychiatry* (Baltimore: Johns Hopkins University Press, 2014). On the mental hygiene movement and its advocates, who helped shape efforts surrounding mental health care in US military and veterans' hospitals, see (in addition to sources listed in the notes to chapter 1) Frankwood E. Williams, "In Memoriam, Dr. Thomas W. Salmon," *Bulletin of the New York Academy of Medicine* 3, no. 11 (1927); Johannes Coenraad Pols, "Managing the Mind: The Culture of American Mental Hygiene, 1910–1950" (PhD diss., University of Pennsylvania, 1997); and Manon Parry, "From a Patient's Perspective: Clifford Whittingham Beers' Work to Reform Mental Health Services," *American Journal of Public Health* 100, no. 12 (2010).

On the history of tuberculosis, in addition to work cited in the introduction, see Christian W. McMillen, *Discovering Tuberculosis: A Global History, 1900 to the Present* (New Haven: Yale University Press, 2015); Helen Bynum, *Spitting Blood: The History of Tuberculosis* (Oxford: Oxford University Press, 2012); Barbara Bates, *Bargaining for Life* (Philadelphia: University of Pennsylvania Press, 1992); Sheila M. Rothman, *Living in the Shadow of Death: Tuberculosis and the Social Experience of Illness in American History* (New York: Basic Books, 1994); Katherine Ott, *Fevered Lives: Tuberculosis in American Culture since 1870* (Cambridge, MA: Harvard University Press, 1996); Michael E. Teller, *The Tuberculosis Movement: A Public Health Campaign in the Progressive Era* (New York: Greenwood, 1988); and Victoria E. Rinehart, *Portrait of Healing: Curing in the Woods* (Utica, NY: North

Country, 2002). On the National Tuberculosis Association and disease advocacy among individuals subsequently involved in planning care for soldiers and veterans, see Richard H. Shyrock, *National Tuberculosis Association, 1904–1954: A Study of the Voluntary Health Movement in the United States* (New York: National Tuberculosis Association, 1957); S. Adolphus Knopf, *A History of the National Tuberculosis Association* (New York: National Tuberculosis Association, 1922), esp. 176–92; William Charles White, "The Plan of the National Tuberculosis Association," *Science* 64, no. 1655 (1926); John Minor, "Memorial: William Charles White, 1874–1947," *Trans American Clinical Climatology Association* 59 (1947); James E. Perkins, "The National Tuberculosis Association: Fiftieth Anniversary," *Public Health Reports* 69, no. 5 (1954); and Robert G. Patterson, "The Evolution of Official Tuberculosis Control in the United States," *Public Health Reports* 62, no. 10 (1947).

The story of the beginning of a veterans' health system is about politics as well as policy. According to Joseph McCartin, "The First World War," in *The American Congress: The Building of Democracy*, ed. Julian E. Zelizer (Boston: Houghton Mifflin, 2004), from 1916 through 1918, President Wilson struggled to gain support for his policies from a contentious, divided Congress. He faced strong opposition from antiwar Democrats and their fiscally conservative, anti-interventionist Republican colleagues. At the same time, he was able to gain support from interventionist Republicans, such as Henry Cabot Lodge, who were long-time proponents of increased military funding. As the war came to a close, there was a growing sense that Democrats had bungled crucial aspects of planning. In the congressional elections of 1918 and 1920, Americans ushered Republicans into the majority in both the House and Senate, thereby declaring their frustration with a variety of Democratic and Progressive policies. The 1918 ascent to power is viewed as one of six "substantial reversals of an established majority" according to James W. Ceasar and Daniel DiSalvo, "Midterm Elections, Partisan Context, and Political Leadership: The 2006 Elections and Party Alignment," *Forum* 4, no. 3 (2006): 6.

Scholars of Warren G. Harding, with rare exceptions, roundly condemn the scandal surrounding the Veterans Bureau and its first director, Charles Forbes, as a symbol of the administration's malfeasance. According to Eugene P. Trani and David L. Wilson, *The Presidency of Warren G. Harding* (Lawrence: Regents Press of Kansas, 1977), Forbes's misdeeds cost taxpayers around $200 million and his appointment constituted "one of Harding's worst misjudgments" (181). See also Carl Sferraza Anthony, *Florence Harding: The First Lady, the Jazz Age, and the Death of America's Most Scandalous President* (New York: William Morrow, 1998), 86; Phillip G. Payne, *Dead Last: The Public Memory of Warren G. Harding's Scandalous Legacy* (Athens: Ohio University Press, 2009), 35; John W. Dean, *Warren G. Harding*, ed. Arthur M. Schlesinger Jr. (New York: Henry Holt, 2004); and Charles L. Mee Jr., *The Ohio Gang: The World of Warren G. Harding* (New York: M. Evans, 1981). A notable and important exception is Rosemary Stevens's *A Time of Scandal: Charles Forbes, Warren G. Harding, and the Making of the Veterans Bureau* (Baltimore: Johns Hopkins University Press, 2016).

On political parties in the interwar years, see Clyde P. Weed, *The Transformation of the Republican Party, 1912–1936: From Reform to Resistance* (Boulder, CO: Lynne Rienner Publishers, 2011); Elliot A. Rosen, *The Republican Party in the Age of Roosevelt: Sources of Anti-government Conservatism in the United States* (Charlottesville: University Press of Virginia, 2014); Robert Mason, *The Republican Party and American Politics from Hoover to Reagan* (Cambridge: Cambridge University Press, 2011); Lewis L. Gould, *Grand Old Party: A History of the Republicans* (New York: Random House, 2003); Kristi Andersen, *The Creation of a Democratic Majority, 1928–1936* (Chicago: University of Chicago Press, 1979); Douglas B. Craig, *After Wilson: The Struggle for the Democratic Party, 1920–1934* (Chapel Hill: University of North Carolina Press, 1992); Alan Ware, *The Democratic Party Heads North, 1877–1962* (New York: Cambridge University Press, 2006); Julian Zelizer, "The Forgotten Legacy of the New Deal: Fiscal Conservatism and the Roosevelt Administration, 1933–1938," *Presidential Studies Quarterly* 30, no. 2 (2000); and James L. Sundquist, *Dynamics of the Party System: Alignment and Realignment of Political Parties in the United States* (Washington, DC: Brookings Institution Press, 1983), esp. chap. 8 and 9.

Regardless of party affiliation, politicians en masse supported legislation granting veterans' entitlements in the interwar years, in part because of the growing power of interest groups like the American Legion and Disabled American Veterans. Sections of this book pertaining to the Committee on World War Veterans' Legislation verify the view that Congress's reliance on committees to formulate policies "works to the advantage of interest groups enabling them to concentrate their lobbyists' work on relatively few legislators and staffers." Jeffrey M. Berry and Clyde Wilcox, *The Interest Group Society*, 5th ed. (New York: Pearson, 2009), 138. Also see John R. Wright, *Interest Groups and Congress: Lobbying, Contributions, and Influence* (Boston: Allyn & Bacon, 1996), 168–71; Jeffrey M. Berry, "Subgovernments, Issue Networks, and Political Conflict," in *Remaking American Politics*, ed. Richard A. Harris and Sidney Milkis (Boulder, CO:

Westview Press, 1989), 239–60; Lael R. Keiser and Susan M. Miller, "The Impact of Organized Interests on Eligibility Determination: The Case of Veterans' Disability Compensation," *Journal of Public Administration Research and Theory* 20 (2010); and Walter Stubbs, *Congressional Committees, 1789–1982* (Santa Barbara, CA: ABC-Clio, 1985).

This book focuses in part on, and cites sources regarding, the experiences of women and African American men, but literature on veterans from a variety of marginalized groups is expanding. Scholars examine the impact of state efforts to influence individuals' perspectives via military service, the tendency of veterans to pursue citizenship rights following their discharges, and an array of other topics, including the health impact of war. The 18 percent of troops serving during World War I who were foreign-born had distinct experiences as service members and veterans. Nancy Gentile Ford, *Americans All! Foreign-Born Soldiers in World War I* (College Station: Texas A&M University Press, 2001), argues that the War Department "turned to Progressive reformers and ethnic leaders to help . . . in training, educating, Americanizing, socializing, and bolstering the morale of [foreign-born] men" (13). Although the American Legion expressed anti-immigrant sentiments throughout the 1920s and 1930s, the group's publications expressed warmth toward American Indian veterans, and its backing helped ensure the 1935 passage of the Nye-Lea Act, which provided for the naturalization of Asian Americans who had served in the military. On the experience of American Indians in this period, see Thomas A. Britten, *American Indians in World War I: At Home and at War* (Albequerque: University of New Mexico Press, 1997); Kristin Erica Lesak, "Soldiers to Citizens: World War I and the Acceleration of the American Indian Assimilation Process" (MA thesis, University of Maryland, 2002); and Thomas Grillot, "Native Americans, America's Colonial Troops," *Books & Ideas*, Sept. 28, 2011, http://booksandideas.net /Native-Americans-America-s.html. On the experience of Asian Americans, see Lucy E. Salyer, "Baptism by Fire: Race, Military Service, and U.S. Citizenship Policy, 1918–1935," *Journal of American History* 91, no. 3 (2004). Even as the American Legion supported citizenship for American Indians and Asian Americans, some of its posts served as bastions for discriminatory practices. One decorated war veteran was infuriated when people of Mexican descent were excluded from the Legion's Fourth of July dance in a small South Texas town: "If shedding my blood for you [Anglo-]Americans does not mean any more than this," he said, "I do not want to ever wear your colors, from now on I am ashamed of having served in your army." José A. Ramírez, *To the Line of Fire!: Mexican*

Texans and World War I (College Station: Texas A&M Press, 2009), 121. There were signs of change following World War II, when two veterans founded the first Legion post for Mexican American members in Arizona, using it as a support network during a successful fight to integrate GI housing in spite of the "fervent protests" of white veterans. Around the same time, in East Chicago, Indiana, an American Legion post that had "led a campaign to repatriate Mexicans . . . welcomed the Mexican American veterans and even had a 'Latin American night.'" F. Arturo Rosales, *Chicano! The History of the Mexican American Civil Rights Movement* (Houston: University of Houston Press, 1996), 97–98. Like black leaders, Mexican American José de la Luz Sáenz imagined that World War I service would propel a larger Mexican American struggle for civil rights. After serving in France, he returned home to found the League of United Latin American Citizens (LULAC). His recently translated wartime diary is a valuable source: José de la Luz Sáenz, *The World War I Diary of José de la Luz Sáenz*, ed. and trans. Emilio Zamora (College Station: Texas A&M Press, 2014). On LULAC's World War I roots, see Cynthia E. Orozco, *No Mexicans, Women, or Dogs Allowed: The Rise of the Mexican American Civil Rights Movement* (Austin: Univesity of Texas Press, 2009).

World War I–era plans for health care and rehabilitation in the United States were influenced by policy makers' and military officials' impressions of the ongoing efforts of other countries. For a World War I–era account of the history and organization of soldiers' and veterans' care in multiple countries before 1919, see Edward T. Devine assisted by Lilian Brandt, *Disabled Soldiers and Sailors Pensions and Training*, ed. David Kinley (New York: Oxford University Press, 1919). Over the last three decades, scholars of the history of France, Great Britain, China, Chechnya, Japan, and other nations have demonstrated that veterans' issues are central to welfare states, imperialism, and the workings of governments. In addition to sources cited elsewhere in this book, see, e.g., Chris Millington, *From Victory to Vichy: Veterans in Inter-war France* (Manchester: Manchester University Press, 2012), and Robert Weldon Whalen, *Bitter Wounds: German Victims of the Great War, 1914–1939* (Ithaca, NY: Cornell University Press, 1984). For a comparative analysis of the treatment of German and British veterans following World War I, see Deborah Cohen, *The War Come Home: Disabled Veterans in Britain and Germany, 1914–1939* (Berkeley: University of California Press, 2001). On Canada's treatment of World War I soldiers and veterans, see Kellen Kurschinski, "Caring for Our Veterans: The History of VAC," *Clio's Current*, Feb. 10, 2014, http://clioscurrent.com/blog/2014/2/10/caring-for-our-veterans

-the-history-of-vac; Peter Neary and J. L. Granatstein, *The Veterans Charter and Post–World War II Canada* (Montreal: McGill-Queen's University Press, 1998); and Desmond Morton and Glenn Wright, *Winning the Second Battle: Canadian Veterans and the Return to Civilian Life* (Toronto: University of Toronto Press, 1987). On the treatment of veterans following World War II in China, see Neil J. Diamant, *Embattled Glory: Veterans, Military Families, and the Politics of Patriotism in China, 1949–2007* (Plymouth: Rowman & Littlefield, 2010). In his study of veterans in post–World War II Japan, *Casualties of History: Wounded Japanese Servicemen and the Second World War* (Ithaca, NY: Cornell University Press, 2015), Lee K. Pennington delves into the World War I era. On West African veterans and imperial France, see Gregory Mann, *Native Sons: West African Veterans and France in the Twentieth Century* (Durham, NC: Duke University Press, 2006). On Chechen veterans in post-Soviet Russia, see Maya Eichler, *Militarizing Men: Gender, Conscription, and War in Post-Soviet Russia* (Stanford, CA: Stanford University Press, 2012), chap. 5. On Australian veterans, see Marina Larsson, *Shattered Anzacs: Living with the Scars of War* (Sydney: University of New South Wales Press, 2009). Recent work demonstrates the potential of cross-cultural analyses of veterans' policies and experiences. See, e.g., Nathalie Duclos, ed., *War Veterans in Postwar Situations: Chechnya, Serbia, Turkey, Peru, and Côte d'Ivoire* (Paris: Palgrave Macmillan, 2012); Martin Crotty and Mark Edele, "Total War and Entitlement: Towards a Global History of Veteran Privilege," *Austrailian Journal of Policy History* 59, no. 1 (2013); and Julia Eichenburg and John Paul Newman, eds., *The Great War and Veterans' Internationalism* (Basingstoke: Palgrave Macmillan, 2013).

　Burdens of War is about how policy, bureaucracy, and veterans' experiences shaped a unique and lasting health system in the interwar years, but there is much work to be done on the early years of veterans' health care. Hospitals, which are the focus of this book, were only one element of a diverse health system that included diagnostic centers, outpatient clinics, and visiting nurse services. Moreover, there were local and regional variations in how soldiers and veterans accessed and experienced care. Compendiums of official documents and policies relating to the Veterans Bureau in this period offer a glimpse of the breadth of the organization's work, and ideas for future historical analyses. In addition to VA annual reports, see, e.g., *Laws Governing the Organization and Administration of the Bureau of War Risk Insurance and the U.S. Veterans' Bureau and the Federal Board for Vocational Education in Its Relation to Veterans of the World War* (Washington, DC: GPO, 1927). Scholars have noted the importance of considering the role of the courts when analyzing the history of the administrative state, and also that the VA was unique among federal agencies because it was not subject to judicial review until 1988. Reuel Schiller, "'Saint George and the Dragon': Courts and the Development of the Administrative State in Twentieth-Century America," *Journal of Policy History* 17, no. 1 (2005). See also multiple relevant articles from James D. Ridgway, including "The Veterans' Judicial Review Act Twenty Years Later: Confronting the New Complexities of the Veterans Benefits System," *NYU Annual Survey of American Law* 66, no. 251 (2010), and Barton D. Stichman, "The Impact of the Veterans' Judicial Review Act on the Federal Circuit," *American University Law Review* 41 (1992). The official ban on judicial review—one lasting measure of Franklin D. Roosevelt's Economy Act—was only put in place in 1933. The *Digest of Legal Opinions Relating to the United States Veterans' Bureau* (Washington, DC: GPO, 1923–26) indicates that throughout the 1920s and early 1930s, veterans' legal claims about their rights—including their rights to health and health care—were addressed not only by the Veterans' Bureau but also by the attorney general and comptroller general of the United States. The cases offer invaluable perspective on perceptions of the veterans' health system and impetuses for change. In short, there are seeds for countless articles, dissertations, and manuscripts about the history of veterans' health care— on topics including changing diagnostic and treatment standards and their connection with perceptions of disability; medical professionalization; the development of research standards and programs; the dynamics of the local administration of a federal health program; and alternatives to institutionally based care.

Index

Page numbers in *italics* indicate figures.